SURGICAL APPROACHES IN PSYCHIATRY

Proceedings of the Third International
Congress of Psychosurgery
August 14th-18th, 1972, Cambridge,
England

SURGICAL APPROACHES IN PSYCHIATRY

EDITORS:

LAURI V LAITINEN, M.D.
Department of Neurosurgery, University Central Hospital, Helsinki, Finland

KENNETH E LIVINGSTON, M.D.
The Wellesley Hospital, Toronto, Ontario, Canada

University Park Press . Baltimore

Published in the USA and Canada by
UNIVERSITY PARK PRESS
University Park Press
Chamber of Commerce Building
Baltimore, Maryland, 21202

> **Library of Congress Cataloging in Publication Data**
>
> International Congress of Psychosurgery, 3d, Cambridge, Eng., 1972
>   Surgical approaches in psychiatry.
>
>   1. Psychosurgery—Congresses. I. Laitinen, Lauri, ed. II. Livingston, Kenneth E., ed. III. Title. (DNLM: 1. Psychosurgery—Congresses. W3IN153 1970s/WL370 1601 1970s)
>   RC480.I57   1972   617'.481   73-12151
>   ISBN 0-8391-0714-5

No part of this book may be reproduced
in any form without permission from the publisher
except for the quotation of brief passages
for the purpose of review

First published 1973
MTP MEDICAL AND TECHNICAL PUBLISHING CO. LTD.
St. Leonard's House
St. Leonardgate
Lancaster, Lancs.
Copyright © 1973 L. Laitinen and K. Livingston

Printed in Great Britain

THE INTERNATIONAL SOCIETY OF PSYCHOSURGERY

OFFICERS
President: William B. Scoville, Hartford, Connecticut, USA
President Elect: Sixto Obrador, Madrid, Spain
Honorary Presidents: Almeida Lima, Lisbon, Portugal
　　　　　　　　　　　Keiji Sano, Tokyo, Japan
Vice Presidents: Geoffrey Knight, London, England
　　　　　　　　　Tom Ballantine, Boston, Massachusetts, USA
Secretary General: Edward R. Hitchcock, Edinburgh, Scotland
Treasurer: Kjeld Vaernet, Copenhagen, Denmark
Editor of Publications: Lauri Laitinen, Helsinki, Finland
Host for the Congress: Walpole Lewin, Cambridge, England

PROGRAM COMMITTEE:
Alfonso Escobar, Mexico City, Mexico
Walpole Lewin, Cambridge, England
Gösta Rylander, Stockholm, Sweden
William Sweet, Boston, Massachusetts, USA
Kenneth Livingston, Toronto, Canada—Chairman

List of Contributors

O J ANDY, M.D.
Neurosurgery Department, University Mississippi Medical Center, Jackson, Mississippi, USA
K AKERT, Institut für Hirnforschung der Universität Zurich, Switzerland
G W ASHCROFT, D.P.M., F.R.C.P.E.
MRC Brain Metabolism Unit, Pharmacology Department, University of Edinburgh, Edinburgh, Scotland
A BEN-SHMUEL, M.D.
Kantonsspital Zürich, Zürich, Switzerland
T BINGLEY, Professor
Karolinska Sjukhuset, Stockholm, Sweden
P K BRIDGES, M.D., Ph.D., M.R.C.Psych.
Regional Neurosurgical Centre, Brook General Hospital, Shooters Hill Road, Woolwich, S.E.18, England
M HUNTER BROWN, M.D.
Senior Neurosurgeon, St John's Hospital and Santa Monica Hospital, Santa Monica, California, USA
J A BURZACO, M.D.
Servicio de Neurocirugia, Hospital Clinico de San Carlos, Madrid, Spain
VALERIE M CAIRNS, M.A.
Department of Surgical Neurology, The Royal Infirmary, Edinburgh, Scotland
MARYSE CHOPPY, M.A.
Clinique de Chirurgie Neurologique, Hôpital de la Salpêtrière, Paris 75013, France
G C COOVER
Stanford University, California, USA
J A N CORSELLIS, F.R.S.P.
Department of Neuropathology, Runwell Hospital, Wickford, Essex, England
J M R DELGADO, M.D.
Servicio Nacional de Neurocirugia, Residencia Sanitaria 'La Paz' de la Seguridad Social, Madrid, Spain
G DIECKMANN, M.D.
Department of Neurosurgery, University of Saarland, Homburg/Saar Federal Republic of Germany

ALFONSO ESCOBAR, M.D.
Department of Neurobiology, National University of Mexico, Mexico City, Mexico

FRANCISCO ESCOBEDO, M.D.
Instituto Nacional de Neurologia, Mexico City, Mexico

MURRAY A FALCONER, F.R.C.S.
Neurosurgical Unit, The Maudsley Hospital, De Crespigny Park, London, England

AUGUSTO FERNÁNDEZ-GUARDIOLA, M.D.
Instituto Nacional de Neurologia, Mexico City, Mexico

P FLOR-HENRY, M.B., Ch.B., M.D.(Edin), ACAD.D.P.M.(London), M.R.C.Psych.
Department of Psychiatry, University of Alberta, Edmonton, Alberta, Canada

MAKRAM GIRGIS, M.D., Ph.D.
Missouri Institute of Psychiatry, St Louis, Missouri, USA

GRAHAM V GODDARD, M.D.
Dalhousie University, Halifax, Canada

E O GOKTEPE, F.R.C.S.
Regional Neurosurgical Centre, Brook General Hospital, Shooters Hill Road, Woolwich, S.E.18, England

ROLF HASSLER, M.D.
Department of Neurobiology, Max-Planck Institute for Brain Research, Frankfurt am Main, Federal Republic of Germany

SADAO HIROSE, M.D., D.M.SC.
Department of Neuropsychiatry, Nippon Medical School, Sendagi, Bunkyoku, Tokyo, Japan

EDWARD R HITCHCOCK, F.R.C.S.
Department of Surgical Neurology, The Royal Infirmary, Edinburgh, Scotland

LEOPOLD HOFSTATTER, M.D.
Missouri Institute of Psychiatry, St Louis, Missouri, USA

O HORNYKIEWICZ
University of Toronto, Toronto, Canada

ALICE B JACK
Department of Neuropathology, Runwell Hospital, Wickford, Essex, England

LOTHAR B KALINOWSKY, M.D.
115 East 82nd Street, New York, N.Y., USA

DESMOND KELLY, Consultant Psychiatrist
St George's Hospital Medical School, Atkinson Morley's Hospital, Wimbledon, England

YONG KIE KIM, M.D.
Department of Neurosurgery, Broughton Hospital, Morganton, N.C., USA

GEOFFREY C KNIGHT, F.R.C.S., F.R.C.Psych.
Psychosurgical Unit, Brook Hospital, London S.E.18, England

LAURI V LAITINEN, M.D.
Department of Neurosurgery, University Central Hospital, Helsinki, Finland

JACQUES LE BEAU, M.D.
Clinique de Chirurgie Neurologique, Hôpital de la Salpêtrière, Paris 13, France

LARS LEKSELL, M.D.
Department of Neurosurgery, Karolinska Sjukhuset, Stockholm, Sweden

S LEVINE, M.D.
Stanford University, California, USA

WALPOLE LEWIN, M.S., F.R.C.S.
Addenbrooke's Hospital, Hills Road, Cambridge, England

KENNETH E LIVINGSTON, M.D.
The Wellesley Hospital, 160 Wellesley Street East, Toronto 5, Ontario, Canada

R B LIVINGSTON, M.D.
University of California, San Diego, USA

WINSTON C MARTIN, M.D.
University of Texas Medical Branch, Galveston, Texas, USA

J G MARTIN-RODRIGUEZ, M.D.
Servicio Nacional de Neurocirugia, Residencia Sanitaria 'La Paz' de la Seguridad Social, Madrid, Spain

MARK L McELHANEY, Ph.D.
University of Texas Medical Branch, Galveston, Texas, USA

C P McGRAW, Ph.D.
University of Texas Medical Branch, Galveston, Texas, USA

DAN C McINTYRE, M.D.
Carleton University, Ottawa, Canada

TURNER McLARDY, M.D.
Myerson Research Laboratory, Boston State Hospital, Boston, Mass., USA

GLENN MEYER, M.D.
Department of Neurosurgery, The Medical College of Wisconsin, Milwaukee, Wisconsin, USA

BJÖRN A MEYERSON, M.D.
Department of Neurosurgery, Karolinska Sjukhuset, Stockholm, Sweden

NITA MITCHELL-HEGGS
St George's Hospital Medical School, Atkinson Morley's Hospital, Wimbledon, England

L G MURRAY, D.P.M.
MRC Brain Metabolism Unit, Pharmacology Department, University of Edinburgh, Edinburgh, Scotland

P NÁDVORNÍK, MUDr.
Research Laboratory for Clinical Stereotaxis, Department of Neurosurgery, Comenius University, Bratislava, Czechoslovakia

H NARABAYASHI, M.D.
Juntendo Medical School, Tokyo, Japan

WALLE J H NAUTA
MIT, Cambridge, Mass, USA

RAYMOND L NEWCOMBE, F.R.C.S.
Maudsley Hospital and Brook Hospital, London, England
SIXTO OBRADOR, M.D.
Servicio Nacional de Neurocirugia, Residencia Sanitaria 'La Paz' de la Seguridad Social, Madrid, Spain
ARMANDO ORTIZ, M.D.
Oakland Medical Center, Michigan Department of Mental Health, Pontiac, Michigan, USA
J POGÁDY, M.D.
Research Laboratory for Clinical Stereotaxis, Department of Neurosurgery, Comenius University, Bratislava, Czechoslovakia
T P S POWELL
Oxford University, Oxford, England
ALAN RICHARDSON, F.R.C.S.
Atkinson Morley's Hospital, Wimbledon, England
GÖSTA RYLANDER, M.D.
Karolinska Sjukhuset, Stockholm, Sweden
WILLIAM BEECHER SCOVILLE, M.D., F.A.C.S.
Department of Neurosurgery, Hartford Hospital, Hartford, Conn., USA
F SHIMA, M.D.
Juntendo Medical School, Tokyo, Japan
CHARLES SHUTE
Cambridge University, Cambridge, England
JEAN SIEGFRIED, M.D.
Department of Neurosurgery, Kantonsspital Zürich, Zürich, Switzerland
J R SMYTHIES
University of Edinburgh, Edinburgh, Scotland
GONZALO SOLÍS, M.D.
Instituto Nacional de Neurologia, Mexico City, Mexico
M ŠRAMKA, MUDr.
Research Laboratory for Clinical Stereotaxis, Department of Neurosurgery, Comenius University, Bratislava, Czechoslovakia
ERIC TURNER, F.R.C.S.
Queen Elisabeth Hospital, Birmingham, England
W UMBACH, M.D.
Department of Neurosurgery, Klinikum Steglitz der Freien Universität, West Berlin, Germany
HOLGER URSIN, M.D.
Institute of Physiology, University of Bergen, Bergen, Norway
JUHANI VILKKI, M.A.
Department of Neurosurgery, University Central Hospital, Helsinki, Finland
N ZIMBACCA*
Clinique de Chirurgie Neurologique, Hôpital de la Salpêtrière, Paris 13, France

* posthumously

Preface

At the conclusion of the Second International Conference of Psychosurgery in August, 1970, it seemed appropriate to plan a subsequent meeting that would attempt to bring into clinical focus some of the recent advances in the basic sciences which contribute insight into brain mechanisms that are particularly relevant to the continuing evolution and refinement of 'Surgical Approaches in Psychiatry'.

The Cambridge Congress was designed with this objective in mind. In terms of the content of formal presentations, more than one-third of the program was devoted to basic science contributions. The general areas selected for emphasis were anatomical relationships, particularly those illuminated by recently developed techniques for following transneuronal degeneration, biochemical relationships, particularly the increasing evidence of anatomical patterning in neurotransmitter systems, and physiological relationships, ranging from recent observations on synaptic behavior at the electron microscopic level to some of the experimental models of seizure excitation in laboratory animals.

In parallel with this analysis of basic neuronal systems that may be functionally disturbed in various forms of psychiatric disease, a relatively unselected view was presented of clinical work currently going on in centers throughout the world concerned with the surgical alleviation of suffering from intractable mental illness. This clinical experience is grouped into several broad areas of interest—the psychiatric aspects of so-called 'Psychosurgery', studies of various types of intervention in the cingulate, orbital, and temporal regions, and a variety of other studies and observations. The important problems of psychological and psychiatric assessment were intentionally not given prime emphasis at this meeting, but we hope that they will represent an area of major attention for the next Congress to be held in Madrid, Spain, in 1975.

The formal presentations represented only a small part of the rich interplay between the basic science and clinical fields that characterized the Cambridge Congress. An important component of the program, unfortunately not reflected in the Proceedings because of quantitative limitations, was the valuable discussion that went on continuously both during and between the formal sessions. The great value of such direct 'transactional' interchange was amply demonstrated. It is the hope of the Officers of the Society and the

Editors of this volume that the publication of these Proceedings will add to the continuing scientific advance along this important human frontier.

Surgical Approaches in Psychiatry reflects a renaissance of psychosurgery, and may interest not only psychiatric and neurosurgical but also psychological and sociological readers. Therefore a short and important comment is necessary. Psychosurgery is not, and must not become, a method for manipulation of the mind. Its only aim is to relieve individual, intractable suffering. It should be applied only when conventional psychiatric methods have not given sufficient help. Even then, psychosurgery must not be such a blunting procedure that it prevents the patient from reacting to his problems in a normal way. If psychosurgery is used wisely, it aims at, and can succeed in, relieving the patient from pathological suffering of the mind and restoring his ability to enjoy and suffer as normal human beings do.

Lauri V. Laitinen and Kenneth E. Livingston

Helsinki and Toronto
May, 1973

Contents

List of Contributors   vii
Preface   xi

PART I—PSYCHIATRIC ASPECTS OF PSYCHOSURGERY

1. The Renaissance of Psychosurgery   3
   GÖSTA RYLANDER

2. Brain Mechanisms and Psychiatry   13
   J R SMYTHIES

3. Attempt at Localization of Psychological Manifestations Observed in Various Psychosurgical Procedures   18
   LOTHAR B KALINOWSKY

4. Psychiatric Syndromes Considered as Manifestations of Lateralized Temporal-Limbic Dysfunction   22
   P FLOR-HENRY

PART II—PRESIDENTIAL ADDRESS

5. Surgical Locations for Psychiatric Surgery with Special Reference to Orbital and Cingulate Operations   29
   WILLIAM BEECHER SCOVILLE

PART III—CINGULATE LESIONS IN THE TREATMENT OF PSYCHIATRIC ILLNESS

6. Stereotactic Cingulotomy with Results of Acute Stimulation and Serial Psychological Testing   39
   GLENN MEYER, MARK MCELHANEY, WINSTON MARTIN & C P MCGRAW

7. The Role of the Limbic Lobe in Central Pain Mechanisms, an Hypothesis Relating to the Gate Control Theory of Pain   59
   ARMANDO ORTIZ

xiv *Surgical Approaches in Psychiatry*

8   Chronic Stimulation of the Cingulum in Humans with Behaviour Disorders 65
    FRANCISCO ESCOBEDO, AUGUSTO FERNÁNDEZ-GUARDIOLA & GONZALO SOLÍS

9   Selective Leucotomy: A Review 69
    WALPOLE LEWIN

10 Observations on the Transcallosal Emotional Connections 74
    L V LAITINEN & J VÍLKKI

PART IV—ORBITO-FRONTAL INTERVENTIONS

11 Anatomical Placement of Lesions in the Ventromedial Segment of the Frontal Lobe 83
    RAYMOND L NEWCOMBE

12 Neuropathological Observations on Yttrium Implants and on Undercutting in the Orbito-frontal Areas of the Brain 90
    J A N CORSELLIS & ALICE B JACK

13 A Review of Patients with Obsessional Symptoms Treated by Psychosurgery 96
    P K BRIDGES & E O GOKTEPE

14 Additional Stereotactic Lesions in the Cingulum Following Failed Tractotomy in the Subcaudate Region 101
    GEOFFREY KNIGHT

PART V—TEMPORAL LOBE

15 Some Properties of a Lasting Epileptogenic Trace Kindled by Repeated Electrical Stimulation of the Amygdala in Mammals 109
    GRAHAM V GODDARD & DAN C MCINTYRE
    Discussion: O J ANDY 115

16 Epileptic Ammonshorn Sclerosis and Schizophrenia: Negative Correlation 118
    TURNER MCLARDY

17 Pathological Substrates in Temporal Lobe Epilepsy with Psychoses 121
    MURRAY A FALCONER

18 The Results of Stereotactic Treatment of the Aggressive Syndrome 125
    P NÁDVORNÍK, J POGÁDY & M ŠRAMKA

19 Which is the better Amygdala Target, the Medial or Lateral Nuclei? 129
    H NARABAYASHI & F SHIMA

20 Fundus Striae Terminalis, an Optional Target in Sedative Stereotactic Surgery 135
    J A BURZACO

21 Long-term Assessment of Stereotactic Amygdalotomy for Aggressive Behaviour   138
J SIEGFRIED & A BEN-SHMUEL

22 Observations on the Development of an Assessment Scheme for Amygdalotomy   142
E R HITCHCOCK, G W ASHCROFT, V M CAIRNS & L G MURRAY

PART VI—MISCELLANEOUS AND MULTIPLE LESIONS

23 Stereotactic Anterior Capsulotomy in Anxiety and Obsessive-Compulsive States   159
T BINGLEY, L LEKSELL, B A MEYERSON & G RYLANDER

24 Technique and Assessment of Limbic Leucotomy   165
DESMOND KELLY, ALAN RICHARDSON & NITA MITCHELL-HEGGS

25 Psychological Changes after Selective Frontal Surgery (especially Cingulotomy) and after Stereotactic Surgery of the Basal Ganglia   174
M CHOPPY, N ZIMBACCA & J LE BEAU

26 Combined Stereotactic Lesions for Treatment of Behaviour Disorders and Severe Pain   182
Y K KIM & W UMBACH

27 Further Experience with Multiple Limbic Targets for Schizophrenia and Aggression   189
B HUNTER BROWN

28 Long-term Evaluation of Orbito-Ventromedial Undercutting in 'Atypical' Schizophrenic Patients   196
SADAO HIROSE

29 Relief of Obsessive-Compulsive Disorders, Phobias and Tics by Stereotactic Coagulation of the Rostral Intralaminar and Medial-Thalamic Nuclei   206
R HASSLER & G DIECKMANN

PART VII—ELECTROPHYSIOLOGICAL STUDIES IN PSYCHOSURGICAL PATIENTS

30 Two-way Radio Communication with the Brain in Psychosurgical Patients   215
J M R DELGADO, S OBRADOR & J G MARTIN-RODRIGUEZ

31 Depth Electrode Investigations of the Limbic System with Radiostimulation, Electrolytic Lesions and Histochemical Techniques   224
LEOPOLD HOFSTATTER & MAKRAM GIRGIS

32 The Concept of Diencephalic Instability   237
ERIC TURNER

xvi *Surgical Approaches in Psychiatry*

PART VIII—BASIC SCIENCES RELATED TO PSYCHO-SURGERY

33 Tentative Limbic System Models for Certain Patterns of Psychiatric Disorders 245
KENNETH F LIVINGSTON & A ESCOBAR

34 Coping with Stress in Rats with Limbic Lesions 253
H URSIN, G C COOVER & S LEVINE

35 Electrophysiological Correlates of Non-Specific Cortical Activation by Electrical Stimulation of the Putamen and Pallidum in Cats 257
G DIECKMANN & R HASSLER

36 Sensory Convergence in the Cerebral Cortex 266
T P S POWELL

37 Cholinergic Pathways of the Brain 282
C C D SHUTE

38 The Subcortical Monoaminergic Systems 293
O HORNYKIEWICZ

39 Connections of the Frontal Lobe with the Limbic System 303
WALLE J H NAUTA

40 Morphological Plasticity of the Synapse 315
KONRAD AKERT & R B LIVINGSTON

Index 331

PART I

PSYCHIATRIC ASPECTS OF PSYCHOSURGERY

CHAPTER 1

The Renaissance of Psychosurgery
GÖSTA RYLANDER

Once upon a time as a young assistant at the Psychiatric University Clinic of Stockholm I gave an account of the just published monograph by Moniz, 'Tentatives Opératoires dans le Traitement de Certain Psychoses', pointing out that anxiety was reduced by this new operation. I proposed that we should try it in selected cases. My chief, Professor Wigert, was horrified and forbade every experiment of that type with human beings. Then I approached Olivecrona, the neurosurgeon. He said definitely no, adding somewhat sarcastically that psychiatrists damaged the brain by electroshock treatment and that there was no reason to destroy part of it in such a doubtful way as Moniz had done.

Later John Fulton told me how uneasy, not to say afraid, he felt when Moniz at the international congress of neurology in 1935 discussed with him the application on human beings of the operations performed on the chimpanzees Lucy and Becky.

Both Freeman and Solomon have described the violent opposition they met when trying to introduce frontal lobe operations.

It may suffice with these memories from the first period of psychosurgery to illustrate the criticism and somewhat aggressive opposition caused by this new type of brain surgery. We are in the same situation today, both in the USA with the Congressional Record where it is said that psychosurgery offends the whole Western ethical tradition of respect for the individual, and in the United Kingdom with a BBC programme on August 4th this year with the title: 'End Psychosurgery Now'. Also in Sweden, mass media have recently taken up the attacks on psychosurgery, mentioning of course the prisoners in California who are said to have been operated upon because of their aggressiveness. I will return to this rather disquieting matter later; I said disquieting for it could obstruct the advancement of psychosurgery and as a result our chances to help chronically ill, mentally tormented human beings.

Moniz' technique or modifications of it was tried out here and there in a tentative fashion, for example by Rizzatti and Bargarello in Italy, and by Lyerly and by Grant in the USA. I doubt, however, that much would have come out of it, had not Freeman and Watts introduced their standard lobotomy. That was a rather daring undertaking for at this time knowledge of the significance of different parts of the frontal lobes and their connections was fragmentary. The concepts of the limbic system and of the visceral brain were not yet born. Papez' epoch-making work, 'A Proposed Mechanism of Emotion' (55) had, it is true, been published 4 years before the first edition of *Psychosurgery* (10) but this idea had not yet taken root and was not mentioned in this monograph by Freeman and Watts.

It is easy to say today that their operation was crude and too extensive. But this, I think, was a factor that, to begin with, made standard lobotomy a success and caused it to be taken up all over the world, for the results were striking. Severely disturbed schizophrenics became calmer, suffered less and were easier to take care of; anxiety tortured patients of other types were relieved. This was the second period of Psychosurgery, that of standard lobotomy. The disadvantages of this empirical and large operation were to be revealed later, contributing to the decline and fall of the psychosurgical empire to use or maybe abuse the title of the famous work by Gibbon.

Freeman sent me his monograph, *Psychosurgery*, and with that in my hand I returned to my superiors. Now they agreed with Olof Sjoqvist, my neurosurgical collaborator, and me that this new treatment was worth trying. I selected some of the most disturbed chronic schizophrenics in the mental hospitals of Stockholm for standard lobotomy. The results were encouraging but very soon I found it difficult to decide whether any undesirable mental changes occurred, because of the concealing effects of the schizophrenic illness. Furthermore, the results of psychological testing could not be relied on, for if the psychotic patient was less disturbed by his schizophrenic symptoms after the operation, he could produce better results, although a reduction of his intellectual faculties might have occurred. Too little regard has been paid to these facts in most studies published at that time. Therefore we decided to select a short series of obsessive-compulsive neurotics whom I tested before and after the operation. The findings showed that a slight but fateful intellectual reduction was caused which sometimes was difficult to demonstrate with ordinary intelligence tests. Particularly abstract thought functions and the ability to plan were hit. Emotionally a flattening of the effect was observed in combination with a tendency to euphoric reactions, i.e. the well-known frontal syndrome.

At the meeting devoted to the frontal lobes in 1946 of the Association for Research in Nervous and Mental Disease (59), I described my findings and warned against applying standard lobotomy, except in serious chronic psychoses. I stressed also as did Penfield, that a smaller operation should be worked out. The appearance of such sequels as I had described was questioned by Sargent and of course by Freeman, a discussion that Fulton later cited in his book *Functional Localization in the Frontal Lobes* (11).

Some trials with small operations had however, already been done by Penfield (51) with gyrectomies and by Pool (20) with topectomies and also by Freeman & Watts (10) with unilateral lobotomies as well as bilateral partial lobotomies, i.e. upper and lower quadrant cuts. Egan (9) supplemented the inferior operation with a horizontal cut from the burr hole forwards to the pole of the frontal lobe. The results seemed less good than after standard lobotomy and undesirable personality changes occurred. Unilateral lobotomy was later tried by several surgeons as well as the lower quadrant cut. Only the latter operation seemed to give promising results.

Summing up the development after the meeting in 1946 I dare say that progress towards selective operations was slow. Standard lobotomy still dominated as a surgical method for many years.

In Sweden, Sjoqvist and I decided to try the inferior cut in severe depressions for reasons I will mention shortly. The results seemed, to begin with, promising. The immediate psychic effects of the operation were similar but less marked than in standard lobotomy. Sjoqvist operated under local anaesthesia so I could follow what happened on the operating table from a mental point of view. The therapeutic results were satisfactory and no personality changes seemed to be caused. Later, however, I found in twothirds of the patients similar defects as after standard lobotomy and therefore we stopped our trials. Later Reitman (56) and Bonner & Cobb (3) made similar observations.

Then two things happened which I consider landmarks on the way of finding how to carry out small operations. At the First International Congress of Psychosurgery in 1948, Scoville (64) described his method of cortical undercutting as a less traumatizing operation than gyrectomy and topectomy. On the basis of clinical and experimental observations he proposed three areas for undercutting—the convex side of the frontal lobes, roughly isolating Broadman's fields 9 and 10, the whole orbital surface, and the medial side, comprising area 24 and 32.

The following year the bold experiment of the Columbia-Greystone Associates was published with ablation of frontal cortex on 24 patients, mostly chronic schizophrenics (7). Only one of the operations was performed in the medial surface and none in the orbital. Decreases of anxiety associated with social improvement seemed to be connected with ablation of areas 9 and 10, in some cases combined with area 46. These findings were confirmed by Heath & Pool (20) after studies of other topectomized patients.

A third event must be mentioned in this connection. At the congress, Spiegel and Wycis (69) related stereotaxic operations in the thalamus using a modernized type of the Horsley-Clark instrument from 1908, hitherto with few exceptions applied only on animals. Thus a seed was planted that slowly would grow and initiate a new type of operation, to a great extent contributing to the renaissance of psychosurgery. The first apparatus constructed by Wycis was, however, too complicated to be accepted for clinical purposes. In Stockholm we decided to wait and see, and to begin with apply cortical undercutting.

We selected anxiety and tension states for superior undercutting in accordance with the suggestions by Scoville, the results of the Columbia-Greystone experiment as well as the findings of Dax, Reitman & Smith (8) who applied lower, middle and superior cuts in the white matter of the frontal lobes.

We applied orbital undercuttings on chronic depressive states for reasons which also had made us try the inferior cut. Already, in 1936, the German neuropsychiatrist Spatz (68) in an excellent article in Zeitschrift fur die Gesamt Neurologie und Psychiatrie, stressed the importance of the basal cortex for emotional life and personality. With basal cortex he meant the parts of the frontal and temporal lobes which lie on the basal part of the cranium. He had a series of Pick's disease histologically examined with atrophic processes starting in these parts of the cortex. Another prominent German of that time, Kleist (27, 28), was of similar opinion, having analysed 300 cases of gunshot wounds of the head from World War I. He thought the orbital cortex which he considered the centre of emotional life was closely related to the cingulum area, where he localized the visceral Ego. Does not this sound very advanced for that time? Furthermore, in my monograph of 1939 (58) on mental changes after operations in the frontal lobes I reported that injuries to the basal part were mostly combined with emotional changes. In Stockholm we also tried the medial side. No therapeutic effect was observed and we abandoned this type of operation, all the more as the reports in the literature at that time were controversial concerning operations in the cingulum.

Cortical undercutting was accepted also in France, where Le Beau (34) and his collaborators had used topectomies according to Pool. In the United Kingdom, undercutting which Knight in 1949 characterized as the most rational procedure, was applied parallel with McKissock's rostral leucotomy, which roughly is the same as Scoville's superior undercutting. Also in Japan undercutting was introduced by Hirose (23).

As time went on, the main interest was more and more concentrated on the orbital surface, for roughly the same reasons which had made us, in Sweden, apply the inferior cut and orbital undercutting. Later, the medial surface aroused the attention of the neurosurgeons and psychiatrists because of the experiments in animals of Smith, Ward and others as well as the growing knowledge of the importance of the cingulum for automatic functions and the mechanisms of the emotions. Cairns (6), Livingston (4), Le Beau (35), Hunter Brown (25) and others reported good results and few side-effects after operations in the anterior part of the cingulum in anxiety states and obsessional neuroses.

Undercutting in the superior surface which had been applied by Scoville, Le Beau, and many others was given up, as operations in this region seemed to interfere with intellectual functions according to the theories of Fulton and Cobb that the superior part of the frontal lobes were of special importance for the integration of intellectual functions. Malmoe (47) showed that a slight intellectual reduction occurred after ablation of areas 9 and 10 in a series of seven cases operated by Penfield. Pool (20) on the other hand as well as the Columbia-Greystone Group denied that intellectual changes followed topectomies in this area and so did Le Beau. In Stockholm we had similar experience concerning undercutting of areas 9 and 10. No significant lowering of the IQ occurred in a series of 17 patients but there was a tendency to give shorter and more concrete explanations of fables and proverbs (60).

I have not been able to find any publications of larger series of undercutting operations in this region, with the patients sufficiently tested before and after operation. Agreement seemed general that no intellectual changes were caused by orbital undercutting (Ström-Olsen & Northfield (70), Rylander (60) and others) or by the cingulate operation (Le Beau & Petrie (33). Undesirable personality changes were lacking or very slight and of no importance.

The selective operations, however, represented a minority. Standard lobotomy still dominated. In Britain for example about 1,000 operations were performed yearly between 1950-54 of which the majority were standard lobotomies (73). This decade was also the digestive period of psychosurgery with a series of important monographs by Partridge (50), by Greenblatt-Solomon (18, 19), by Petrie (52), by McDonald Tow (72), by Le Beau (34), by Robinson & Freeman (54) and by Lewis, Landis & King (38).

And then psychosurgery faded away under the influence of the disappointing experience with standard lobotomy and the introduction of the psychotropic drugs, as well as group therapy, community therapy and behaviour therapy. The list of psychosurgical publications compiled by the Library of the Royal Society of Medicine beautifully illustrates this. Between 1936 and 1941 there was less than a dozen publications a year. The number increased during the following decade to a maximum of approximately 300 a year in 1951 and 1952, then decreasing to less than a dozen annually during the 1960s. Also from 1965 the chapter 'Psychosurgery' was excluded from the annual Review *Progress in Neurology and Psychiatry*.

One may say that death sentences were also passed on psychosurgery. In 1960 for example a symposium on psychosurgery in the Royal Society of Medicine was closed with the words that it might be a historic meeting, the last one in which the surgery of mental disorder was presented for review and discussion. However, in February this year I attended a symposium on psychosurgery at the Royal Society, so this subject has been taken up again. Neither was psychosurgery abandoned in Great Britain after 1960. Knight (30) performed orbital undercutting and Sargent (62, 63) was a warm spokesman for selected operations in serious psychoneurotic disorders. In the USA, Ballantine (1) and Hunter Brown (25) applied anterior cingulectomy. In Sweden superior and orbital undercutting were performed but in a decreasing number and Leksell applied anterior stereotaxic capsulotomy until 1957 (22), inspired by Alfred Meyer's anatomical findings.

It was a pity that psychiatric surgery —a term I prefer to the inadequate and ill-famed name of psychosurgery—was dying out in most countries for new possibilities had in the meantime emerged.

An imposing amount of anatomical and physiological knowledge had been collected concerning the complex relationship within the limbic system as well as its connections with frontal and temporal neocortex and with the hypothalamus. In some countries, these new facts were partially applied. I am thinking of Grantham's bimedial operation (17) cutting the ventromedial projection, which Fulton in 1951 called the most important new technique of lobotomy. Still more influenced by recent research findings is Knight's (31) restriction of orbital undercutting, first to the medial and then to the post-medial part of the orbital surface, intending to cut fibres from the posterior orbital cortex, anterior cingulate and amygdaloid areas in the substantia innominata. I should also mention the orbito-ventro medial cut applied by Hirose (24) which aims at the thalamic fibres to the orbital cortex. A similar operation was performed by Busch (5) but touching less of the orbital surface than was the case in Hirose's operation and more of the medial side. Finally, Greenblatt and Solomon (19) tried the bimedial operation, cutting the fibres close to the anterior cingulate because of the findings of Smith (67), Ward (75) and Yakovlev (78) concerning its autonomic functions and role for emotional expressions.

The renaissance of psychiatric surgery started slowly in the end of the 1960s mainly thanks to three factors, two of which I have already touched upon. The rapid development of the stereotaxic methods provided a means of making small restricted lesions at selected points also in deeper parts of the brain. Thanks to improved instruments and technique, elaborated during the 1950s by Talairach (72), Leksell (36, 37), Lister & Sherwood (39), and many others, stereotaxic operations became a clinically useful method. The expanding insight into the central mechanisms underlying emotional activity and behaviour as well as the increased knowledge of the limbic system and its interplay with subcortical nuclei and neocortex had opened up new ways of attacking certain mental disorders. In this connection I would like to remind you of the important work of Fulton and his group (13), McLean (43-46), Livingston (41, 65), Girgis, (14-16) and many others (2, 49, 53). The limitations of drug therapy and other modern psychiatric treatments have finally revived the interest in psychiatric surgery. The Second International Congress (46) showed this clearly with 41 papers from 11 different countries. Promising is the close contact between neurophysiology and other branches of brain research and psychiatric surgery which this congress so well demonstrates.

Twenty years ago, Alfred Meyer said as a warning that there was a plethora of brain operations for mental disorder, an opinion which seems even more justified today. Operations are carried out in the hypothalamus (61), the thalamus, in the amygdaloid nucleus (77), in the corpus callosum (32) in different parts of the cingulum, in the fornix (61) in the temporal lobes, in the frontal lobes, and nearly all give results in the same or in different pathological states; a fact which can give rise to hours of discussion.

Very promising are the new possibilities to unmask the neurological basis of behaviour, opened by psychiatric surgery, by anatomy and by neurophysiology (14, 42-46, 48, 49, 53, 79), by deep electrodes (21, 66) and by biochemistry.

I shall not go into details, the Congress may speak for itself but I cannot refrain from making a small selection among the most fascinating subjects and findings. I will start with the deeper understanding of psychosomatic mechanisms obtained through the new knowledge of the limbic system with its two major circuits and the frontal cortex occupying the apex of them, and its role in the harmony (or disharmony) through interplay between mechanisms situated on different levels of the CNS for producing autonomic and emotional phenomena. Secondly, the so-called pleasure-pain bundle, which when stimulated electrically in certain spots causes feelings of well-being and pleasure in man and self-stimulation (which can be stopped with chlorpromazine and be increased with amphetamine) until exhaustion occurs in animals, opens wide perspectives (21). The finding that narcotic drugs give rise to special electrical phenomena in these pleasure spots can throw some light upon the addicts' drive to take the drug in spite of the risks for health and life and may pull together the pharmacodynamic action of drugs with structural functional relationships which have emerged following behind the advances in psychiatric surgery. Finally, the operations in the amygdala system for pathologic aggressiveness (61, 77) and in hypothalamus (57) for sexual deviations must not be forgotten. Except in the articles just referred to, you can find descriptions of these different types of operations in the recently published proceedings of the Conference on Psychosurgery in Copenhagen (65).

In closing I come back to my hints about the attacks on psychiatric surgery. I think everybody here should read the Congressional Records (of February 24th and March 30th 1972) irrespective of what misconceptions and errors they contain. Referring to their content I must stress that in Sweden brain operations as psychiatric treatment of prisoners are out of the question. I think we should thoroughly discuss such uses of psychiatric surgery. The question of operating on children ought also to be taken up as well as the borderline between treatment and experimental research. I am thinking of the implantation of deep electrodes in the human brain. If their function is to find the right location for the lesion—well, then the use of these electrodes is part of the treatment.

BIBLIOGRAPHY
1. Ballantine HT, Cassidy W, Flannagan NB & Marino R (1967). Stereotaxic anterior cingulotomy for neuropsychiatric illness and untractable pain. *J. Neurosurg.*, **26**, 488
2. Ban T (1966). The septo-preoptico-hypothalamic system and its autonomic function. *Progress in Brain Research*, **21A**. Elsevier Publ, Comp. Amsterdam.
3. Bonner T, Cobb C, Sweet WH & White JC (1952). Frontal lobe surgery in treatment of pain with consideration of postoperative psychological changes. *Psychosom. Med.*, **14**, 383
4. Brazier M (1971). Modern advances in the use of depth electrodes. *Surgical Control of Behavior*, **5**. Springfield, Ill.: Charles C. Thomas.
5. Busch E (1957). Orbitomedial undercutting. *Handbuch der Neurochirurgie VI*, **137**. Heidelberg-Göttingen-Berlin: Springer.
6. Cairns H, Duffield JE, Tow PM & Whittey CW (1952). Anterior cingulectomy in the treatment of mental disease. *Lancet*, **i**, 4, 75
7. Columbia-Greystone Associates (1949). Selective partial ablation of the frontal cortex. New York: Harper & Brothers
8. Dax EC, Reitman F & Radley-Smith J (1949). Investigation into clinical problems and prefrontal leucotomy. *1st International Conference on Psychosurgery*, **167**. Lisbon: Livraria Luso-Espanhola.
9. Egan G (1949). Results of isolation of the orbital lobes in leucotomy. *J. Ment. Sci.*, **95**, 115
10. Freeman W & Watts JW (1942). *Psychosurgery*, 2nd ed. 1950. Springfield, Ill.: Charles C Thomas.

10   *Surgical Approaches in Psychiatry*

11. Fulton J (1949). *Functional Localisation in the Frontal Lobes and Cerebellum.* Oxford: Clarendon Press.
12. Fulton J (1951). *Frontal Lobotomy and Affective Behavior.* New York: Norton & Co.
13. Fulton J (1954). Recent advances in neurophysiology. *J. Neurosurgery*, **11**, 1
14. Girgis M (1966). The Limbic system of the brain and psychosomatic medicine. *Southern Med. J.*, **4**, 82
15. Girgis M (1970). The 'Rhinencephalon'. *Acta Anat.*, **76**, 157
16. Girgis M (1971). The Orbital surface of the frontal lobe of the brain and mental disorder. *Acta Psychiat. Scand.* Suppl., 222
17. Grantham E (1951). Prefrontal lobotomy for relief of pain. *J. Neurosurg.*, 8, 405
18. Greenblatt M & Solomon HC (1950). *Studies of Lobotomy.* New York: Grune & Stratton.
19. Greenblatt M & Solomon HC (1950). *Frontal Lobes and Schizophrenia.* New York: Springer.
20. Heath RG & Pool JS (1948). Bilateral fractional resection of frontal cortex for the treatment of psychoses. *J. Nerv. Ment. Disl*, **107**, 411
21. Heath RG (1971). Depth recording and stimulation studies in patients. *Surgical Control of Behavior*, **5**. Springfield, Ill.: Charles C Thomas.
22. Herner T (1961). Treatment of mental disorder with frontal stereotaxic thermolesions. *Acta Psychiat. Neurol. Scand.*, Suppl., **36** 158
23. Hirose S (1958). Evaluation of prefrontal lobotomy in schizophrenia. A study of 280 patients followed two to eleven years. *Psychiat. Neurol. Jap.*, **60**, 1341
24. Hirose S (1965). Orbito-ventromedial undercutting 1957-63. Follow-up of 77 cases. *Amer. J. Psychiat.*, **121**, 1194
25. Hunter Brown M & Lighthill JA (1968. Selective anterior cingulotomy: a psychosurgical evaluation. *J. Neurosurg.*, **29**, 513
26. Kelly DHW, Walter CJS & Sargent, TW (1966). Modified lobotomy assessed by forearm bloodflow and other measurements. *Brit. J. Psychiat.*, **112**, 871
27. Kleist K. (1934). Kriegsverletzungen des Gehirns. *Handbuch der ärtzl.* Erfahrungen im Weltkriege, Leipzig.
28. Kleist K (1938). Bericht über die Gehirnpatologie in ihrer Bedeuting für Neurologie und Psychiatrie, *Zbl. Ges. Neurol Psychiat.*, **158**, 159
29. Knight GC & Fredgold RF (1955). Orbital leucotomy. A review of 52 cases. *Lancet*, **i**, 981
30. Knight GC (1960). 330 cases of restricted orbital undercutting. *Proc. Roy. Soc. Med.*, **53**, 728
31. Knight GC (1969). Bifrontal stereotactic tractotomy. *Brit. J. Psychiat.*, **115**, 257
32. Laitinen LV (1972). Stereotactic lesions in the knee of the corpus callosum in the treatment of emotional disorders. *Lancet*, **i**, 472
33. Le Beau J & Petrie A (1953). A comparison of the personality changes after 1. prefrontal selective surgery for the relief of intractable pain and for the treatment of mental disorder. 2. Cingulectomy and topectomy. *J. Ment. Sci.*, **99**, 53
34. Le Beau J (1954). *Psychosurgery et Fonctions Mentales.* Paris: Masson et Cie.
35. Le Beau J (1954). Anterior cingulotomy in man. *J. Neurosurg.*, **11**, 268
36. Leksell L (1949). A stereotaxic apparatus for intracerebral surgery. *Acta chir. Scand.*, **99**, 229
37. Leksell L (1971). *Stereotaxis and Radiosurgery. An operative system.* Springfield, Ill.: Charles C Thomas.
38. Lewis NDL, Landis C & King HE (1956). *Studies in Topectomy.* London: Grune & Stratton.
39. Lister WC & Sheerwood SL (1955). A lightweight stereotaxic instrument. *Electroencephalogr. Clin. Neurophysiol.*, **7**, 311
40. Livingston KE (1951). Cingulate cortex isolation for the treatment of psychoses and psychoneurosis. *Res. Publ.*, **31**, A.R.N.M.D., 374
41. Livingston KE (1969). The frontal lobes revisited. The case for a second look. *Arch. Neurol.*, **20**, 90

42. MacLean PD (1949). Psychosomatic disease and the visceral brain. *Psych. Som. Med.*, **11**, 338
43. MacLean PD (1959). The limbic system with regard to two basic life principles. The Central Nervous System and Behavior. New York: Jos. Macy Jr. Found., 19
44. MacLean PD (1952). Some psychiatric implications of physiologic studies on frontotemporal portion of limbic system (visceral brain). *Electroencef. Clin. Neurophysiol.*, **4**, 407
45. MacLean PD (1954). The limbic system and its Hippocampal formation. *J. Neurosurg.*, **11**, 29
46. MacLean PD (1960). Psychosomatics. *Handbook of Physiology*. Neurophysiology, Vol. III, 1723
47. Malmoe RB (1948). Psychological aspects of frontal gyrectomy and frontal lobotomy in mental patients. *Res. Publ.*, **27**, A.R.N.M.D., 537. Baltimore: Williams & Watkins.
48. Meyer A & Beck E (1954). Prefrontal leucotomy and related operations. *Anatomical Results of Success and Failure*. Edinburgh and London: Oliver & Boyd.
49. Nauta WJH (1964). Some efferent connections of the prefrontal cortex in the monkey. *The Frontal Granular Cortex and Behavior*. New York: McGraw-Hill, 399
50. Partridge M (1950). *Prefrontal Leucotomy*. Oxford: Blackwell Scientific Publ.
51. Penfield W, Cameron D, Prados M & Malmoe R (1948). Symposium on gyrectomy. *Res. Publ.*, **27**, A.R.N.M.D., 519
52. Petrie A (1952). *Personality and the Frontal Lobes*. London: Routledge & Kegan Paul.
53. Pribran KH, Ahemada A, Hartog J & Ross L (1964). A progress report on the neurological processes disturbed by frontal lobe lesions in primates. *The Frontal Granular Cortex and Behavior*. New York: McGraw-Hill, 28
54. Robinson Fr M & Freeman W (1954). *Psychosurgery and the Self*. New York and London: Grune & Stratton.
55. Papez JW (1937). A proposed mechanism of emotion. *Arch. Neurol. Psychiat.*, **38**, 725
56. Reitman F. (1948). Evaluation of leukotomy results. *Amer. J. Psychiat.*, **105**, 86
57. Roeder F (1966). Stereotaxic lesion of the tuber cinereum in sexual deviates. *Confin. Neurol. (Basel)*, **27**, 102
58. Rylander G (1939). Personality changes after operation on the frontal lobes. *Acta Psych. Neurol. Scand.*, Suppl. XX. London: Oxford University Press.
59. Rylander G (1948). Personality analysis before and after frontal lobotomy. *Res. Publ.*, **27**, A.R.N.M.D., 691
60. Rylander G (1957). Mental symptoms and therapeutic results after different types of frontal lobe operations in mental disorder. *Brain Nerve (Tokyo)*, **9**, 67
61. Sano K (1966). Sedative stereoencephalotomy: fornicatomy, upper mesencephalic reticulotomy and posteromedial hypothalatomy. *Progress in Brain Research*. Amsterdam: Elsevier Publ. Comp., **21B**, 350
62. Sargent W (1953). Ten years clinical experiences of modified leucotomy operations. *Brit. Med. J.*, **2**, 80
63. Sargent W (1962). The present indications for leucotomy. *Lancet*, **i**, 1197
64. Scoville WB (1949). Proposed methods of cortical undercutting of certain areas of the frontal lobes as a substitute for prefrontal leucotomy. 1st International Conference on Psychosurgery. Lisbon: Livrario Luso-Espanhola, 91
65. Second International Conference on Psychosurgery (1972). Springfield, Ill.: Charles C Thomas.
66. Sem-Jacobsen CW (1968). *Depth-electrographic Stimulation of the Human Brain and Behavior*. Springfield, Ill.: Charles C Thomas.
67. Smith WK (1945). The functional significance of the rostral cingular cortex as revealed by its responses to electrical stimulation. *J. Neurophysiol.*, **8**, 241
68. Spatz H (1937). Über die Bedeutung der basalen Rinde. *Ztschr.f.d.ges.Neurol. Psychiat.*, **158**, 208

69. Spiegel EH & Wycis HT (1949). Physiological and psychological results of thalatomy. *Proc. Roy. Soc. Med. Suppl.*, **142**, 84
70. Ström-Olsen R & Northfield DWC (1955). Undercutting of orbital cortex in chronic neurotic and psychotic tension states. *Lancet*, **i**, 986
71. Ström-Olsen R & Carlisle G (1971). Bifrontal stereotactic tractotomy. A follow-up study of its effects on 210 patients. *Brit. J. Psychiat.*, **118**, 14
72. Tailarech J (1952). Étude stéréotaxique des structures encéphaliques profondes chez l'homme. Technique intérèt physiopathologique et thérapeutique. *Presse méd.*, **60**, 605
73. Tooth GC & Newton MP (1961). *Leucotomy in England and Wales 1942–54.* London: HM Stationery Office.
74. Tow MacDonald P (1955). *Personality Changes following Frontal Leucotomy.* London: Oxford University Press.
75. Ward A (1948). The cingulate gyrus: area 24. *J. Neurophysiol.*, **13**
76. Ward A (1948). The anterior cingulate gyrus and personality. *Res. publ.*, **27**, A.R.N.M.D., 438
77. Vaernet K & Madsen A (1970). Stereotaxic amygdalectomy and basofrontal tractotomy in psychotics with aggressive behavior. *J. Neurol. Neurosurg. Psychiat.*, **33**, 858
78. Yakovlev P (1948). Motility, behavior and the brain. Stereodynamic organization and neural co-ordinates of behavior. *J. Nervous Mental Disease*, **107**, 313
79. Yakovlev P (1954). Anatomical studies in frontal leucotomies II: cortical origin of the frontopontin tract and organization of the thalamus-frontal projections. *Trans. Amer. Neurol. Assoc.*, **53**

CHAPTER 2

Brain Mechanisms and Psychiatry
J R SMYTHIES

INTRODUCTION
The brain mechanisms I shall be discussing in this paper are mainly at the biochemical level. This is really because one of the major problems in science today is communication between disciplines owing to the exponential growth of knowledge in all fields. The gap that I am concerned with is between thinking going on currently in biological psychiatry about the aetiology of psychiatric illness, and the thinking in psychosurgery about the strategy of deciding which particular tracts or nuclei one should operate on.

Clearly it would be advantageous in psychosurgery if one had some understanding of the aetiology of the conditions one is operating on. I am going to concentrate particularly on schizophrenia.

It is generally agreed that the term schizophrenia covers a variety of different diseases with quite a wide range of aetiologies. It would be surprising if this were not so since the diagnosis of 'schizophrenia' is based entirely on symptoms, and we know from the progress of general medicine that no 'disease' defined only by two symptoms ever turns out to have a single aetiology.

Rosenthal & Kety (1969) have produced good evidence that one can distinguish quite clearly between chronic process schizophrenia and acute schizophreniform reactions on the basis of their genetics. The former has a marked genetic component while the latter has not. This indicates that a defect in some enzyme, or a collection of enzymes, is involved for almost all genetically determined diseases, which usually are due to very weak enzymes—only few are due to over-active ones. So the odds are that schizophrenia is associated with one or more enzymes which are defective. These enzymes may well be located in areas of the brain strategically concerned with reactions to stress, or areas organizing perception, thinking, affect or other systems that go wrong in schizophrenia, or in some more basic organizational system the function of which is to co-ordinate other brain mechanisms. Of course different cases of schizophrenia may depend on lesions in different biochemical systems as it is well known that different genotypes commonly yield very similar phenotypes.

METHIONINE AND PSYCHOSIS
In the last few years some genuine data have been obtained about

physiological abnormalities in schizophrenia, after some 50 years of innumerable false claims and red herrings. I want to discuss very briefly what these findings are because I will submit that they may give us some indication about the basic mechanisms of schizophrenia. I refer here to what we might call the methionine effect, the histamine effect, and the mechanisms of action of antipsychotic drugs. Taking these in turn: Dr Kety's group (Pollin, Cardon & Kety, 1961) found that methionine, the ordinary constituent of diet if given in dosage of 10–20 g of L-methionine a day, will produce in some 40% of chronic schizophrenics an acute toxic, florid psychotic reaction. The other 60% of schizophrenics do not show any change. Kety and his co-workers were interested in amines and gave their patients different amino acids with iproniazid, a MAO inhibitor, to try to raise the level of the amines in the brain. One of the amino acids they gave was L-methionine.

The only amino acids which produced any abnormality were methionine and tryptophane. Tryptophane produced a non-specific euphoria without psychotic features, while the methionine caused a quite florid psychosis which had some features of an acute schizophrenic reaction superimposed on the chronic one and some features of an acute delirium. They reported that the effect was so obvious that one could not possibly miss it. Their finding has now been confirmed by five other groups of workers and it has been shown that the MAO inhibitor is not necessary, i.e. the effect is caused by methionine.

Why does methionine produce this change in behaviour? Firstly we can say that the schizophrenics can be grouped into two different categories—'methionine-sensitive' and 'methionine-insensitive' patients and the distinction is absolute. Patients either react to methionine with an acute psychosis or they do not react at all. There is no 'in between' kind of reaction. The hypothesis commonly held to explain the methionine effect has been based on the fact that methionine is the main methyl donor in the body. One of the theories of the biochemical basis of schizophrenia is the transmethylation hypothesis which suggests that toxic compounds like dimethyltryptamine could be produced in the brain. It has been recently demonstrated that the enzyme necessary for making hallucinogenic dimethyltryptamine and destroying it is present normally in the brain. This leads to an interesting problem of what the brain is doing with such hallucinogenic compounds in it. It seems possible that administration of methionine raises the level of dimethyltryptamine in the brain which of course produces a psychosis. This has been the standard explanation for the methionine effect.

We have recently done some work on the behavioural mechanism of methionine. It is interesting that no one has ever done a thorough study of its effect on normal people. We would like to know what would happen to normal people when given 20 g of L-methionine a day. Dr Kety has done a few experiments and reported that he did not find any behavioural changes. At the moment, a study is going on using this dose of methionine in normal people to see if it produces changes in thinking or other aspects of behaviour.

ANIMAL EXPERIMENTS

It is possible to reproduce these changes in animals. Dr Carranza of Mexico City gave methionine to mice and after some days, the animals developed behavioural disturbances. Usually methionine was given along with amphetamine to see if one could raise the level of methoxylated derivatives of amphetamine which was thought to be at the basis of the amphetamine psychosis. In one of the controls methionine was administered alone and after 2 days the mice developed behavioural changes very similar to those induced by amphetamine, i.e. overactivity, stereotyped behaviour and disruption of grouped behaviour. Dr Carranza used a very simple ethological test. The mice were placed in a cage. Normally these mice like to live in groups—they spend much of their time in a pile in one corner. He measured the number of times in half an hour that the mice were away from the home corner. Normally he obtained a very low count. But if he gave amphetamine the mice started dispersing and he found eventually the mice walking around on the ceiling and the walls of the cage. Methionine produced a very similar effect.

The methionine effect takes some time to develop, but the reaction after 3 and 4 weeks is marked and then it takes a long time—up to 5 weeks—to get back to normal. Serine has an opposite action to methionine and causes increased grouping. But when serine administration is stopped there is a rebound reaction similar to many compounds which induce tranquillization. A combination of methionine and serine might result in a disappearance of the effect; the one would increase the dispersing effect while the other would decrease it. But in fact a profound potentiation of the effect is obtained and the animals on methionine and serine together become wildly disordered. They swing around on the roof of the cages doing all sorts of acrobatics and showing all sorts of weird stereotyped behaviour. They have piloerection and look very much as though they had had a large dose of amphetamine.

Nicotinamide potentiates the methionine effect just as serine does. This is directly contrary to the transmethylation theory because nicotinamide is a potent methyl acceptor. Therefore giving methionine together with nicotinamide, one would expect, according to the transmethylation theory, that they would cancel each other out because the nicotinamide would mop up all the excess methyl groups.

The next experiment I want to describe uses rats as the experimental animal. Here we have a more sophisticated measure of behaviour (Sidman avoidance) which we have been using for the past 5 years to distinguish between the mescaline-like and amphetamine-like compounds. I would like to describe this very briefly. The rats are placed in a Skinner box for 20 s in the dark. At 20 s a light comes on and at 30 s they get shocked (0·5 s). The shock is repeated every 10 s until the rat presses the lever. A lever press will recycle the programme to the beginning. A rat soon learns that the optimum time to press the lever to avoid shocks is somewhere in the middle of the 'light-on' period so that the animals will start emitting most of their responses during the period about between the 25th and 28th second of the schedule. This is a very sensitive test for drugs which disrupt behaviour.

The responses emitted too early are called 'premature' and those during the shock 'late' responses. If the rat is given amphetamines the 'premature' responses increase. Hallucinogens like LSD will increase both 'premature' and 'late' responses. If the rat gets drugs like chlorpromazine it will emit almost all 'late' responses. This is a good way of distinguishing between amphetamine-like compounds, mescaline-like compounds, tranquillizers and so on. Using this test with L-methionine (25 mg/kg) three rats showed a response to only one dose equivalent to 1 mg/kg amphetamine and one rat a response equivalent to 25 mg/kg of mescaline.

DISCUSSION

We have thus the interesting fact that methionine by itself (25 mg/kg) produces an effect in some schizophrenics like schizophrenia, and in rats an effect sometimes like amphetamine and sometimes, like mescaline. It is well known that amphetamine itself can produce in chronic users a typical paranoid type of psychosis indistinguishable from schizophrenia.

How can we tie all this together? I would suggest the hypothesis shown in Figure 2.1 which has nothing to do with transmethylation at all. This is one way one can connect the potentiation of the methionine effect by serine and nicotinamide. This involves the one-carbon cycle whereby methionine gives up its methyl group to a methyl acceptor (e.g. nicotinamide) and becomes homocysteine. Homocysteine plus serine together form cystathionine which in turn then breaks down to cysteine and various other compounds.

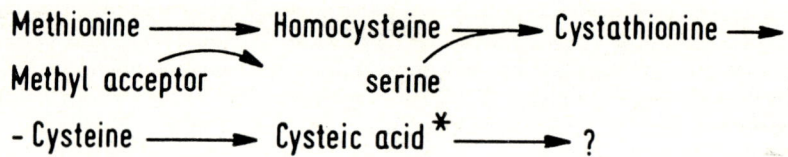

Figure 2.1 Part of the one carbon-cycle. The lesion in some cases of schizophrenia may be at the locus*.

Brune & Himwich (1963) found that cysteine produces the same effect as methionine in schizophrenics. Workers from Professor Bradley's group in Birmingham, England, giving cysteine intraventricularly to cats found that it produced overactive behaviour. Also there is an inborn error of metabolism—cystathionuria—where one gets high levels of cystathionine in the brain. This is entirely asymptomatic so the lesion cannot be due to a defect in the enzyme metabolizing cystathionine. We suggest that the lesion may be 'downstream' from cysteine. Cysteine can form cysteic acid which is an excitatory amino acid like glutamate. Maybe the production of excited behaviour is due to some disarrangement in cysteine or cysteic acid function.

The next data I am going to mention is the effect of histamine. Schizophrenics have been shown by many workers to be more resistant to histamine than normals. If one injects histamine into the skin, one would normally get a wheal. The wheal produced by histamine in schizophrenics is smaller than normal, and it increases as they get better. We do not know the significance of this reaction, but any theory of schizophrenia has to explain it. The last relevant fact is the effect of the antischizophrenic drugs such as the phenothiazines, butyrophenones and pimozide. The phenothiazines of course act on a large number of systems but they are mainly antiadrenergic and antidopaminergic. Pimozide is a specific blocker of dopamine receptors. It has no action on serotonin receptors and it has no action on noradrenaline. We have tried pimozide clinically and found that it seems to act on a different kind of schizophrenia than chlorpromazine does. The latter acts particularly on violent combative schizophrenics with many positive symptoms, hallucinations, delusions and so on. Pimozide can make such patients worse but it can produce a very good response in chronic withdrawn flat and energic schizophrenics—as though these people were suffering from an overactive dopamine system.

I leave you with two thoughts. One is: what is the possible relationship between the one-carbon cycle and the dopamine system? Secondly, since many schizophrenias are the result of overactive dopaminergic and adrenergic systems in the brain, a surgical lesion which would depress the action of the dopaminergic ventral limbic system might be of therapeutic benefit in schizophrenia.

ACKNOWLEDGEMENT

The experiments described were conducted in conjunction with John Beaton, Ronald J. Bradley and William F. Bridgers and represent a contribution of the Neuroscience Program, University of Alabama.

REFERENCES

Brune GC & Himwich HE (1963). *Recent Advances in Biological Psychiatry*. New York: Plenum Press.
Pollin W, Cardon PV & Kety SS (1961). Effects of aminoacid feedings in schizophrenic patients treated with iproniazid. *Science*, **133**, 104
Rosenthal D & Kety SS (1969). *The Transmission of Schizophrenia*. London: Pergamon Press.

CHAPTER 3

Attempt at localization of psychological manifestations observed in various psychosurgical procedures
LOTHAR B KALINOWSKY

INTRODUCTION
Twenty-five years of psychiatric experience with a variety of psychosurgical procedures should permit certain conclusions regarding the mode of action of these therapeutic approaches. While none of the somatic treatments in psychiatry has a clear rationale, psychosurgery actually has a better theoretical foundation than the other forms of therapy. Many discrepancies, however, remain to be clarified. Therefore, an attempt at localization of psychopathological manifestations observed in psychosurgery seems to be indicated.

LOCALIZATION OF PSYCHOLOGICAL ILLNESS IN THE BRAIN
Since the times of Wernicke and Kleist, localization of psychopathological changes in certain parts of the brain has been tried, but their failure led to discreditation of this approach. Initially, psychosurgery seemed to confirm the doubts in this direction. Here the attempts of the comprehensive Columbia–Greystone Project (1949) regarding topectomy in certain areas of the frontal cortex should be mentioned. This research done in an excellent multi-disciplinary setting negated a localization of mental symptoms in the surgical target area. The more widely used leucotomies in the white matter of the frontal lobes did not contribute more to a localization. They rather suggested a quantitative principle, namely that the degree of therapeutic effect as well as the appearance of undesirable personality changes depended on the quantity of destroyed brain substance. Rostral leucotomy produced less psychopathological changes because it left a part of the fronto-thalamic fibres intact. However, already before the present stereotactic era it was noticed that operations in the medial and orbital part of the frontal lobes gave better results than lateral targets, and this suggested a greater interest in the limbic system.

The first stereotactic operation, thalamotomy devised by Spiegel & Wycis (1962) had a well-thought-out anatomical localization in the dorsal medial nucleus of the thalamus. If the results were not entirely convincing, and if the operation was not generally accepted, the reason could be that fibres from the frontal lobe go partly beyond this area into the hypothalamus, and, therefore, remain intact. This would be in accordance with the expectation of many of us that if one day the localization of psychiatric disorders becomes possible, it will be found in the deeper structures of the limbic and reticular systems. In this area many authors had described tumours, particularly around the third ventricle which were characterized by schizophreniform and manic-like syndromes (Malamud, 1967). Closest to an operation in this area of the brain comes Sano from Japan, who operates in the posteromedial hypothalamus (Sano, 1962). It remains difficult to explain why the positive results of this operation in such deep parts of the brain hardly differ from the results of operations in higher regions. This is well demonstrated by Obrador who for 25 years operated in the frontal lobe and the limbic system including amygdala and gyrus cinguli, and who found that Sano's operation in the hypothalamus produces the same amount of reduction of anxiety, psychomotor excitement and emotional reaction to psychiatric symptoms as his previous operations (Obrador, 1972).

MECHANISMS OF PSYCHOSURGERY
Psychopathologically the common feature of all the various interventions may be defined as diminished reaction and vigilance of the brain to unpleasant sensations. This poses the question to the neuroanatomists how identical psychopathological changes can be explained by operations in so many different structures. Comparative investigations by the same clinician on material operated on with different procedures, are few. Most impressive is the material of Knight who operated on 600 cases by orbital undercutting and later on 450 patients stereotactically by means of radioactive yttrium implanted into the substantia innominata. The clinical effects were identical, but it appears that the postoperative side-effects were missing in the latter operations (Knight, 1964).

Too little attention has been paid to the immediate psychopathological changes occurring after psychosurgery. They are unpredictable but hardly differ from those after other brain operations or traumatic brain injury. They have manifold characteristics of a brain syndrome with Korsakoff-like symptoms and emotional blunting, often followed by euphoria. Loss of initiative can be extreme even in patients who later become rather overactive. Usually these symptoms are reversible. However, they are disturbing, and they make the immediate postoperative care very difficult. Their usual absence after stereotactic operations should be a decisive factor in favour of these latter procedures.

The psychopathological changes seen in psychosurgery can be best described by using concepts developed by Manfred Bleuler. He made a clean distinction between diffuse and localized brain damage. In diffuse brain damage one must distinguish between an acute and a chronic psychosyndrome. In psychosurgery an acute syndrome characterized by such symptoms as clouded sensorium, disorientation, apathy, is only seen in the immediate postoperative period and it does not differ from the psychopathology of other brain traumata or operations. It lasts only days or weeks and seems to be largely absent in smaller stereotactic lesions. Contrary to this acute psychosyndrome of diffuse brain damage, a chronic diffuse brain syndrome, characterized by intellectual impairment, intellectual fatiguability and emotional dullness, does not manifest itself after psychosurgical intervention. The psychopathology in psychosurgery corresponds to the picture of the local organic psychosyndrome. In the older literature a psychopathological frontal-lobe syndrome, as also a psychopathological brain-stem syndrome, was described. It was later realized that the psychopathology of the brain-stem syndrome and of the frontal-lobe syndrome hardly differ. It is this experience that may explain why the lasting effects of psychosurgery, both therapeutic and side-effects, are identical, irrespective of whether the operation is performed in the frontal lobes or in the deeper parts of the brain. The local organic psychosyndrome has always been known to leave the intellectual functions intact, and is mainly characterized by diminished drive and a decrease of interest, tact and responsibility. This local organic psychosyndrome is more pronounced in larger lesions. These patients have also been known to have sudden mood swings which may explain occasional suicides after psychosurgery as reported by Freeman (1972). The one psychiatric change which is the whole purpose of psychosurgical procedures is the diminished concern. Thus, the concern over obsessive fears, compulsive thinking or a concern regarding delusions, hallucinations, hypochondrical and depressive thoughts is therapeutically desired, while reduced concern about human inter-relationships and the impression made on others is undesirable. Another definition of the effect of these operations is reduced vigilance of the brain regarding both pleasant and unpleasant sensations. Aggressiveness is reduced as an exaggerated reaction to disturbing factors, and there can also be a reduction of normal and desirable goal-directed aggression in a competitive world.

How far this effect of surgery influences the total personality depends also on such factors of the individual personality as degree of differentiation, attitude, tendencies and general behaviour. These factors also contribute to the final outcome of the operation which is obviously not decided alone by the site and extension of the lesion. The optimal site or sites for this type of brain surgery should be decided by the minimum of acute postoperative changes and a minimum of undesirable side-effects. At this point it would be desirable that the neurosurgeons, in co-operation with psychiatrists who are experienced in this therapeutic approach, agree on an optimal site acceptable by all concerned. Of course the specificity of certain operations like the ones by Hassler & Dieckmann (1973) and by Laitinen (1972) must be investigated further. The same can be said for claims that different operations are superior in different psychiatric diseases.

REFERENCES

Columbia-Greystone Association (1949). *Selective Partial Ablation of the Frontal Cortex*. New York: Columbia-Greystone Association.

Freeman W (1972). Frontal lobotomy in early schizophrenia. Long follow-up in 415 cases. In: *Psychosurgery* (Eds Hitchcock, Laitinen & Vaernet), p. 311. Springfield, Ill.: Charles C Thomas.

Hassler R & Dieckmann G (1973). Relief of obsessive-compulsive disorders, phobias and tics by stereotactic coagulation of the rostral extralaminar and medial thalamic nuclei. In: *Surgical Approaches in Psychiatry* (Eds Laitinen & Livingston). Lancaster: MTP.

Knight GC (1964). The orbital cortex as an objective in the surgical treatment of mental illness. The results of 450 cases of open operation and the development of the stereotactic approach. *Brit. J. Surg.*, **51**, 114

Laitinen LV (1972). Stereotactic lesions in the knee of the corpus callosum in the treatment of emotional disorders. *Lancet*, **1**, 472

Malamud N (1967). Psychiatric disorders with intracranial tumors of limbic system. *Arch. Neurol. (Chicago)*, **17**, 113

Obrador S (1972). Observations and reflections on psychosurgery at different levels. In: *Psychosurgery* (Eds Hitchcock, Laitinen & Vaernet), p. 83. Springfield, Ill.: Charles C Thomas.

Sano K (1962). Sedative neurosurgery. *Neurologia. med.-chir.*, **4**, 112

Spiegel EA & Wycis HT (1962). *Stereoencephalotomy*, Part II. Clinical and physiological applications. New York: Grune & Stratton.

CHAPTER 4

Psychiatric syndromes considered as manifestations of lateralized temporal-limbic dysfunction
P FLOR-HENRY

An increasing number of investigations in recent years converge to suggest that, to a remarkable degree, the psychiatric syndromes can be correlated with definite cerebral regions. The efficacy of prefrontal leucotomy in chronic depressive states and the characteristic euphoric disinhibition encountered in the frontal lobe syndrome both suggest that the orbital surface of the frontal lobes is intimately related to affect. That the non-dominant temporal-limbic structures are particularly related to the affective state is demonstrated by: (*a*) the characteristic euphoria associated with lesions in the non-dominant hemisphere (Hecaen & Ajuriaguerra, 1952); (*b*) the preponderance of lesions in the non-dominant hemisphere in dysphoric states occurring after penetrating head injuries (Lishman, 1966); (*c*) the characteristic euphoria produced by intracarotid injections of amytal into the non-dominant, but not into the dominant hemisphere (Hommes & Panhuysen, 1971), and (*d*) the therapeutic equivalence of bilateral and unilateral ECT of the non-dominant hemisphere, as opposed to the diminished effectiveness of ECT of the dominant hemisphere only (Giacomo D'Elia, 1970). In addition, data from epileptic studies (Flor-Henry, 1969) relate neurotic types of depression and manic-depressive psychosis to non-dominant temporal lobe epilepsy. Similarly a substantial and coherent body of evidence is accumulating which links the schizophrenic and paranoid psychoses to dominant temporal-limbic dysfunction. This evidence is derived from neurological studies, studies of organic psychoses associated with cerebral tumours and other cerebral pathology (Davidson & Bagley, 1969), studies of schizophrenic psychoses associated with epilepsy (Flor-Henry, 1969), studies of perceptual ability and of lateral preference in schizophrenia, as well as neurophysiological investigations (Walker & Birch, 1970; Puskina, 1971).

For example, Hillbom (1960) investigated soldiers who had suffered head injuries during World War II in Finland, and found that dominant temporal pathology was positively correlated with psychotic manifestations. Similarly Lishman (1966), in a very large and detailed investigation of British soldiers with head injuries, also sustained in World War II, found that psychic sequelae after penetrating head injuries was correlated with dominant temporal pathology, whereas affective disturbance was correlated significantly with non-dominant hemispheric pathology, notably with non-dominant frontal pathology. Further, Davidson & Bagley (1969), reviewing the international literature on schizophrenia-like psychoses associated with organic disorders, found statistically significant associations between 'lesions of the left cerebral hemisphere, and particularly temporal lobe lesions with primary delusions and catatonic symptoms, whilst diencephalic lesions correlate with auditory hallucinations and brain stem lesions with thought disorders and Schneider's symptoms of the first rank'. Revitch & Zallanski (1969), reviewing 2,335 hospitalized psychotic veterans, found 126 cases with an anterior temporal focus. Sixty-eight of these were seizure-free and 58 had seizure manifestations. In both the epileptics and the seizure-free groups there was a marked preponderance of left-sided foci. Similarly, Vinar & Skalickova (1965), studying 100 schizophrenic patients and 20 manic-depressive patients, whom they compared with 220 healthy controls, found neurological evidence showing that their schizophrenic population was characterized by pathology of the dominant hemisphere. This was statistically highly significant. Mefford, Lester, Willand, Falconer & Pokorny (1969), testing 26 schizophrenics and 26 controls matched for age, intelligence, sex, education, race and auditory acuity, found that schizophrenics significantly failed to reproduce stimulus words, irrespective of whether distraction was employed or not. Again this observation strongly suggests a disturbance of function in the dominant temporal region. Of very great interest are the studies on lateral preference and dichotic stimulation carried out in dyslexics and schizophrenics. Unexpectedly, dextrals in the dyslexic group exhibited left-ear, instead of the expected crossed, right-ear superiority (Zurif & Carson, 1970). Moreover, in schizophrenic children, as compared with normal children, development of right-left preference and awareness are impaired: thus functional impairment of the dominant hemisphere is suggested in both groups, at the level of language for dyslexics and at the level of thought for schizophrenics. Further, neurophysiological evidence indicates that limbic dysfunction with a dominance shift occurs in the course of certain schizophrenias and in deep depression. In the laboratory of neurophysiology of the Institute of Psychiatry of the Academy of Medical Sciences of the USSR, Moscow, Puskina (1971) showed by toposcopic analysis of interareal responses to serial light-flashes that in paranoid-hallucinatory schizophrenia 'the temporal lobe is locked out of the unitary (cerebral) functional system'. Further, it was demonstrated by interareal analysis of in-phase alpha synchronization, that, whereas in normal subjects there is a preponderance of alpha synchronization of the dominant over the non-dominant hemisphere, this was reversed in paranoid schizophrenia, and reduced in the paranoid-hallucinatory phase of the illness. Alterations of cerebral dominance have also been demonstrated in depression. Hommes & Panhuysen (1971) at the Catholic University of Nijmegan, studying depression and cerebral dominance by means of bilateral intracarotid amytal injections in 11 patients, found that amytal injections on the side of the non-dominant hemisphere produced elevation of mood in both normal and depressed patients, but that whereas in normals injections into the dominant hemisphere tended to lower mood, in depressed patients they had the opposite effect. The authors conclude that in 'depressed patients both hemisphere appear to have the organizational structure of the non-dominant hemisphere'. They found a close negative relationship between depth of depression and level of left speech dominance. These observations may perhaps be explained by the extension of the non-dominant cerebral dysfunction to bitemporal dysfunction as the depression becomes more intense. The possibility that reduced cerebral dominance may be a feature of early schizophrenia is suggested by Oddy & Lobstein (1972), who report that 140 patients with schizophrenia and without known cerebral lesions show a significant excess of cross-dominance as compared with a normal population.

There is evidence that the obsessional syndrome is anatomically dependent on the central, midline structure of the limbic system—its anterior thalamic-cingular gyrus axis. Multifocal thermocoagulation of the cingulate gyrus is

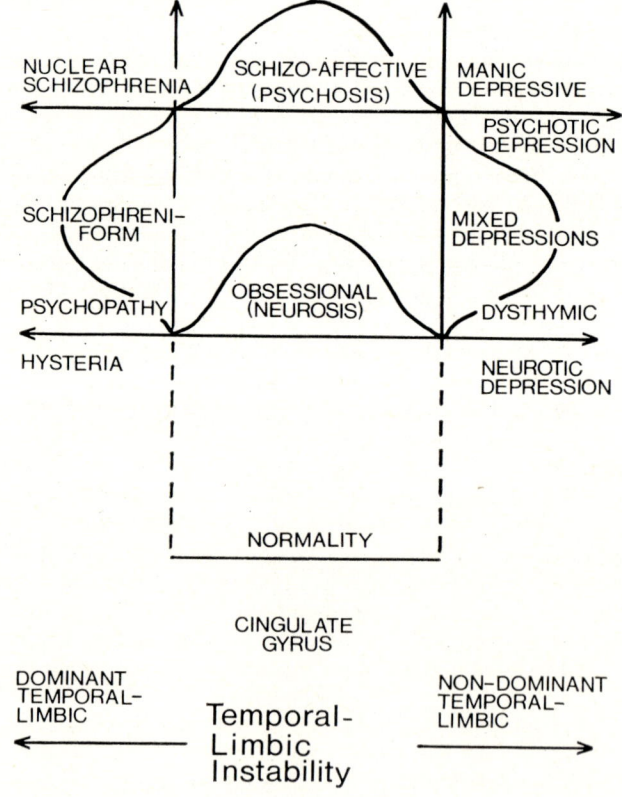

Figure 4.1 Schematic illustration of lateralized temporal-limbic dysfunction.

effective therapeutically, but a similar procedure directed at the mesial frontal regions principally alleviates anxiety-depressive states. Thus the dorsomedial thalamic-orbital frontal axis appears to be specifically associated with affect. The clinical counterpart of this neuronal organization is reflected by the fact that the obsessional syndrome is, in a sense, intermediate between the schizophrenic and depressive syndromes, waxing and waning, intensifying or disappearing with the former, and positively correlated with the latter. Neuropathological investigations also demonstrate that schizophrenic or manic-depressive presentation of frontal lobe tumours hinge on anterior limbic perturbation, since these occur essentially with orbito-frontal lesions, and not with involvement of the lateral surface, which is associated with dementia. Similarly, neuropathological studies in temporal lobe epilepsy (Falconer & Taylor, 1968) confirm the importance of temporal-limbic dysfunction in psychotic states associated with epilepsy, since in mesial temporal sclerosis, (where the hippocampus is the structure predominantly affected), psychotic complications are rare or absent, although in lesions of other areas of the temporal-limbic system they are common.

In addition, there is reason to believe that the affective psychoses and schizophrenia fall at opposite poles of a normal distribution for psychosis (Kendell & Gourlay, 1970), intermediary or schizo-affective forms with features common to both predominating, and since there is data from epileptic studies (Serafetinides, 1965) demonstrating that psychopathy is associated with dysfunction of the dominant temporal lobe, and neurotic types of depression with dysfunction of the non-dominant temporal lobe, a neurological model for the psychiatric syndromes emerges and is presented heuristically.

CONCLUSIONS

According to this hypothesis, predominantly unilateral dominant temporal-limbic neuronal disorganization (or bilateral temporal-limbic dysfunction) is associated with the schizophrenic syndrome, whereas predominantly unilateral non-dominant temporal-limbic dysfunction (with bilateral involvement of the orbito-frontal extension of the limbic system) is associated with the affective psychoses (Figure 4.1). Asymmetrical dysfunction of the limbic system as a whole would explain the atypical depressions with paranoid symptomatology. Lesser degrees of dominant temporal limbic disturbance would similarly lead to psychopathy and of non-dominant to 'neurotic' types of depression. Disorganization of the central (anterior–thalamic–cingulate gyrus) limbic axis, according to this model, would be the neuronal basis underlying the obsessional syndrome.

REFERENCES

Davidson K & Bagley CR (1969). Schizophrenia-like psychoses associated with organic disorders. In: *Current Problems in Neuro-psychiatry* p. 150. London: The Royal Medico-Psychological Association.

Falconer MA & Taylor DC (1968). Surgical treatment of drug resistant epilepsy due to mesial temporal sclerosis: Etiology and significance. *Arch. Neurol.* (*Chicago*), **19**, 353

Flor-Henry P (1969). Psychosis and temporal lobe epilepsy. A controlled investigation. *Epilepsia (Amst.)*, **10**, 363

Giacomo D'Elia (1970). Unilateral electroconvulsive therapy. *Acta Psychiat. Scand.* Suppl., **215**, 97

Halliday AM, Davidson K, Browne MW & Kreeger LC (1968). A comparison of the effects on depression and memory of bilateral ECT and unilateral ECT to the dominant and nondominant hemisphere. *Brit. J. Psychiat.*, **114**, 997

Hecaen H & Ajuriaguerra J de (1952). *Meconnaissances et Hallucinations Corporelles.* p. 63. Paris: Masson et Cie.

Hillbom E (1960). After-effects of brain injuries: research on the symptoms causing invalidism of persons in Finland having sustained brain injuries during the wars of 1939-40 and 1941-44. *Acta Psychiat. Scand.*, **35**, Suppl. **142**, 195

Hommes OR & Panhuysen LHHM (1971). Depression and cerebral dominance. *Psychiat. Neurol. Neurochir.*, **74**, 259

Kendell RE & Gourlay J (1970). The clinical distinction between the affective psychoses and schizophrenia. *Brit. J. Psychiat.*, **117**, 261

Lishman WA (1966). Brain damage in relation to psychiatric disability after head injury. *Brit. J. Psychiat.*, **114**, 373

Mefford RB, Lester JW, Willand BA, Falconer GA & Pokorny AD (1969). Influence of distraction on the reproduction of spoken words by schizophrenics. *J. nerv. ment. Dis.*, **149**, 504

Puskina (1971). *Modern Perspectives in World Psychiatry.* (Ed Howells), Chapt. XIX, 'The Pavlovian theory in psychiatry, some recent developments' by KK Monakhov (transl. Dr R Pos, Univ. Toronto), p. 531. New York: Brunner-Mazel.

Oddy HC & Lobstein TJ (1972). Hand and eye dominance in schizophrenia. *Brit. J. Psychiat.*, **120**, 331

Revitch E & Zallanski Z (1969). Slow anterior temporal foci in a mental hospital population. *Behavioural Neuropsychiatry*, **9**, 8

Serafetinides EA (1965). Aggressiveness in temporal lobe epileptics and its relation to cerebral dysfunction and environmental factors. *Epilepsia (Amst.)*, **6**, 33

Vinar J & Skalickova O (1965). Neurologicke Hodneceni Schizofrenniho Onemocneni. *Ceskoslovenska Psychiatrie*, **61**, 373

Walker HA & Birch HG (1970). Lateral preference and right-left awareness in schizophrenic children. *J. nerv. ment. Dis.*, **151**, 341

Zurif EB & Carson G (1970). Dyslexia in relation to cerebral dominance and temporal analysis. *Neuropsychologia*, **8**, 351

PART II

PRESIDENTIAL ADDRESS

CHAPTER 5

Surgical locations for psychiatric surgery with special reference to orbital and cingulate operations
WILLIAM BEECHER SCOVILLE

Mental surgery, popularly known as psychiatric surgery, received great impetus in the late 1940s and 1950s, following the pioneer work of Fulton on chimpanzees (Fulton & Jacobsen, 1935) and Egas Moniz (1936) on humans although Burckhardt (1890) of Switzerland and Puusepp (1937) of Esthonia made largely unrecognized operations at the turn of the century. Early operations were limited to gross cutting of most of the connections from the prefrontal lobe to the thalamus. Even such crude operations offered dramatic benefit to the sick thoughts and feelings of the mentally ill but at a cost of considerable blunting of higher sensitivities. Following the excessive early enthusiasm for surgical attack on the mind, interest faded in the late 1950s and early 1960s because of electric shock therapy and then drug therapy. All three approaches gave therapeutic benefit and great advances in the knowledge of brain physiology. In recent years there has been a resurgence of interest by a whole new generation of psychiatrists because of the failure of both shock therapy and drugs to adequately improve some of the more intractable psychoses and psychoneuroses. In fact shock therapy, when used in excess, has been shown to cause as much blunting as the more radical surgical procedures. Throughout all these years psychiatric surgeons have sought to develop ever more selective operations which would specifically lessen the diseased mental functions but not the normal mental output.

Such operations should rest on the following criteria:

(1) Symptomatic benefit
(2) Preservation of intact personality
(3) Sufficient quantitative precision to permit exact duplication of tract interruptions in successive cases
(4) Determination as to whether there is anatomical specificity for various types of mental disease. In other words, is there a specific area in the brain linked to depressions, schizophrenia or neuroses?

In a search for selective operations satisfying the above criteria two major schools, which I call the 'orbital' and 'cingulate', have developed, interrupting respectively connections from these areas to the thalamus and limbic lobe. I early introduced both approaches with my 'undercutting' procedures, carrying out ultimately 50 cases of operations in each of the three areas (Scoville, 1949) and in the late 1940s I communicated my results to Eduard Busch in Denmark, Hugh Cairns at Oxford, and Le Beau in Paris (Figures 5.1,2). All three enthusiastically developed these operations with somewhat differing conclusions from myself. My own findings indicated that rostral cingulate undercutting, limited to the cingulate complex itself, gave less benefit to psychiatric symptoms while severance of connections from the superior convexity and the orbital surface resulted in more benefit. There

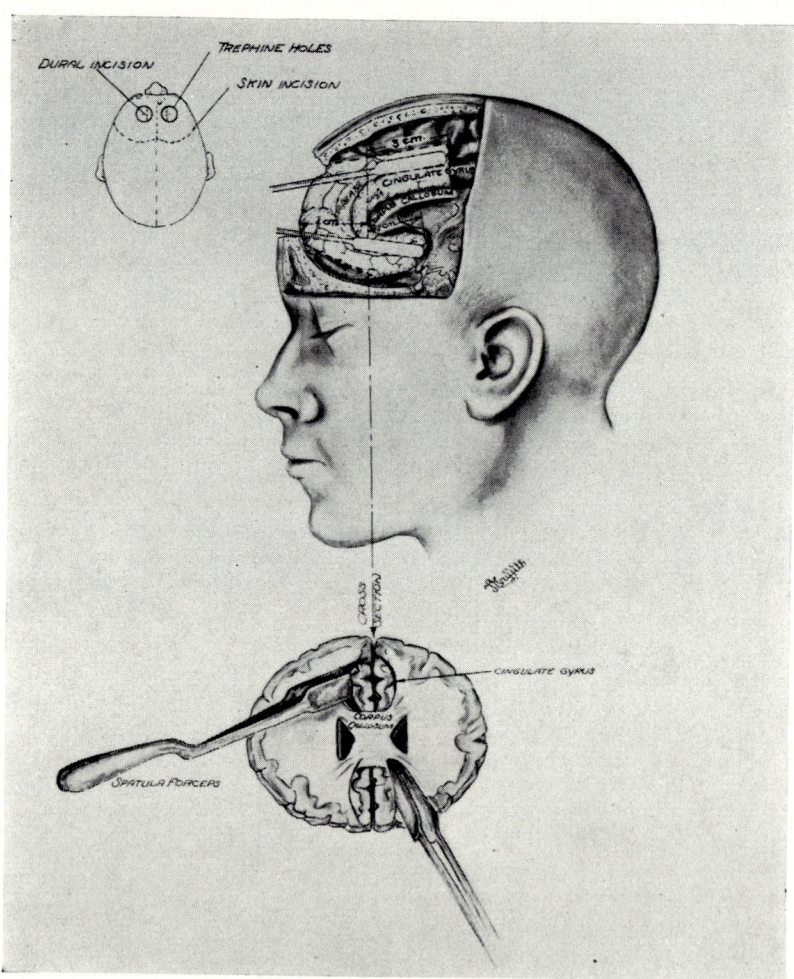

Figure 5.1 Sketch of rostral cingulate undercutting as carried out by the writer in the 1940s.

seemed little specificity in their effect upon depressions versus neuroses except for considerable personality blunting in the superior convexity undercutting; hence I have discontinued the latter and utilize orbital undercutting for all forms of mental disease.

Since then cingulate operations have been described by Cairns (1952), Le Beau (1954), Livingston (1953), Foltz (1962), Ballantine (1967) and an increasing number of younger men with frequent stress on their benefit in the psychoneuroses.

There have been many other operations described as selective leucotomies and lobotomies which probably all interrupt connections from one or the other area, the most important of which have been bimedial inferior leucotomies as developed by McKenzie (1964), Greenblatt & Poppen (1952,) Grantham (1951), Mayfield (1954) and McKissock (1949). By and large the English school, excepting Cairns' group (Whitty, Duffield, Tow & Cairns, 1952), has favoured severance of orbital connections by knife and isotopes as proposed by Tow & Lewin (1953) and Knight (1964).

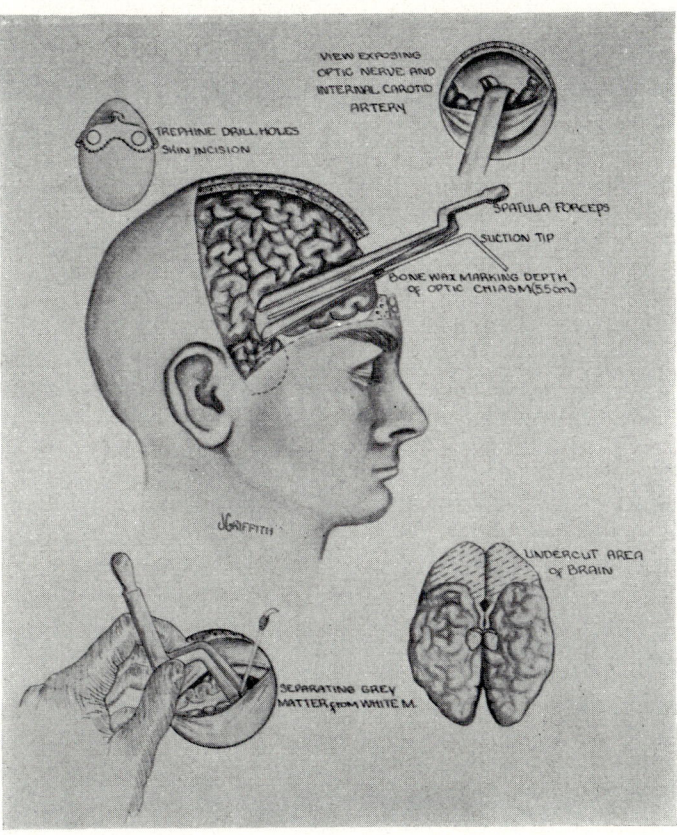

Figure 5.2 Scoville's orbital undercutting.

There is no question that all present operations satisfy the first two criteria although to a varying degree of symptomatic benefit and preservation of an intact personality. There is some evidence that cingulate operations frequently require repeated procedures to get sufficient symptomatic benefit to restore the patient to society.

But let us turn to the third criterion of quantitative precision. It is my belief that the rostral cingulate complex itself is not an important area affecting mental disease, but rather the adjacent white matter lying between the cinguli and the frontal horns of the cerebral ventricles which contain converging fibres from both the orbital and superior convexity en route to the thalamus and limbic lobe. Cingulotomies are generally performed through stereotactic or 'closed' approaches spilling into the concentrated white matter. Hence is this a true cingulotomy operation or rather a bimedial leucotomy? Perhaps cingulate leucotomy would be a more appropriate term. But more important is the impossibility of quantitative precision in most of the present cingulotomy operations making it impossible to exactly duplicate tract interruptions in successive cases. This is particularly important at this time inasmuch as we are not yet certain as to what areas are best suited for surgical attack on specific mental illnesses. When we cannot directly measure areas interrupted by either direct vision or microscopic counting of fibres we cannot know whether varying results are due to our case selection or the number of white fibres cut.

I want to bring up this problem because many psychiatric surgeons today are concentrating on one or the other approach without personally having tried both. I have tried both and have found my orbital operations yield better results than my cingulate leucotomies as well as permitting precise measurement of the area interrupted under direct vision in terms of centimetres. A plea is made to present surgeons who are doing a sufficient number of cases to be of statistical value, to alternate the two approaches in their own clinics. This is the only objective way to determine which area is the more important in effecting a cure.

Are there other areas than the superior convexity, the medial cingulate and the orbital areas of the frontal lobes which will affect mental disease? Certainly Yakolev (1948), Nauta (1972) and Powell (1972), and others have shown that the medial surface of the temporal lobe is closely connected to the posterior orbital surface as well as to the limbic lobe and connects both frontal and temporal lobes to the deeper midline structures of the diencephalon and telencephalon. It is these limbic and hypothalamic areas which undoubtedly contain the basic elements of emotional colouring and the seeds of mental aberration. I have been intrigued for years with such areas and attempted at our last Conference of Copenhagen to describe how lesions in such midline structures may cause clinical pictures exactly similar to schizophrenic psychoses. Unfortunately it is easier to cause than to cure them. Chemical alterations and stimulation therapy may be of more future benefit than surgical ablations. Data of great interest has been collected by stereotactic lesions or electrode implants in these deeply hidden areas of the brain. Sano (1962) is directly attacking the

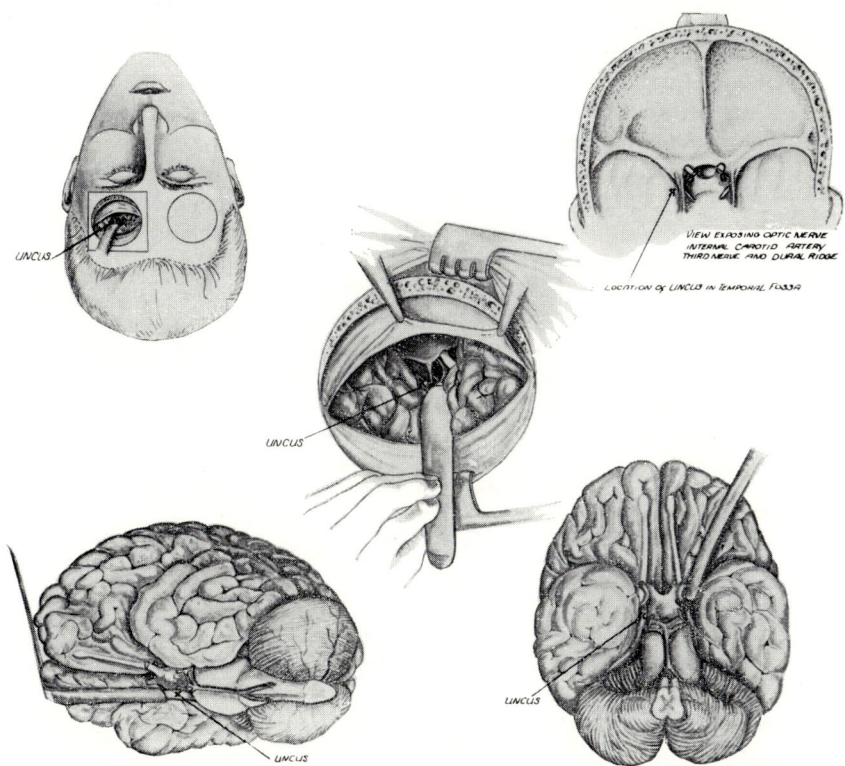

Figure 5.3 Combined uncotomy and amygdalotomy as carried out by Scoville in the 1950s.

hypothalamus and pulvinar surgically. Heath (1971), Delgado & Obrador (1971), and Sem-Jacobsen (1972) have stimulated such areas and I (Scoville, 1971), with Lindquist and Norlen (1966), have shown that haemorrhages of anterior communicating aneurysms, cysts in the floor of the third ventricle, malformations of Galen's vein, can all cause profound psychic changes. To date thalamic and hypothalamic lesions have proved of more benefit in pain syndromes than in mental disease.

Are surgical lesions limited to the temporal lobes important in psychiatric surgery? Certainly medial temporal lobe epilepsy causes behavioural and psychic changes and in the presence of seizure disorders surgery has been of great benefit. But in non-epileptic patients suffering from schizophrenia, cyclical depressions or psychoneuroses, surgical lesions have shown little benefit. Obrador (1948) was the first to make temporal lesions for functional mental disease without impressive result, and Scoville, et al., carried out twenty-two cases of bilateral medial ablations including the uncus, the amyedala and finally the temporal hippocampal complex in schizophrenic patients

34 Surgical Approaches in Psychiatry

(Figure 5.3). They found little change in behaviour. Stimulation caused seizure formation, respiratory arrest and loss of consciousness (Scoville, 1959). Scoville & Milner (1954) proclaimed the dangers of bilateral surgical ablations in the hippocampus resulting in a permanent loss of recent memory (Figure 5.4). Hence temporal lobe surgery in my experience has been of little benefit in functional mental disease. There has been one exception: bilateral removal of the uncus and amygdala has confirmed Klüver and Bucy's observations of a gentling effect. This has been demonstrated on 200 monkeys by Correll and myself and recently utilized on extreme behaviour problems in retarded children by Andy & Jurko (1972) and Narabayashi, Nagao, Saito, Yoshido & Nagahata (1963) and again reported in this Congress. Further research must be done as there is a definite risk of other behavioural deficits when such lesions are done in children of normal IQ and without epilepsy and extreme care must be taken to leave intact the hippocampal complex bilaterally, at least on one side.

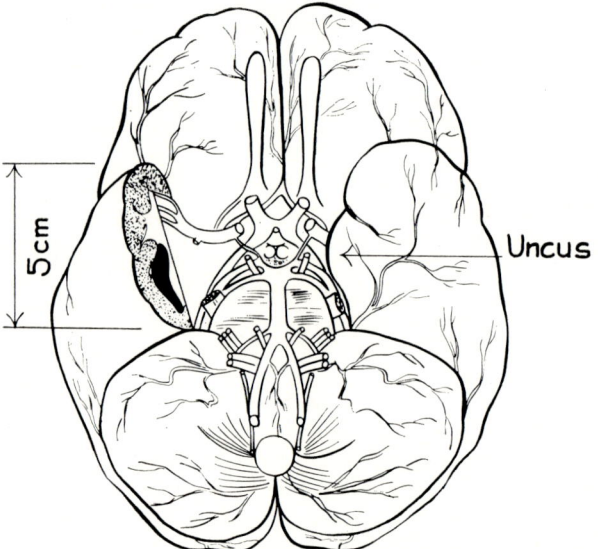

Figure 5.4 Combined uncotomy, amygdalotomy and hippocampectomy carried out by the writer in the 1950s resulting in memory loss.

In conclusion, I wish to mention those types of mental and behavioural diseases which are not benefited by surgical lesions. They are criminals, constitutional psychopaths and possibly sex perverts. I have seen no alterations in sexual behaviour in the orbital, cingulate, or temporal lesions except for an increased libido in orbital undercutting possibly from a lessening of anxiety and tension. The work to date indicates that functional mental disease is benefited by surgical lesions only when they exhibit an excess or exaggeration of normal feelings or thoughts. In other words, there must be an excess of guilt; of depression; of incoming sensory stimuli causing hallucinations of sight or sound; or an excess of anxiety and of neurotic fixations. This exaggeration of normal feeling tone or sensory input can be benefited by surgical lesions resulting in a lowering of such excess down to a normal level. Because of these observations I believe that psychosurgery of the prefrontal lobes does have a blunting effect, hopefully of a selective nature, on those thought processes and feeling tones which are grossly exaggerated above the normal. Hence psychosurgery should be done only on patients suffering from an excess in those modalities, and in simplistic terms the patient must be acutely suffering with an intense desire to get well and have character integrity. The majority of criminals and psychopaths are constitutionally or genetically lacking in these characteristics and surgical ablations will make them worse rather than better. For this reason I am alarmed by the present trend of questions asked us by both politicians and news reporters as to whether mental surgery will benefit criminals, rebels and social misfits. Mental surgery will never restore social conscience, character defects or infantile sexual arrest. These are matters for genetic metabolic and environmental therapy.

REFERENCES

Andy OJ & Jurko MF (1972). Thalamotomy for hyperresponsive syndrome. In: *Psychosurgery* (Eds Hitchcock, Laitinen and Vaernet), p. 127. Springfield, Ill.: Charles C Thomas.
Ballantine HT (1967) Stereotaxic anterior cingutotomy for neuro-psychiatric illness and intractable pain. *J. Neurosurg.*, **26**, 5. 488
Burckhardt G (1890). Ueber die Rindenexcisionen als Beitrag zur Operationstherapie der Psychosen. *Allg. Zschr. Psychiat.*, **47**, 463.
Delegado J & Obrador S (1971). Behavior control conference on the physical manipulation of the brain. Tarrytown, New York, (Institute of Society, Ethics and the Life Sciences)
Foltz E (1962). Pain release by frontal cingulotomy. *J. Neurosurg.*, **19**, 89
Fulton JF & Jacobsen F (1935). The functions of the frontal lobes. A comparative study in a monkey, chimpanzee and man. *II Internat. Neurol. Congr.*, London, p. 70
Grantham EG (1951). Prefrontal lobotomy for relief of pain, with a report of a new operative technique. *J. Neurosurg.*, **8**, 405
Heath RG (1971). Depth recording and stimulation studies in patients. In: *Symposium on the Surgical Control of Behavior* (Ed Winter). Springfield, Ill.: Charles C Thomas
Knight GC (1964). Neo-orbital cortex as an objective in the surgical treatment of mental illness. *Brit. J. Surg.*, **51**, 114
Le Beau (1954) *J. Psycho-chirurgie et fonctions mentales*. (Eds Masson et Cie). Paris
Lindquist G & Norlén G (1966). Korsakoff's syndrome after operation of ruptured aneurysm of anterior communicating artery. *Acta Psychiat. Scand.*, **42**, 24
Livingston KE (1953). Cingulate cortex isolation for the treatment of psychoses and psychoneuroses. *A.R.N.M.D.*, **31**, 374
Mayfield FH & McIntyre H (1954) Ventromedial quadrant coagulation in the treatment of the psychoses and neuroses. *Amer. J. Psychiat.*, **3**, 2
McKenzie KG & Kaczanowski G (1964). Prefrontal lobotomy: A five year control study. *Canad. Med. Ass. J.*, **9**, 1193
McKissock W (1949). Recent techniques in psychosurgery. In: *Anglo-American Symposium. Proc. of the Royal Society of Medicine*, **42**, Supplement. p.13.

Moniz E (1936). Les premières tentatives opératoires dans le traitement des certaines psychoses. *Encéphale*, **91**, 1

Narabayashi H, Nagao T, Saito Y, Yoshida M & Nagahata M (1963). Stereotaxic amygdalotomy for behavior disorders. *Arch. Neurol. Chicago*, **9**, 11

Nauta WJH (1972). Afferent and efferent relationships of the frontal lobe with the limbic system. In: *Proc. of the III World Congress of Psychosurgery*. Cambridge, England

Obrador S (1948) *Amer. Psychiat.*, **105**, 467

Poppen JL & Freshwater DB (1952). Symposium on orthopedic surgery and neurosurgery: Lobectomy for intractable pain—progress report on 64 patients. *Surgical Clinics North America*, **32**, 787

Powell TPS (1972). Sensory convergence on the cerebral cortex. In: *Proc. of the III World Congress of Psychosurgery*. Cambridge, England

Puusepp L (1937). Alcune considerazioni sugli interventi chirurgici nelle malattie mentali. *Gior. roy. Accad. med. Torino*, **100**, 3

Sano K (1962). Sedative neurosurgery. *Neurologia, med.-chir.*, **4**, 112

Scoville WB (1949). Selective cortical undercutting as a means of modifying and studying frontal lobe function in man. *J. Neuorosurg.*, **6**, 65

Scoville WB (1959). Observations on consciousness and seizure formation following stimulation of septal and uncal areas in man. *First Internat. Congr. Neurol. Sci. Brussels*, 1957.

Scoville WB (1971). The effect of surgical lesions of the brain on psyche and behavior in man. In: *Symposium on the Surgical Control of Behavior* (Ed Winter). Springfield, Ill.: Charles C Thomas.

Scoville WB, Dunsmore RH, Liberson WT, Henry CE & Pepe A (1953). Observations on medial temporal lobotomy and uncotomy in the treatment of psychotic states. In: *Psychiatric Treatment, XXXI Proc. A.R.N.M.D.* Baltimore: Williams and Wilkins.

Scoville WB & Milner B (1957). Loss of recent memory after bilateral hippocampal lesions. *J. Neurol. Neurosurg. Psychiat.*, **20**, 11

Scoville WB, Wilk EK & Pepe AJ (1951). Selective cortical undercutting. Results in new method of fractional lobotomy. *Amer. J Psychiat.*, **107**, No. 10

Sem-Jacobsen CW & Styri OB (1971). Depth-electrographic stereotaxic psychosurgery. In: *Proc. of the II International Conference on Psychosurgery*, Copenhagen, Denmark. Springfield, Ill.: Charles C Thomas

Tow PM & Lewin W (1953). Orbital leucotomy. *Lancet*, **2**, 644

Whitty GWM, Duffield GE, Tow PM & Cairns H (1952). Anterior cingulectomy in the treatment of mental disease. *Lancet*, **1**, 475

Yakovlev PI (1948). Motility, behavior and the brain: Stereodynamic organization and neural coordinates of behavior. *J. nerv. ment. Dis.*, **107**, 313

PART III

CINGULATE LESIONS IN THE TREATMENT OF PSYCHIATRIC ILLNESS

CHAPTER 6

Stereotactic cingulotomy with results of acute stimulation and serial psychological testing
GLENN MEYER, MARK McELHANEY,
WINSTON MARTIN & C P McGRAW

INTRODUCTION

Since the introduction of cingulum and/or cingulate gyrus lesions by Cairns (Lewin, 1961) and Le Beau (Le Beau & Petrie, 1953) in 1947 there has been a slowly increasing interest in controlled destruction of this area in patients suffering from disabling mental illness and intractable pain. This development was noted with great interest at the University of Texas Medical Branch because of the strong, organic orientation of the Department of Psychiatry. As evidence of this orientation, more than 500 lobotomies of various types were performed during the past several decades. Because of dissatisfaction with the occasionally disabling side-effects of the earlier radical operations, most of these lobotomies performed since 1950 were of the Grantham type (limited coagulation lobotomies; Grantham, 1951).

As an extension of this background, stereotactic cingulotomies were first performed at the UTMB in 1968. The initial eight patients operated upon were all deteriorated, chronic alcoholics selected from a large population of alcoholics treated at the US Public Health Service Hospital in Galveston. After approximately 18 months stereotactic cingulotomy became the standard initial lesion for intractable psychiatric illness of several types.

In addition to a standard report of methods and results we wish to describe two, somewhat unique features of this study. Firstly, there are the results of acute electrical stimulation of the cingulum area in 75 consecutive patients who were fully awake or very lightly sedated. Secondly, a detailed report is made of the results of serial pre- and postoperative psychological tests selected specifically for this purpose and performed on 30 patients.

METHODS
Patient population
The present series of cases consists of 75 patients in whom 89 bilateral operations were performed; 12 patients were operated on twice, and one intractable pain patient was operated on three times. There was only one

major complication and no deaths in the total group (Figure 6.1.). The surgery in three-fourths of these cases was performed by one of the authors during the past $2\frac{1}{2}$ years.

I. IMMEDIATE COMPLICATIONS
  Cases
  5   Confusion ($\times$ 4 days–2 weeks)
  2   Seizures (1 with prior history)
  2   Scalp infections
  1   Temporary increase in psychotic symptoms
  1   Acute sub-dural (after burr holes)
II. LATE COMPLICATIONS
  3   Suicides
  1   Increased organic symptoms

Figure 6.1 The immediate and late complications of 89 bilateral cingulotomies.

Of the 75 patients 71 were Caucasian and 4 were Mexican-American. Thirty-three were male and 42 female. The age distribution was as follows: 1 patient in the second decade of life, 14 in the third decade, 30 in the fourth, 18 in the fifth, 8 in the sixth and 4 in the seventh decade. The mean education level was high school graduation. There were 26 who had at least some college education, and among these, four held doctorates.

Clinical Evaluation
In most instances the patients were referred from a psychiatrist outside the medical centre after failure of all conventional forms of therapy. Case summaries and resumés of treatment given were supplied for almost all patients. All but seven of the patients were given psychiatric evaluations by one of the authors which included a detailed psychosocial history. Based on this evaluation, all patients were placed in a major psychiatric diagnostic category. If a patient was thought perhaps to be a suitable candidate for cingulotomy, he was then further subjected to a battery of seven psychological tests.

At this juncture, if the psychiatrist and clinical psychologist members of the team agreed that the patient might benefit from psychosurgery, referral was made to the neurosurgeon member of the team who made a complete neurological history and physical examination. In all instances, the patient had preoperative skull x-rays, electroencephalography and echoencephalography. If there were any significant abnormalities in the basic neurological workup, additional appropriate diagnostic procedures were carried out. As a result of this approach, about one-fourth of the patients had a preoperative angiogram or pneumoencephalogram.

A small group of patients were given a different battery of psychomotor tests. It included such tests as multiple limb co-ordination, tapping rates, pursuit rotor tests, reaction times, response orientation, critical flicker fusion rates, the Barratt impulsiveness scale, and the manifest anxiety scale. There are insufficient numbers in this group to make any definite statement about the results of this testing, and as expected, the limited ability of these patients to persevere with these tasks proved to be a barrier to adequate data collection.

Part III—Cingulate Lesions 41

Placement of burr holes
In all cases bilateral burr holes were made in the operating room, usually the day before the stereotactic procedure. Most patients underwent general anaesthesia for burr hole placement. The burr holes were centred $2\frac{1}{2}$ cm from the midline and $10\frac{1}{2}$ cm posterior to the nasion. The dura mater was opened with a cruciate incision and pial vessels were coagulated. Often major superior cerebral veins were spared and their position noted to avoid damaging them during the stereotactic procedure.

Stereotactic procedure
All procedures were performed 1–3 days after burr hole placement under sterile conditions in a specially prepared x-ray diagnostic room. In some instances, moderate doses of preoperative sedative drugs were given, but

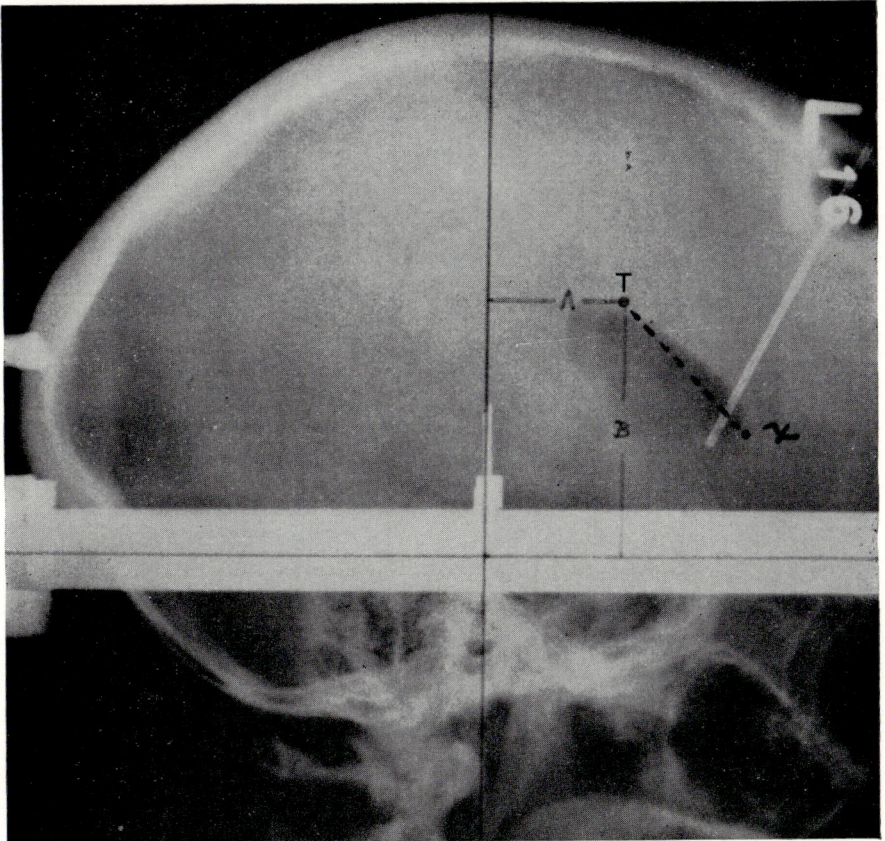

Figure 6.2a Lateral roentgenogram showing the cingulotomy target (T) above the roof of the frontal horns. The tip of the right frontal horn is cannulated and 15 cc air insufflated.

42 *Surgical Approaches in Psychiatry*

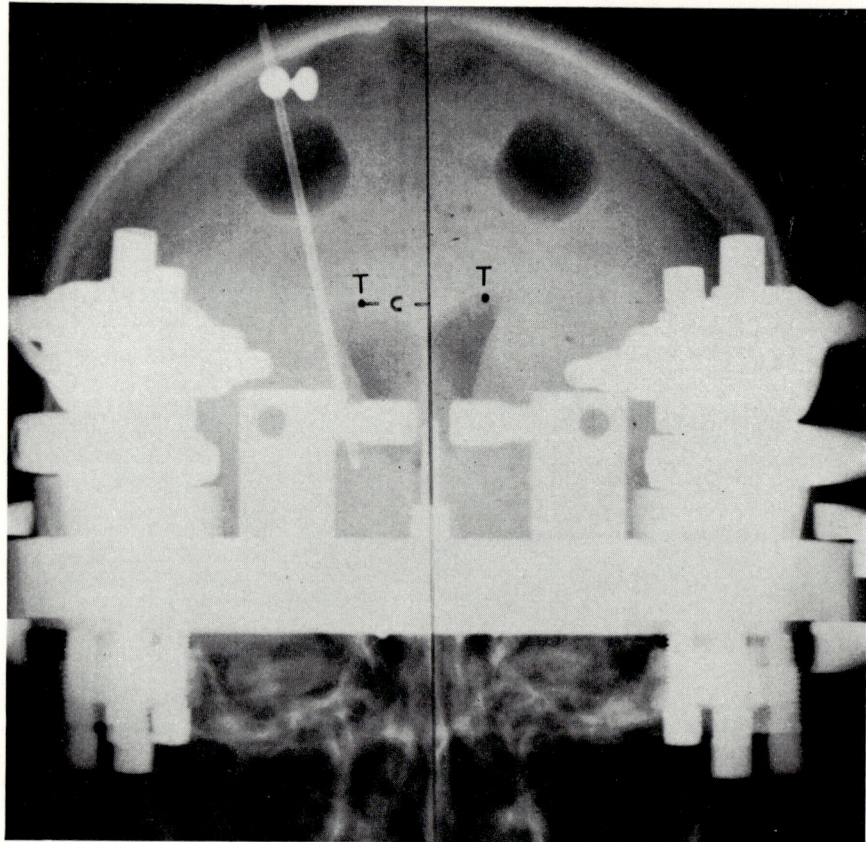

Figure 6.2b Anteroposterior view. Laterality of the bilateral targets (T) was initially 10 mm and now 8 mm.

most patients required no sedation. After local anaesthesia of the scalp the patients were affixed to the base ring of a Riechert stereotactic apparatus with two frontal and two occipital skull pins (Riechert & Mundinger, 1959). In all instances a filtered room air ventriculogram was performed to allow adequate visualization of the anterior portions of the third and lateral ventricles.

The stimulation and lesion targets were selected as follows. The most anterior extent of the frontal horn of the lateral ventricles was identified in the lateral plane (Figure 6.2a). A straight line was then drawn posteriorly to a point on the roof of the lateral ventricles 25 mm from the frontal horn reference. Currently, this distance has been increased to 35 mm. In the AP the plane (Figure 6.2b) 10 mm lateral to the midline was the initial lateral co-ordinate. More recently, this distance has been decreased to 8 mm. In those cases where an unsatisfactory result necessitated a repeat procedure, one or two additional lesions were placed in each hemisphere 15–25 mm from the most anterior extremity of the lateral ventricle and 8–10 mm from the midline. In all cases the lesion was made with a radio frequency probe heated to 75 °C for 90 s three separate times. The first coagulation was made at the co-ordinates given. The probe was then serially elevated 4 mm before each of the next two lesions. In those cases where anatomical confirmation of the lesion exists, a 9 × 16 mm cylindrical area of coagulation was formed. The lesion lay obliquely in the coronal plane with the dorsolateral end 3–4 mm more lateral then the ventromedial end (Figure 6.3). The lesion underlay and

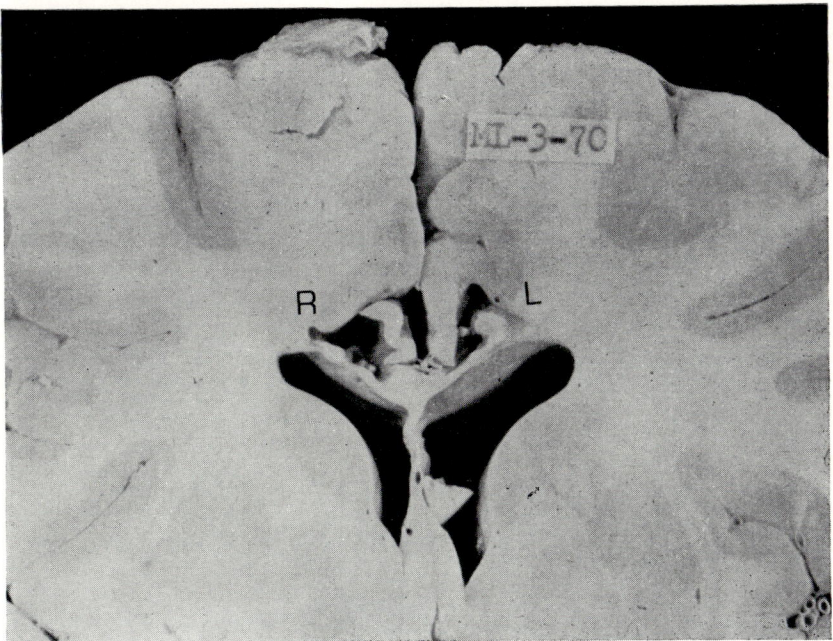

Figure 6.3 Coronal section through the cingulum lesions. Both lesions encroach upon the corpus callosum. The destruction is not quite complete in the left cingulum (L).

encroached upon area 24 of the cortex. Adjacent areas of the corpus callosum and colloso-marginal gyrus were most likely damaged as well. In general, our target selection conformed to the methods previously reported by Foltz & White (1962) and Ballantine, Cassidy, Flanagan & Marino (1967).

Stimulation methods
Stimulation was carried out using a standard Grass stimulator (model S4-G) and isolation unit (SIU-4B), connected to a concentric bipolar electrode. The

outside pole of the pair is 1.5 mm in diameter and the centre pole is 1 mm in diameter with an interelectrode distance of 6 mm. Both electrodes are stainless steel, insulated except for the distal 2 mm. A 60 Hz unidirectional square wave of 1 ms duration was used. Effective stimulation voltage varied from 5–25 V.

Patient care
All patients were hospitalized in the psychiatric wards and returned there immediately postoperatively. The patients were seen by the neurosurgeon member of the team on two or three preoperative occasions and the procedures were thoroughly and frankly discussed. All patients either requested operation or consented to it. Both the psychiatrist and neurosurgeon members of the team followed the patient for approximately one week postoperatively, after which time follow-up was primarily by the psychiatrist.

STIMULATION RESULTS
As will be apparent, a great variety of effects was seen after stimulation, and in the author's opinion, this reflects the dozen or more components of the cingulum bundle. Our pre-study bias had been that the interelectrode distance of 6 mm would allow us to stimulate a major portion of the cingulum each time. We therefore expected more uniform results.

Some effect was observed in 65 of the 75 cases and no response was seen in 10 (Table 6.1). In each instance, when no effect was observed the entire stimulating apparatus was rechecked to ensure optimal function. The 65 responses were categorized into the following five main headings: A. altered speech, B. temporal lobe symptoms or altered state of consciousness, C. affective responses, D. specific sensory-motor responses and E. other.

Speech responses
Speech was tested by having the patient proceed with a repetitive speech task, which was in most instances retrograde counting from 100. A few patients were unable to do this and they were asked to count antegrade or recite some overlearned material. Of the 36 patients having some change in speech, 24 had marked dysphasia or aphasia. Nine patients perseverated to varying degrees. In most instances they only repeated a number twice, but several patients repeated a number or phrase many times, or until stimulation ceased. Ten patients gave the more subtle response of simply having a change in the rate or volume of speech when stimulated. Two patients spoke characteristic phrases with each stimulation. One stated repetitively, 'hello, I will be speaking to you about a word.' The other, whose response the operator found most upsetting, stated in a loud voice, 'Father forgive them for they know not what they do.'

Temporal lobe or altered consciousness effects
Thirty-nine patients had one or more stimulation result in this group. Nineteen picked at the bed clothing, usually with both hands. Nineteen had

Part III—Cingulate Lesions 45

momentary confusion, most commonly manifested by difficulty in thinking of the next number in a retrograde series, while being able to state overlearned material such as name, address, etc. Another 16 had lip smacking movements that were very reminiscent of those seen as an automatism in temporal lobe seizures. Nine patients rubbed the face and eyes, and appeared to the operator to have paraesthesias, but in all instances they denied the occurrence of any

Table 6.1 The effects of electrical stimulation of the cingulum.

	Number of patients		Per cent
I. *Responses to stimulation*	(65)		87%
A. *Speech*	(36)		55%
1. Dysphasia	(24)	37%	
2. Perseveration	(9)	14%	
3. Change in rate or volume	(29)	45%	
B. *Temporal lobe or altered consciousness*	(39)		60%
1. Picking at bedclothes	(19)	29%	
2. Confusion	(19)	29%	
3. Fixed gaze	(17)	26%	
4. Lip smacking	(16)	25%	
5. Rubbing face and eyes	(9)	14%	
6. Akinetic mutism	(1)	2%	
C. *Affective responses*	(20)		31%
1. Intense fear	(11)	17%	
2. Pleasure	(8)	12%	
3. Agitation	(6)	9%	
D. *Specific sensory motor response*	(22)		34%

	Bilateral	Unilateral
Legs	6	0
Arms	5	2
Face	0	1
All extremities	7	
Unilateral extremities	2	
Hemisensory phenomenon	1	

	Number of patients		Per cent
E. *Other responses*	(15)		23%
1. Pain	(3)	5%	
2. Amnesia	(8)	12%	
3. Generalized structure	(2)	3%	
4. Nausea	(2)	3%	
II. *No response*	(10)		13%

particular sensory phenomenon. One patient who had a 'staring episode' with aphonia, is listed as akinetic mutism.

Affective response
Twenty patients showed some change in affect, the most common form of which was intense fear in 11 cases. Another 6 appeared only moderately agitated, while 8 reported that the perceived sensation was pleasurable. Six of the 11 patients having a fear response, reported that the fear was 'overwhelming', and two described an intense feeling of oppression. One stated that he had the feeling that death was imminent.

Specific sensory-motor responses
Twenty-two patients displayed some characteristic motor response during stimulation. As can be seen in Table 6.1, there was no particular pattern manifest. Six patients moved both legs, 5 moved both arms and 2 moved one arm while 1 blinked the contralateral eye. Hemilateral extremities were moved in 2 patients, and in 7 others, all four extremities were moved each time the stimulus was applied. Only one patient reported a hemisensory phenomena, which consisted of tingling paraesthesia.

Other responses
Fifteen patients were placed in this group. Three of the 15 reported pain. In two instances this was headache, and in the third it consisted of generalized body pain. Two had generalized seizures and two reported nausea. Eight patients exhibited amnesia. Two of these ceased a retrograde counting task immediately when the stimulus was applied, and manifested an apparent alerting response. They were able to relate overlearned material, but appeared to be totally unable to think of the next number of a retrograde series. These two patients began counting again exactly where they had left off after stimulation ceased. When they were interrupted and asked to describe what sensations they had experienced during the time they could not count, they both stoutly maintained that nothing had happened and that they had never stopped counting.

CORRELATION OF STIMULATION RESULT WITH CLINICAL FOLLOW-UP
General evaluation
Intensive effort was made to achieve as close to 100% follow-up as possible. In 30 of the 68 cases we were able to achieve optimal follow-up with serial batteries of psychometric tests and outpatient visits. In 31 there was psychiatric outpatient follow-up only. The result in seven cases was evaluated by a letter from the referring psychiatrist only, and seven others were too recently operated on to evaluate. The maximum follow-up time is $4\frac{1}{2}$ years and minimum 5 months; the average follow-up is 18 months and the median 12 months. Three patients were evaluated at least once and then were lost to further follow-up.

Table 6.2 The clinical results in the six diagnostic categories. (eval = evaluated; av. impr. = average improvement).

	Total	Eval.	Significant +3 Well	Improvement +2 Marked	+1 Moderate	Insignificant −1 Slight	−2 None	−3 Worse	Av. impr.
Schizophrenia	28	26	5	6	5	6	4	0	0.7
Depression	24	22	2	9	8	1	2	0	1.2
Alcoholism	13	12	3	2	1	1	1	4	−0.1
Obsessive-Compulsive	5	3	1	1	1	0	0	0	2.0
Pain	4	4	0	0	3	1	0	0	0.5
Anxiety	1	1	1	0	0	0	0	0	3.0
Total	75	68	12	18	18	9	7	4	0.8

To rate the clinical results, a conference was held with two or more members of the team, and the patients were assigned to one of six categories (see Table 6.2). The best category was labelled 'well', which implied that the patients now took no medication, functioned normally in their usual life setting, and received only very infrequent psychiatric follow-up for purposes of our study. The next best category is labelled 'marked improvement' and includes those patients who were now taking only small amounts of medication. In some instances, they were receiving some supportive psychotherapy, but these patients were functioning quite normally in their prior position. The third category, labelled 'moderate improvement', includes those patients who have shown very significant improvement in their clinical condition and in most instances return to employment. The patients in category 4 showing 'slight improvement' are those who, in general, continue tranquillizer therapy and/or psychotherapy on a regular basis. Several patients in this group remain institutionalized. The last two categories are those showing no change and those who were judged to be worse following cingulotomy (see Figure 6.4).

Of the 75 patients in this series, 68 have reported postoperative results. In these 68 patients, the primary diagnostic categories are as follows: 22 psychotic depression, 26 schizophrenia, 12 alcoholic, 4 intractable pain, 1 anxiety neurosis and 3 obsessive-compulsive neurosis. The overall results in these 68 patients showed that 12 are well, 18 demonstrate marked improvement, 18 moderate improvement, 9 slight improvement, 7 no change and 4 patients were worse (see Figure 6.4).

Therapeutic failures
Individual descriptions of those 4 patients judged to be worse are necessary. There was nothing characteristic about the stimulation results in these patients. Three of the 4 were in the original group of 8 chronic alcoholic men.

48 *Surgical Approaches in Psychiatry*

The first was a 40-year-old male Caucasian, depressed, chronic alcoholic. At 8 months postcingulotomy his psychometrics were much improved and he was sober and employed. He did well for 2½ years until suffering a low back injury, which led to several lumbar spine operations in a local hospital, and marked marital problems. He died of a self-inflicted gunshot wound to the head 2 years and 8 months after cingulotomy.

The second case was a 38-year-old Caucasian alcoholic with agitated depression. At 15 months after cingulotomy his IQ remained high at 129 and

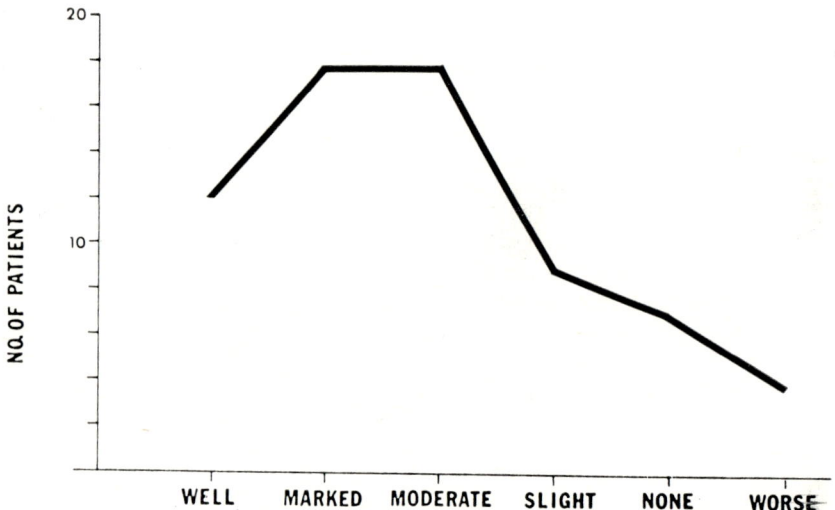

Figure 6.4 Clinical effect of cingulotomy in 68 patients.

psychometrics showed a general slight improvement. He was not drinking and was out of hospital but unemployed and having continued marital discord. He died of a self-inflicted gunshot wound to the head 20 months postoperatively.

The third was a 52-year-old Puerto Rican, male alcoholic with a long history of agitated depression and 'schizophrenic potential'. He had had alcoholic seizures, and several years previously had a coagulation type frontal lobotomy. Precingulotomy psychometrics showed a full-scale IQ of 102 and 'mild organicity'. Repeat tests 2 weeks postoperatively showed an IQ of 109 and slight general improvement. Seven months later the IQ was 94 and organicity was 'severe'. He had stopped drinking but was unemployed. He died under mysterious circumstances 2 years postoperatively. Autopsy showed massive haemorrhagic gastritis, portal cirrhosis and pulmonary fibrosis.

The fourth and final case was a 43-year-old Caucasian housewife with severe depression, drug abuse, alcoholism and multiple suicide attempts. All conventional forms of psychiatric treatment were unsuccessful. Preoperative psychological tests showed an IQ of 78 with organicity and marked anxiety. Postoperative testing showed no change but slight clinical improvement persisted for 8 months. A second more anterior set of cingulum lesions were placed after 1 year with only slight transitory improvement. She died 5 months after the second operation of a self-administered barbiturate overdosage.

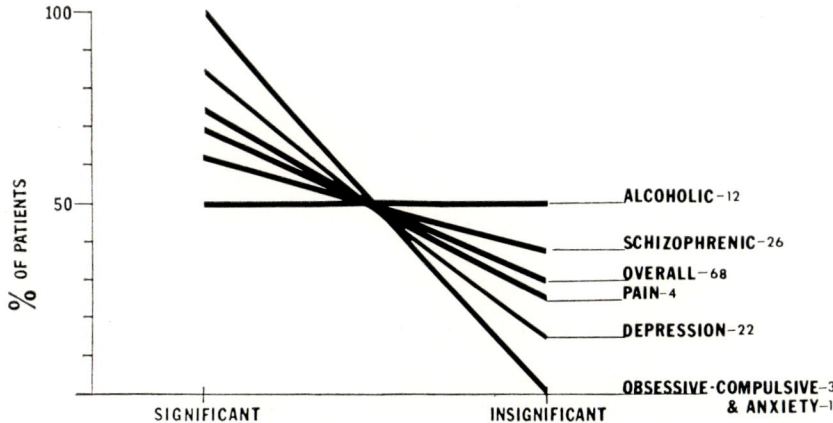

Figure 6.5 Percentage of significant and insignificant improvement in different diagnostic categories. The 'overall' line shows that of the 68 patients 70% were markedly improved, while 30% did not benefit significantly from cingulotomy.

Diagnostic categories
Figure 6.5 graphically depicts the results by primary diagnostic category. Seventy per cent of the total patients had significant improvement, while only 50% of the alcoholic group did well. Approximately 60% of the schizophrenic group improved significantly while the pain, depression and obsessive groups all did better than the overall average.

Stimulation categories
Figure 6.6 shows the correlation of stimulation effects and final results. It is interesting that the percentage of significant improvement in those having an affective response is the same as that for the overall group. Those 35 patients showing some change in speech during stimulation did decidedly better, while for some unexplained reason those having a motor response did even better. The 7 patients in whom a miscellaneous response was

obtained did decidedly less well than the other groups, but of course they do not represent a significant sample. Also, those with a temporal lobe type response did less well than the average.

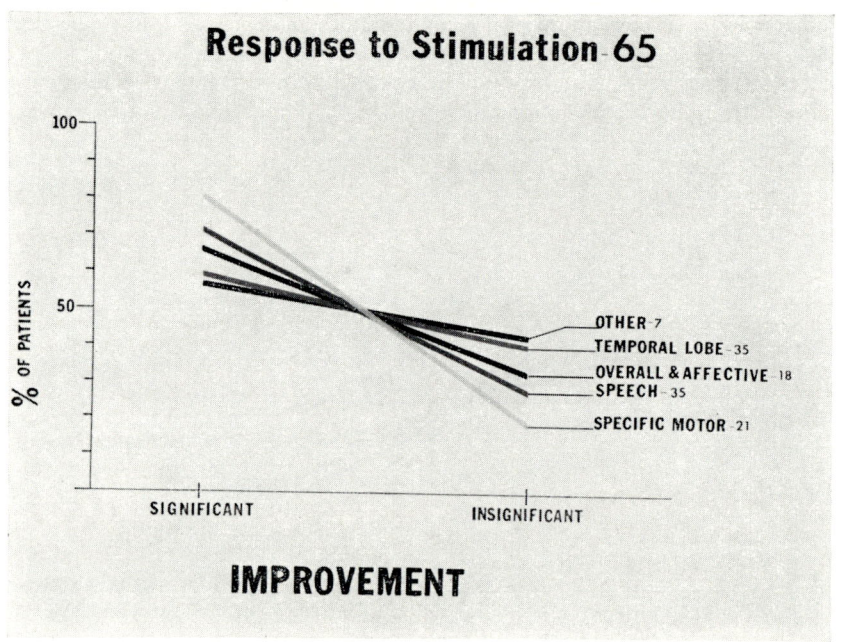

Figure 6.6 The relationship between the response type to electrical stimulation of the cingulum and the clinical improvement. It can be seen that affective responses did not predict a favourable result of surgery.

CORRELATIONS OF MAJOR SYMPTOMS WITH CLINICAL FOLLOW-UP

By means of a system of punch cards a large number of correlations were readily made. Only the most interesting and possibly significant ones are mentioned. Table 6.3 is a list of the major symptoms in 75 patients. It indicates the number of patients having one or more symptoms within the five somewhat arbitrary groups of symptoms. Also indicated are the numbers of patients showing individual symptoms. The following comments about results within each symptom grouping are based only on those 68 of the 75 patients for whom adequate follow-up data is available.

Inadequate personality symptoms

The interesting feature of this group is a comparison of the results in 22 patients with alcoholism. Twelve of these patients (55%) showed significant improvement while 11 of the 13 patients having chronic drug abuse (85%) improved significantly.

Table 6.3 The number of patients having various symptoms.

	Number of patients	
I. *Inadequate personality symptoms*	62	
A. Hostility		(31)
B. Dependency		(26)
C. Alcoholism		(24)
D. Inadequate interest		(27)
E. Mental immaturity		(19)
F. Low frustration tolerance		(19)
G. Unstable		(18)
H. Chronic drug abuse		(13)
I. Unco-operative		(13)
II. *Affective symptoms*	70	
A. Recurrent depression		(66)
B. Chronic anxiety		(58)
C. Frequent crying		(29)
D. Feeling of worthlessness		(24)
E. Feeling of despair		(18)
III. *Psychotic symptoms*	53	
A. Paranoia		(32)
B. Suicidal conversation		(26)
C. Suicidal attempts		(25)
D. Hallucinations		(19)
IV. *Somatic symptoms*	58	
A. Insomnia		(46)
B. Anorexia		(30)
C. Polysurgery		(22)
D. Hysteria		(17)
V. *Obsessive-compulsive symptoms*	16	

Affective and psychotic symptoms
There was no symptom group within either of these two categories showing results markedly different from the overall results. The authors' preconception was that those patients with one or more of the four psychotic symptoms would do less well. This did not prove to be the case since several patients with both paranoia and hallucinations did very well.

Somatic symptoms
Of the 21 patients (20 females) who had polysurgery prior to cingulotomy, only 11 (55%) showed significant improvement. Conversely, 14 of the 17 (86%) of those with hysterical symptoms had a significant improvement.

Obsessive-compulsive symptoms
The results in this group were excellent and also in those patients having this symptom as their primary diagnosis. Of the 12 patients who were evaluated in the obsessive symptom group, 11 (92%) had worthwhile improvement.

Other characteristics

Consistent with several other reports, the 38 females (75% improved) did better than the 30 males (60% improved) in our series. Also as expected, those with more than a high school education did better by about the same margin.

Those 15 patients in the series who had prior frontal lobotomies of various types did less well than the average. Nevertheless, 50% of them showed significant improvement, which was a most gratifying result in this most difficult group of patients. Another gratifying feature of the study was that those 17 patients diagnosed as having some degree of organic mental syndrome, either clinically or by psychological testing, did just as well as the overall average. The 45 patients who had prior shock treatment also did as well as the average.

Finally, those 13 patients who underwent a second operation had a final result which was just as good as the average. Only two of the 14 had shown even temporary significant improvement after the first procedure.

PSYCHOLOGICAL TESTS

Purpose

The purpose of the psychological measures obtained from the patients undergoing psychosurgery for emotional problems was to determine the relationship between the risks and benefits involved in the operation. The tests were designed to measure, qualitatively and quantitatively, what intellectual and emotional changes, if any, may take place in each patient following stereotactic brain surgery (Gilbert, 1969). Evaluation was made of the following: (1) the level of intellectual ability and efficiency, (2) the degree of anxiety and depression, (3) the amount of hostility, (4) the presence and severity of organic brain damage and (5) the self-concept.

In addition to the above variables, the psychological measures were expected to identify the presence or absence of psychosis, psychotic potential and neurosis. The psychological tests, in conjunction with interview material, provided the measures of the intellectual and emotional effects of psychosurgery upon the individual.

The psychological test battery

1. The Wechsler–Bellevue Scale for Adolescents and Adults or the Wechsler Adult Intelligence Scale. These tests measure the intelligence quotient and they are also useful for identifying such pathology as psychosis and brain damage.
2. The Rorschach Test. This projective device enabled the clinician to assess anxiety, depression, hostility, inadequacy and psychosis.
3. The Bender–Gestalt Test. This served to discover brain damage, and provided documentation of hostility and emotional instability.
4. Wechsler Memory Scale. This helped to determine the degree of recent memory loss and identified learning disabilities.
5. The Draw-A-Person Test. This projective test helped to identify such qualities as immaturity, anxiety, hostility, psychosis and brain damage.

6. The Minnesota Multiphasic Personality Inventory. This test is 566 statements to be designated by the patient as true or false. It provides a quantitative measure of the depression-anxiety level, degree of hostility and amount of defensiveness.
7. The Adjective Self-Inventory. This test consists of a number of adjectives from which the patient selects those that describe him. It provides a quantitative measure of the self-concept and the degree of depression.

Test validity
The tests used in this study are well known, validated tests. Examiner bias was compensated for in two ways. Firstly, the same examiner gave almost all of the tests. Secondly, tests such as the MMPI, the Figure Drawing Test (McElhaney, 1969) and the Adjective Self-Inventory are minimally, if at all, influenced by the examiner. The schedule which the authors endeavoured to follow was: (1) a preoperative testing, (2) a postoperative test battery at approximately 3–6 months following surgery, and (3) a postoperative test at yearly intervals for an indeterminate period of time.

Quantitative measures
To quantitate the amount of change three tests amenable to quantitative measures were selected. These were the Wechsler–Bellevue Intelligence Test, and MMPI and the Adjective Self-Inventory. The Wechsler–Bellevue also provides a numerical IQ score. The MMPI Test provides a profile sheet that indicates standard deviations above and below the 'normal' or mean score. The test furnishes a convenient rating of such variables as the anxiety-depression level and the degree of hostility of a particular patient. A score on the anxiety-depression scale one standard deviation above normal limits was for the purpose of this study defined as 'mild'. Two standard deviations was considered 'moderate'. Three standard deviations above normal limits was regarded as 'severe'.

Corresponding scores on the Pd scale, which measures the level of hostility that a patient manifests, were defined for the purpose of this study as 'moderate', 'high', 'extreme' and 'uncontrolled'. A significant change in the level of hostility or of anxiety-depression was a change of one standard deviation or more.

A quantitative measure for the self-concept was devised by analysing a list of adjectives selected by the patient to describe himself. The percentage of complimentary adjectives that the patient felt described himself was compared to the percentage of uncomplimentary adjectives in the following way: (1) 60% or more of complimentary adjectives was defined for the purpose of this study as 'normal', (2) 51–59% was defined as 'relatively poor', (3) 26–50% was considered 'poor', (4) 5–25% was regarded as 'very poor' and (5) no complimentary adjectives was defined as 'extremely poor'.

The patient sample
Of the 75 patients treated, some lived at such distance that they were unable

to return for follow-up psychological assessment. Some, because of their own objection or that of their families, were not given the psychological test battery before surgery. Others had received the surgery so recently that sufficient time had not elapsed for a re-test. This left a sample of 30 patients who received pre- and postoperative tests.

The sample of patients who had stereotactic cingulotomies comprised three general categories.

1. Alcoholics. Empirically, alcoholics present a constellation of problems that might be classified as 'the alcoholic syndrome'. This syndrome usually combines the following characteristics: anxiety; depression; hostility; dependency; immaturity; emotional instability; a poor self-image.
2. Depressed patients
3. Chronic psychotics

The sample of 30 patients who received pre- and postoperative psychological tests was composed of 6 alcoholics, 9 psychotics and 15 neurotic depressives. None of these patients had responded to conventional treatment.

RESULTS
1. Behavioural Changes
Although this study is primarily concerned with results that can be measured on the psychological tests, the matter of most vital concern is change that occurs in the behaviour of the patients. The patient was interviewed independently by three of the doctors involved in this investigation. There was almost perfect correlation between reported changes in behaviour on the part of the patients and the clinicians' assessment of changes that had occurred and those changes shown by the results of the psychological tests.

The following are examples of behavioural changes. One alcoholic in this study was completely disabled by the emotional problems that caused his compulsive drinking. He reported that he had terrible nightmares and that he had 'one hell of a time getting along with people'. Three years after surgery he reported that his anxiety, his depression and his nightmares were gone and that he had stopped drinking and was working every day.

One patient in this sample was practically immobilized by an agitated depression, and she seriously considered committing suicide. Eight months after surgery she reported, 'I do not believe that I would be alive today if I had not had this operation. I think that I would have killed myself.' Today her behaviour can be described as normal.

One patient was so troubled by a preoccupation with 'sin' that she filled several notebooks with answers to questions that she had directed to her priest regarding what did and did not constitute a sin. She ruminated for days over whether it was or was not a sin to leave a particle of food on her dinner plate. Five months after her surgery she reported that these questions no longer bothered her.

A college English professor stated that she had become unable to face her classes because of intense anxiety. She spent her weekends drinking in a fruitless attempt to allay her anxiety so that she could get through the following week. Eight months after her surgery, she reported that she could teach her classes without feeling anxious and no longer required either tranquilizers or alcohol.

2. Psychological tests

Table 6.4 indicates the results obtained from the psychological examinations. Fourteen patients showed excellent improvement, 6 experienced slight improvement, and 3 patients apparently remained unchanged. Excellent improvement was defined for the purpose of this study as a significant improvement in four or more of the following six: (1) the IQ score; (2) the presence or absence of organic brain damage; (3) the anxiety-depression level; (4) the level of hostility; (5) the self-concept and (6) the presence or absence of psychosis or of a psychotic potential.

Table 6.4 Results of serial psychological testing.

Number of patients (total 30)

Excellent improvement	Moderate improvement	Slight improvement	No improvement
14	7	6	3

Moderate improvement is defined for the purpose of this study as a significant improvement in two or three of the variables that are being measured. Slight improvement indicates minimal improvement in two or three variables or significant improvement in only one variable.

Organic brain damage—An extremely important variable measured by the psychological tests is the presence or absence of brain damage, and the test battery selected was very sensitive for this purpose. Of the 30 patients, 12 were found to have some indication of organic brain damage. Only one patient showed evidence of brain damage in her postoperative test but showed no organicity in the preoperative test. However, in this case, the only preoperative test was given 23 years before her surgery. Further, the indicated damage was in the parietal lobe, which was not directly involved in her surgery.

In the remaining eleven patients, nine had indications of brain damage which remained unchanged. In two patients, the brain damage actually appeared to be less severe after surgery. In no case was there any evidence that the psychosurgery damaged any part of the brain that is involved in 'frontal lobe' processes.

Psychosis—Eleven patients revealed evidence of psychosis or of a psychotic potential in their preoperative tests. In the postoperative tests, three of these patients were free of symptoms indicating psychosis. Six of the patients revealed some remission of their psychotic symptoms.

Intelligence—The IQ score of 15 patients in the sample used in this study revealed an increase of five or more IQ points. One patient's IQ score increased by 33 points. The IQ scores of 12 of the patients remained the same. A variation of less then five IQ points was considered to be due to chance. Three patients revealed a decline in IQ score of five or more points. However, in none of these 3 patients was there any evidence that the decline in IQ score was attributable to the surgery.

Depression-anxiety—Nineteen patients in this sample showed a significant improvement in their level of anxiety and depression when their preoperative and postoperative test records were compared. Two patients manifested no change in their anxiety and depression. One patient in this sample of 30 revealed an increase in the level of anxiety and depression.

Hostility—Twenty patients in this sample showed a significant improvement in the degree of hostility when their postoperative test battery was compared to their preoperative records. Nine patients revealed only a slight amount of hostility on their preoperative tests. One patient revealed an increase in hostile feelings as shown by his psychological tests.

DISCUSSION

The authors have been encouraged by the results in the first 75 patients. The one life threatening, operative complication (acute subdural haematoma) was successfully eliminated and resulted in no permanent neurological deficit. It is felt that this amount of morbidity is acceptable in this very ill group of patients whose most common single dominant symptom was a suicide attempt. Those staff psychiatrists at this institution who have had extensive experience with various types of frontal lobotomies, have indicated that the patients in whom the best results occurred are very comparable in both the cingulotomy and lobotomy groups. They noted that the major advantages of cingulotomy is the absence of the psychologically crippling side-effects, i.e. loss of inhibition, motivation etc.

It is felt that better evaluation methods and longer follow-up are clearly needed. This became apparent as our methods evolved extensively during the past few years while experience was gained. The group experience has been that within limits, neither evidence of 'organicity' nor schizophrenia are absolute contraindications to surgery. Several patients with 'schizo-affective' psychosis have done spectacularly well, in some cases with the help of therapeutic modalities, which had been totally ineffective before cingulotomy.

Several groups of patients who did better than the average are those with chronic drug abuse, hysterical symptoms, and those with disabling obsessive-compulsive neuroses. All three of the patients having obsessive-compulsive neuroses as the primary diagnosis are well.

The biggest disappointment was in the alcoholic group. Eight of the 13 patients in this group were the first patients in the series and therefore long-term follow-up is available. Two of the four relapsed after an initial gratifying improvement. Two of the three who committed suicide, did so with no prior attempts and no documented prior suicidal rumination. In contradistinction, it is interesting that while most of the psychotically depressed patients had a number of preoperative suicidal attempts, there have been no successful postoperative attempts, and only several attempts or gestures of any kind. Adequate post mortem examination of two of the four deceased patients was made. In one the lesions were perfectly placed (see Figure 6.3), destroying almost the entire cross-sectional area of the cingulum. In another the lesion on one side was too laterally placed and only nicked the cingulum bundle. We feel that more work should be done with the hopeless alcoholics. Part of the problem in our estimation, is the heterogeneity of psychopathology in this group, with at least two distinct types of alcoholics in our case material. Better psychological and psychophysiological test procedures are clearly necessary for more adequate case selection.

Our results are in accord with the opinions expressed by Ballantine *et al.* (1967) who stated that re-operation of the unimproved patients should be definitely considered. Our re-operated group has done as well as the average. This represents more evidence against the placebo theory as proposed by some to explain the effectiveness of psychosurgery.

It is the hope of the authors that this study might serve to incite better controlled clinical research efforts, which will focus the expertise of a variety of neuroscientists on this potentially rewarding area. We do not feel that our stimulation results allow clinically useful predictions of the eventual outcome of an individual. We feel that this part of the study deserves further emphasis and the use of more advanced devices and rigorously controlled technique.

ACKNOWLEDGEMENT

We wish to acknowledge the efforts contributed to this study by Doctors John Coe, Charles Borne, Hamilton Ford and George Tindall. We are particularly indebted to Doctor Ernest Barratt and his staff.

REFERENCES

Ballantine HT, Cassidy WL, Flanagan NB & Marino R (1967). Stereotaxic anterior cingulotomy for neuropsychiatric illness and intractable pain. *J. Neurosurg.*, **26**, 488

Foltz EL & White LE (1962). Pain 'relief' by frontal cingulotomy. *J. Neurosurg.*, **19**, 89

Gilbert J (1969). *Clinical Psychological Tests in Psychiatric and Medical Practice* Springfield, Ill.: Charles C Thomas.

Grantham EG (1951). Prefrontal lobotomy for relief of pain. *J. Neurosurg.*, **8**, 405

Le Beau J & Petrie A (1953). A comparison of the personality changes after (1) prefrontal selective surgery for the relief of intractable pain and for the treatment of mental cases (2) cingulectomy and topectomy. *J. ment. Sci.*, **99**, 53

Lewin W (1961). Observations of selective leucotomy. *J. Neurol. Neurosurg. Psychiat.*, **24**, 37

McElhaney M (1969). *Clinical Psychological Assessment of the Human Figure Drawing.* Springfield, Ill.: Charles C. Thomas.

Riechert T & Mundinger F (1959). Stereotaxic instruments. In: *Introduction to Stereotaxis with an Atlas of the Human Brain* (Eds Schaltenbrand and Bailey), **1**, 437. Stuttgart: G. Thieme.

CHAPTER 7

The role of the limbic lobe in central pain mechanisms, an hypothesis relating to the gate control theory of pain
ARMANDO ORTIZ

INTRODUCTION
The surgical procedures directed at interruption of pain pathways at central or peripheral nervous system levels have often failed in the treatment of intractable pain.

Open surgical procedures or closed stereotaxic surgical procedures which interrupt pain pathways in the brain, such as thalamotomies (Mark, Ervin & Yakovlev, 1962) or mesencephalic tractotomies, had a questionable degree of success.

Anterior cingulotomy, an operation directed to non-specific pain pathways, and carried out either as a stereotaxic or open procedure, alleviates intractable pain with marked degree of success (Ballantine, Cassidy, Flanagan & Marino, 1967). Since the procedure is also utilized for the treatment of mental illnesses of the type of affective psychosis, the effect on pain has been interpreted as suppressing the 'affective' component of pain. The surgical procedure is simple, morbidity negligible, and the degree of success has helped to establish it as a procedure of choice in properly selected cases for the treatment of chronic intractable pain.

As the knowledge of the limbic lobe and its connections increases, the rationality of cingulotomy is better understood. Nevertheless, that knowledge is incomplete and its understanding in relation to pain makes the analysis of the surgical cases, the lesions, and the physiology of the limbic lobe worthwhile to review frequently.

PATIENTS
This report deals with 20 cases of pain, treated by bilateral stereotaxic radio-frequency cingulotomy. They were all adults. Only 3 patients with intractable pain had psychiatric backgrounds. One patient had been committed to a mental institution. The cause of his pain was carcinoma of the tongue with metastasis. The duration of the pain varied in patients. One patient was operated upon with recent onset of pain due to carcinoma of the breast with metastasis to the head and neck. The remaining patients have had long-standing problems of pain due to benign conditions and are still alive.

SURGICAL TECHNIQUE

The surgical procedure was carried out in the operating room. Under preoperative medications with mild sedation of atropine and innovar, a lumbar pneumoencephalogram was carried out prior to induction. After the injection was completed, the patient was anaesthetized and burr holes were made. The head was then fixed in the Todd-Wells stereotactic frame. Preliminary films were taken for target localization. The target point selected was 2·5 cm from the tip of the anterior horn of the lateral ventricles, 13–15 mm from the midline according to the degree of atrophy of the lateral ventricles if any, and 5 mm above the roof of the lateral ventricles (Figures 7.1–3).

The electrode was inserted and R.F. coagulation, at a temperature of 75 °C for a period of 120 s, was carried out.

After the coagulation was completed, the patient's wounds were closed and he was returned to the ward. Minor analgesics were used thereafter.

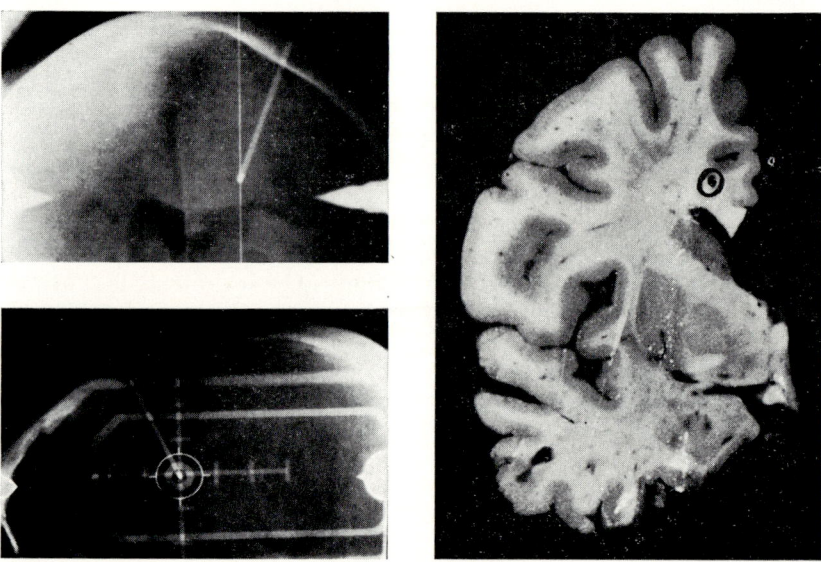

Figure 7.1 Anteroposterior roentgenogram showing the electrode in position, 15 mm from the midline.

Figure 7.2 Lateral view. The target lies 2·5 cm posterior to the tip of the frontal horn and 5 mm above the roof of the lateral ventricle.

Figure 7.3 Postmortem localization of a lesion in the cingulum.

RESULTS

We were impressed by the immediate cessation of pain and the absence of a narcotic withdrawal reaction postoperatively. Only one patient failed to experience postoperative relief of pain, and underwent a repeat insertion of electrode 3 days later. The period of confusion mentioned in other studies has not been found in our series. Headache has been a fairly constant complaint. In only one case was its severity more than average and lasting for several days. The pain returned in 8 patients and three re-operations were done within 8 weeks. The pain was relieved transiently again. Five patients experienced a return of pain from 3–6 months postoperatively.

DISCUSSION

The understanding of the central neurophysiological mechanism of pain remains a matter of controversy (Mehler, 1962). To the two theories of pain, specificity of impulses and transmission and patterning of impulses and summation, has been added the gate control theory (Melzack & Wall, 1965). This theory has increased our understanding of the neurophysiological mechanisms of pain and the symptom itself.

The aim of this paper is to postulate that the study of the relief of pain which is obtained with cingulotomy, and the recurrence of the symptom, adds to our understanding of the central mechanisms of pain in the light of the gate theory.

Specific pain receptors from free nerve endings of the A-delta and C unmyelinated fibres carry the stimulus to the lateral spinothalamic projecting system and to the specific centres in the thalamus, which result in sensation and behaviour correlates of pain. There was an assumption of a direct type of 'telephone line' connection and pathways of peripheral receptors to the brain. The specificity of the receptors was preserved through the activity of the neural networks, always resulting in pain conduction.

The theories of patterning of a stimulus are based on studies showing that stimulus intensity and central formation of the stimulus along spatio-temporal patterns over non-specific routes are the neurophysiological basis for pain. The theories ignored the specificity of receptors and conduction, the physiological specialization, but added central mechanisms of summation, inhibition and facilitation (Noordenbos, 1959), and input modification of certain patterns of activity (Livingston, 1943).

The gate control theory for the understanding of pain takes into account physiological specialization and patterning of stimulus, with central summation and input control. Based on new understanding of spinal mechanisms, it introduces a concept of integration, with central mechanisms playing a definite role for co-ordination of input.

We would like to postulate that within the framework of this theory, and based on the studies and observation of patients who have undergone cingulotomy, the limbic lobe may well constitute a central trigger mechanism of the gate theory of Melzack & Wall.

The substantia gelatinosa of Rolando acts as a gate control system, modulating afferent input of peripheral nerve fibres to central cells. Terminals of large nerve fibres and small unmyelinated fibres converge on the substantia gelatinosa. The activity of cells in substantia gelatinosa is determined by the total number of active fibres, the frequency of the inputs that they transmit, and the balance of activity of the large and small fibres (Melzack & Wall,

1965). The transmission of the first sensory neuron of the spinal cord in the dorsal horn would be modified by an afferent input control, based on accepted physiological mechanisms of reticular-spinal inhibition and facilitation. This control may be exercised through the gate control system. Activities such as emotional states, distraction and memories of past experiences are said to modify the sensory input. As originally proposed by Melzack & Wall (1965), the manner in which the mechanism takes place is 'a problem'.

The limbic lobe has been integrated as a pathway with sensory input from sensory cortices, hippocampus, amygdala, and with afferent pathways to the hypothalamus, thalamus and midbrain (Mehler, 1962). It plays a role in emotions by its rich autonomic connection and may have influence on central mechanisms of inhibition and excitation by its reticular formation connection (Nashold, Wilson & Slaughter, 1969). Through reticular efferent influences, it is likely that an integrated system may exert control of the neurons in the gate at the substantia gelatinosa. As it is related to the hippocampus it may add a dimension of previous memories and experiences for the recollection of pain.

Connected to the thalamus, and projected through thalamic nuclei to the sensory-motor cortex and association cortices, it may add the dimension of awareness of the pain.

The two ascending afferent systems of transmission, the medial spino-reticular system and the anterolateral path, project into the mesencephalon to relay stimulus to Nauta's limbic midbrain area, a relationship which was interpreted by Mehler as providing for a polysynaptic path which could relay noxious stimulus into the limbic system.

The limbic lobe thus integrated would set the physiological stage for transmission to be recognized. The two conditions, recognition and patterning of the stimulus on spatial and temporal summation, would be indispensable

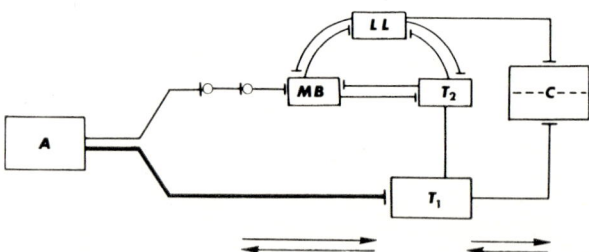

Figure 7.4 Model of pain mechanisms related to the limbic lobe (LL) integration, with specific and non-specific pathways. In the action system a specific pathway projects to the ventrolateral nucleus of the thalamus, which in turn projects to the cortex (C) through specific and non-specific projections. Non-specific pathways project to the midbrain (MB), and non-specific thalamic nuclei (T2) (dorsomedial nuclei). The arrows point to a bi-directional flow, in keeping with mechanisms of inhibition and facilitation. Lesions at LL, MB, T2 and C would not prevent the patient from recognizing pain. Recurrence of pain after lesions in the non-specific pathways may be due to new synaptic activity, new neural connections or reactivation of initially suppressed mechanisms.

for the recognition of pain. Projection alone to the thalamus would not by itself be giving rise to awareness of pain sensation.

The action system of the gate control theory may reside in the thalamus and in its projections to the sensory cortex, association cortex and limbic lobe (Figure 7.4).

The 'pain centre' in the thalamus may be negated in the light of present physiological evidence. Pain is not effectively suppressed with destruction of the VPL and VP nuclei of the thalamus. But the 'trigger system' of the limbic lobe may influence this 'pain centre' and may drive it.

RATIONALITY OF THE CONCEPT

The paradoxical effects of cingulotomy have joined those of all other operations directed to the interruption of central or peripheral pain pathways.

The best examples of surgical procedures aimed to a specific pathway, which have failed to relieve pain in one degree or another, are, thalamotomy, directed to the ventroposterior nuclei, mesencephalic tractotomy, posterior rhizotomy of cranial nerves, medullary tractotomy, trigeminal tractotomy, posterior spinal rhizotomy and neurectomy. All are surgical procedures aimed at a specific pathway of pain in the central or peripheral nervous system.

Operations such as posterior central gyrectomy, prefrontal lobotomy, dorso-medial and intralaminar thalamotomy, hypophysectomy and cingulotomy are surgical procedures which relieve pain, without interfering with so-called specific pain pathways.

Cingulotomy has the advantage of interfering with physiological events without the resultant personality changes seen in dorsomedial thalamotomy or prefrontal lobotomy (Faillace, Allen, McQueen & Northrup, 1971; Mark, Ervin & Yakovlev, 1962). Yet cingulotomy gives adequate relief of pain. This relief concerns only long-standing chronic pain. Pain of new modality, which is related to situations that usually 'hurt', such as headache, pin prick, and pain of any other nature which is new to the patient, is felt adequately with normal behaviour correlates. In our experience, depersonalization of the patient has not been observed.

When the chronic pain returns, it has the same characteristics as previously. The relapse develops usually after a few weeks or months.

The recurrent pain seems to have the same pattern, and gradually the same intensity, as before cingulotomy. We have had patients in whom cordotomy has failed to relieve the pain, and the pain subsided after cingulotomy. The emotional state of the patient is satisfactory, and there are no psychiatric disturbances.

The return of pain may mean that the memory for the pain was disturbed for some time postoperatively. The peripheral input had continued, since we did not interfere with the mechanisms of spinal transmission. It is possible that a new relearning experience is gradually taking place, until patterning and summation of the stimulus is such that pain becomes apparent again as a newly formed experience, which can then be compared to the past experiences and to previously stored sensory perceptions. Whether there has been repatterning, or whether there are new synaptic connections, is difficult to say. It is tempting to hypothesize that the hippocampal formation plays a role in the relearning process.

The fact is that when the patient feels pain again, it has the same characteristics as before surgery. This would speak in favour of re-establishing neuronal circuits with the adequate functional stimulus in the peripheral receptor of pain. If the gate was not changed by direct surgical means, the physiology of the pain cannot be understood except in terms of a change in the central mechanism. The direct pathway to thalamic projection remains intact and so does the sensory cortical projection. Yet pain is absent after cingulotomy. It would, therefore, be possible to postulate that limbic integration and control of the gate system by limbic reticular projections may be changed by interference in a 'central trigger' control system.

Although the brain as a whole does not respond to the modality of the sensations, called pain, the postulate would be that the limbic system would integrate the sensory input and the brain mechanism to obtain such a response. This may give us a better understanding of the phenomenon of pain, and the rationality for denying a pain centre in the brain.

REFERENCES

Ballantine HT Jr, Cassidy W, Flanagan NB & Marino R Jr (1967). Stereotaxic anterior cingulotomy for neuropsychiatric illness and intractable pain. *J. Neurosurg.*, **26**, 488

Faillace LA, Allen RP, McQueen JD & Northrup B (1971). Cognitive deficits from bilateral cingulotomy for intractable pain in man. *Dis. nerv. Syst.*, **32**, 171

Folts EL & White LE Jr (1966) Rostral cingulotomy and pain 'relief'. In: *Pain: Henry Ford Hospital International Symposium* (Eds Knighton & Dumke), p. 11. Boston: Little Brown Co.

Livingston WK (1943). *Pain Mechanisms.* New York: McMillan.

Mark VH, Ervin FR & Yakovlev PI (1962). The treatment of pain by stereotaxic methods. *Confin. neurol.*, **22**, 238.

Mehler WR (1962). The anatomy of the so-called 'pain tract' in man: An analysis of the course and distribution of the ascending fibres of the fasciculus anterolateralis. In: *Basic Research in Paraplegia* (Eds Fench & Porter). Springfield, Ill.: Charles C Thomas.

Melzack R & Wall PD (1965). Pain mechanisms: A new theory. *Science*, **150**, 971

Nashold BS Jr, Wilson WP & Slaughter SG (1969). Sensations evoked by stimulation of midbrain in man. *J. Neurosurg.*, **30**, 14

Noordenbos W (1959). *Pain Problems Pertaining to the Transmission of Nerve Impulses which give Rise to Pain.* Amsterdam: Elsevier.

CHAPTER 8

Chronic stimulation of the cingulum in humans with behaviour disorders
FRANCISCO ESCOBEDO, AUGUSTO FERNÁNDEZ-GUARDIOLA & GONZALO SOLÍS

INTRODUCTION
Current interest in the limbic system has increased considerably within the last few years. The responses to chronic electric stimulation of the cingulum in human beings with behavioural disorders about to undergo cingulotomy were recorded as a means of studying the 'emotional circuit' and its effects upon normal functions or altered behaviour.

TECHNICAL PROCEDURE
For bilateral stimulation of the cingulum in patients before cingulotomy electrodes are implanted under intratracheal anaesthesia with sodium pentothal combined with fluothane supplemented with nitrous oxide. Immediately before the operation, a lumbar pneumoencephalogram is made with 40–50 ml of air. The patient is in the supine position with the head elevated 15 degrees above the horizontal plane and fixed in the midposition.

Through a stab incision, two drills 3 mm in diameter are placed at either side, 3 cm lateral of the midline and 1 cm in front of the coronal suture.

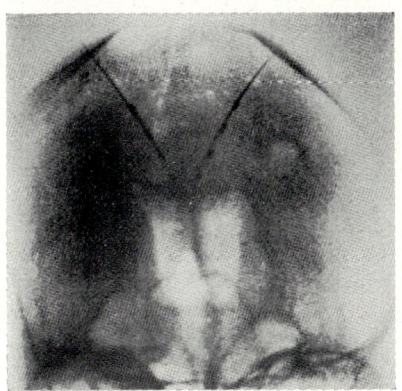 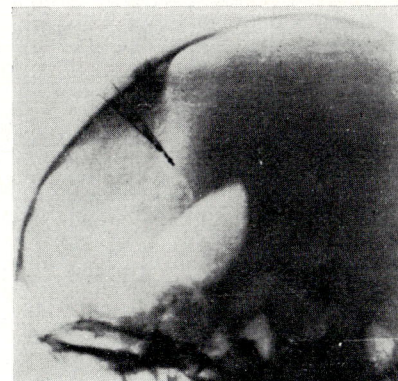

Figure 8.1 Anteroposterior x-ray showing the position of the chronic electrodes.

Figure 8.2 Lateral x-ray.

Surgical Approaches in Psychiatry

After the opening of the dura with a needle and electrocoagulation, the electrodes are introduced and positioned with their tips 5 mm lateral of the midline 1 cm above the roof of the frontal horn of the ventricle and in the posterior part of the rostral third of the corpus callosum.

The position of the electrodes is accurately determined with the aid of x-rays (Figure 8.1,2).

The electrodes are fixed to the scalp with sutures and remain in place for a period of 2–3 weeks while stimulation and recording are done.

Each electrode consists of a polythene tube 1 mm in diameter. This is pierced by four holes, which correspond to four stainless steel cylinders 3 mm long, arranged in the tube with 3 mm spaces between them, and attached to insulated copper wires. These lead into a special socket, which is connected to the stimulus generator or electroencephalograph (Figure 8.3).

Before any stimulus was applied, basal records of pulse rate, respiratory rate, blood pressure and surface EEG were obtained, as well as depth recording and behavioural patterns.

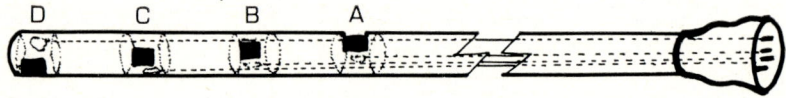

Figure 8.3 Construction of the four-polar electrode.

Bipolar stimuli with square waves (1 ms and 50 Hz), were applied to corresponding points, starting with low voltage, and the current was gradually increased. Stimulation was stopped at the moment when the voltage increase elicited electrical or clinical epileptic seizures or when electrical postdischarge was recorded.

PATIENTS

This technique was used in two patients; right-handed males, 17 years old, with mental retardation (IQ 60–70), who from the ages of seven and nine had had generalized epileptic seizures which were psychomotor at times and demonstrable clinically and electrically; the behaviour of these patients was as a rule destructive and aggressive.

RESULTS

Electric stimulation of the cingulum produced the following effects:

(a) *Vegetative responses:*
Increase of blood pressure from 110/80 to 180/120 mmHg. Marked respiratory slowing with periods of complete arrest for 30 to 40 s.
Swallowing,
Yawning,
Sensation of hunger,
No perceptible changes in pulse rate were recorded.

(b) *Motor responses:*
Semi-elaborated movements in contralateral limbs, mainly in the legs,
Restlessness,
Closing the eyes.

(c) *Psychological responses:*
Confusion. Inability to explain the feeling of 'As if I were blind . . .',
Auditory hallucinations,
Taste hallucinations (savour of mango, grapefruit, chocolate).

(d) *Behavioural responses:*
Sleepy,
Negativism,
Insistent (on smoking),
Screaming,
Psychomotor activity (when electric current had been greatly increased).

With stimulation in neighbouring areas, more laterally and dorsally (Figure 8.4), the results showed certain differences. In general the responses elicited were better integrated and more elaborated; auditory hallucinations were well integrated: 'I hear my father's voice . . . he is telling me where the money is and how I can become rich', and so were visual and taste hallucinations: 'There is a banana and a mango on the wall . . . I have eaten the mango, it is sweet, I want some more.'

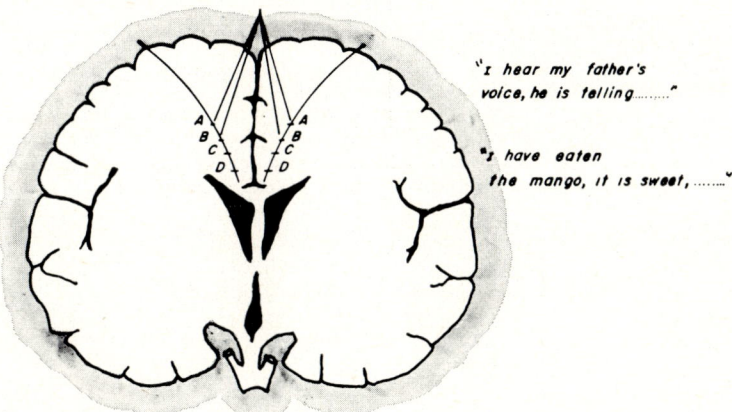

Figure 8.4 Well-integrated auditory, visual and gustatory hallucinations were obtained with stimulation through electrodes A and B.

In case 1, after bipolar stimulation of the first two external electrodes (Figure 8.4, A and B) immediate erection of the penis occurred. However, we cannot state that this area corresponds strictly to the cingulum.

DISCUSSION

With these patients we have obtained results similar to those reported many years ago by Smith (1945) after electric stimulation of the rostral cingulate cortex in the monkey, by Kremer (1947) in dogs, and by Pool & Ransohoff (1949) after acute electric and mechanical stimulation of the rostral portions of the cingulate gyrus in man:— that is, autonomic responses, motor effects and suppressor action with marked respiratory slowing and stopping for periods of up to 25 s, accompanied with a marked fall and occasional rise in blood pressure.

We must emphasize the results obtained in some psychological and behavioural responses, which may be due to stimulation of the cingulum not only at the level of the cortex. These results suggest that we are chiefly stimulating the fibres that connect this area with the temporal lobe, hypothalamus and other structures of the limbic system.

No significant differences were seen after stimulation of the dominant and non-dominant hemispheres; however, the fact that both the patients described in this paper had significant brain damage must be borne in mind.

These results lead us to believe that this area of the cingulum, as part of the limbic system, is one of the higher centres controlling emotional and autonomic responses and, particularly, the exteriorization of acts and performances. Thus it is able to regulate behaviour through its influence over the temporal lobe, hypothalamus, thalamus, frontal lobe and other structures of the limbic system.

Nevertheless, the cingulum does not seem to participate in the integration of higher and more elaborate functions.

REFERENCES

Kremer WF (1947). Automatic and somatic reactions induced by stimulation of the cingulate gyrus in dogs. *J. Neurophysiol.*, **10**, 371

Pool JL & Ransohoff J (1949). Autonomic effects on stimulating rostral portion of cingulate gyri in man. *J. Neurophysiol.*, **12**, 385

Smith WK (1945). The functional significance of the rostral cingular cortex as revealed by its responses to electrical excitation. *J. Neurophysiol.*, **8**, 241

CHAPTER 9

Selective leucotomy: A review
WALPOLE LEWIN

INTRODUCTION
Over the last 20 years two sites for selective leucotomy have been established for the relief of mental illness, one in the cingulate area and the other in the white matter beneath the posterior orbital cortex. Lesions in these sites have produced encouraging and substantially similar results from several centres, as reported at the Conference in Copenhagen 2 years ago (Hitchcock, Laitinen & Vaernet, 1972). We may agree with the statement from a recent review article on this subject that 'individual results are so strikingly good that this time there can be no turning back' (*Lancet*, 1972). As an introduction to this Symposium, I would like to comment on some aspects of selective leucotomy, and in particular on operations in the cingulate area, in the light of our experience of open operations by orbital undercutting and cingulectomy since 1948.

The year 1947 was a watershed in the development of psychosurgery. It saw sufficient major reviews of the results of standard prefrontal leucotomy to show that there was benefit to be derived from surgical procedures, but equally, that a more selective approach should be sought if adverse side-effects were to be avoided. It was in that mood that there appeared on the programme of the meeting of the Society of British Neurological Surgeons in Glasgow on November, 1947, a paper by Professor John Fulton, entitled 'Bilateral Lesions Restricted to the Orbital Surface of the Frontal Lobes'. In the discussion that followed, Professor Fulton was asked where seemed to be the most promising site for a local lesion in the frontal lobe to produce a favourable result. In reply he said that were it feasible in man, cingulectomy would appear to be an appropriate place for limited leucotomy. He developed this thesis further in his Withering lectures of 1948 and in the Salmon lectures which were published in book form entitled 'Frontal Lobotomy and Affective Behaviour' (Fulton, 1951).

In Oxford, under the direction of Sir Hugh Cairns, we began our programme of selective leucotomy with the view that we should adopt open selective procedures, not only in an attempt to improve the results, but to see to what extent there was localization of function within the frontal lobes. In July, 1948 the first open anterior cingulectomy was performed and the first series reported in 1952 (Whitty, Duffield, Tow and Cairns, 1952). Similar work took place in France (Le Beau & Pecker, 1949) and in Canada

(Livingston, 1953). Our earlier results from patients with schizophrenia showed that although cingulectomy benefited those with aggressive states and obsessional symptoms, it was inadequate for the overall illness. Subsequently, therefore, the operation was restricted to those patients with affective disorders showing these features. On the other hand, patients with anxiety and tension within a schizophrenic illness or with affective illnesses predominated by depression, were treated by open orbital leucotomy, following the lead given by Scoville in his report of the operation in 1949 (Scoville, 1949; Tow & Lewin, 1953). Later the opportunity was taken to review this work at Oxford and to record the results of 113 patients treated by one or other of the open operations during the years 1948–59 (Lewin, 1961). The results were encouraging. In that report it was stated that 'the results from various centres together with the experimental evidence on which these operations are based, make cogent arguments for directing surgery to the orbital for symptoms of anxiety and depression, and to the cingulate gyrus for aggression and obsessional disorder'.

That paper reported on seven patients with aggressive states who were treated by cingulectomy. Considerable improvement was shown in five cases. Of the four patients who also suffered from epilepsy, the number of such attacks decreased in two. These findings supported the earlier reports of Le Beau (1952, 1954). It may be further discussed at this meeting that, where aggression is the dominant symptom, operations on the amygdala will be an alternative approach in the future.

RECENT EXPERIENCE

In the last 10 years at Cambridge we have continued with these two open operations and a further 59 patients have been treated. The results are similar to the first series and in line with the results from other centres, most of which were reported at the Copenhagen conference.

With regard to surgery for affective disorders dominated by depression and with or without tension, it would seem that the results according to present tests, are similar whether one operates by open orbital undercutting or uses a stereotactic approach with the lesion in the presubstantia innominata, as has been described by Geoffrey Knight (Knight, 1964, 1972).

I would, however, like to comment further on cingulectomy. It will be recalled that the operation of open bilateral cingulectomy is restricted to area 24 over a length of 4 cm to remove the cingulate gyrus on each side, extending into the white matter for up to 1 cm. The significance of this area is seen by the demonstration of a 'Korsakoff-like' syndrome in the early postoperative period. This emphasizes the connections with the hypothalamus, and the autonomic effects shown in some patients (in whom operation in earlier years was conducted under local analgesia to facilitate the approach) by stimulation of the cingulate gyrus unilaterally and bilaterally. This operation yielded a satisfactory improvement in primarily obsessional disorders and also in some cases of a pure tension state of aggression. However, attention was drawn quite early on to the fact that where depression was a main symptom the result was not as good. Indeed in the 1961 (Lewin, 1961) paper, a patient was referred to who presented primarily obsessional symptoms but also suffered some depression; after cingulectomy he did well for 4 years and then relapsed with a pure depressive illness which subsequently responded dramatically to orbital leucotomy. Our policy, therefore, was to prefer orbital leucotomy whenever there were depressive symptoms present.

Over the last decade, however, there has been renewed interest in the cingulate area. Foltz & White (1962), using a stereotactic approach, concluded that cingulectomy gave the best results with anxiety and/or depression. This was followed by a report from Ballantine, Cassidy, Flanagan & Marino (1967). Using a stereotactic approach, they reported 22 useful improvements out of 40. These included several patients with depressive illnesses. In the light of this I questioned whether our earlier view should not be revised, particularly as the results of psychological testing of our patients before and after operation had shown that although adverse personality changes were mild in all cases, they were at their least after cingulectomy. One was therefore anxious to extend the indications for this operation if it were practicable. Accordingly, two patients underwent cingulectomy as a first procedure. In these cases obsessional symptoms were predominant but there was also a very definite depressive element or frank illness parallel with it or in the past. There was a satisfactory early improvement in both patients, but then relapse within a year with marked depressive symptoms accompanying the obsessionalism and necessitating orbital leucotomy. The early results of this second operation are encouraging.

In this recent series we have also reversed the order of these two operations. In a patient with an overt obsessional illness but with depressive features and some suggestion of a schizophrenic background we elected to perform an orbital leucotomy in the first instance. He was able to return to work 6 months after this operation, having previously been totally incapacitated. He remained relatively well for 2 years, but then relapsed with an almost pure obsessional illness. It was equally noteworthy that the earlier symptoms of depression and anxiety had been considerably relieved by the first operation, and this still remained so. His IQ of 132 at this stage was higher than before the orbital leucotomy. Four years after the first operation cingulectomy was performed. Six months later he pronounced himself completely relieved of his obsessional symptoms and since then—$4\frac{1}{2}$ years ago—he has been on full work. Objectively, obsessional symptoms and some tension are easily apparent to the observer, but from a practical point of view there has been substantial relief from these two groups of symptoms since the two operations.

These observations have therefore made me reluctant to change the original view, that open cingulectomy, as we perform it, is not an effective operation when depressive symptoms are paramount. Wherein then lies the difference between this operation and its apparent modern version by a stereotactic approach? It should be noted that in a later report Ballantine has laid considerable stress on the stereotactic lesion being placed right on to the corpus callosum so as to make certain that the cingulum bundle is interrupted

(Ballantine, Cassidy, Brodeur & Giriunas, 1972). But where exactly is this cingulum bundle, and how extensive is it in man? In our operations, after removing the cingulate gyri by suction, it has not been possible to see clearly in the white matter just above the corpus callosum proper, any identifiable band which could be called a cingulum, whatever its appearance in the fixed brain may be. It is likely, therefore, that this tract is wider and more diffuse than we had been led to suppose from the anatomic textbooks. It should also be remembered that much of it consists of short connecting fibres within the medial limbic system. It also has connections with area 32, the posterior orbital cortex and other frontal areas as well. It is possible that it is because of these connections that the results of stereotactic procedures differ from our results of open cingulectomy. Our operation is virtually a pure removal of area 24, and although part of the cingulate bundle must obviously be taken, this is not an essential part of the procedure. Also, when one looks at the cingulate gyri at operation, they so often meet and fuse at the midline and are grey and diffluent, so it is unlikely that ordinary stereotactic procedures can be relied on to destroy the cingulate gyri selectively. Indeed the primary object of these stereotactic operations may be the destruction of the white matter with its cingulate fibres just above the corpus callosum. This may explain why it appears to be a more effective operation for a greater range of illnesses than does the formal cingulectomy. At the same time, however, there is a risk that with its more diffuse effect it may prove in the long run to be a less effective operation for the purely obsessional illness than the open cingulectomy, and also inferior to orbital leucotomy or a stereotactic lesion in the presubstantia innominata for the primarily depressive illness. A similar interpretation could be placed on ventral cingulotomy (Laitinen & Vilkki, 1972), where the pathways from the posterior orbital cortex into the anterior part of the cingulum bundle must be destroyed.

THE NEXT PHASE
The next phase in selective leucotomy will demand a much closer collaboration between the various disciplines concerned. From the psychiatrists we shall need to have as precise a diagnosis as it is possible to make so that a decision as to the most effective operation can be taken. As surgeons we have not only to be clear as to what we think we are doing, but also to seek proof as the opportunity presents itself, of what we have actually done. The apparent differences already referred to between open and stereotactic procedures on the cingulate gyrus draw attention to the error that may arise if one prematurely groups various operations together on the assumption that they are all interrupting the same areas. In fact it already seems to be emerging from newer anatomic knowledge and from clinical results that this is not so. This has obvious implications for future clinical indications. The surgeons, together with anatomists and physiologists, must continue to examine very carefully the site of these lesions and their anatomic consequences.

Finally, one should mention the assessment of the results. Selective leucotomy is producing worthwhile clinical improvement with apparently minimal adverse effects. But are we judging the effects adequately or do we lack sufficiently fine and precise psychological tools to measure the effects of these more limited operations? Psychological testing seems to have become a very highly personal performance with no general agreement amongst psychologists as to what should be tested and how it should be done. It becomes difficult, therefore, for surgeons to compare the results from different centres except in the crudest way. Therefore, one is tempted to suggest that if the target of these limited operations is to be fully evaluated, the time has come to seek for an agreed form of pre- and postoperative assessment.

CONCLUSIONS

In conclusion it would appear that until advances in biochemistry, or in some other field, render surgery for mental illness unnecessary, the results to date suggest that selective leucotomy does alleviate suffering for some patients, and for the present should have a place in therapy. But whilst this is so, it is our duty in the immediate future to refine our psychiatric diagnosis, our surgical intent and the appraisal of our results.

REFERENCES

Ballantine HT, Cassidy WL, Brodeur J & Giriunas I (1972). Frontal cingulotomy for mood disturbance. In: *Psychosurgery* (Eds Hitchcock, Laitinen & Vaernet), p. 221. Springfield, Ill.: Charles C. Thomas.
Ballantine HT, Cassidy WL, Flanagan NB & Marino R (1967). Stereotaxic anterior cingulotomy for neuropsychiatric illness and intractable pain. *J. Neurosurg.*, **26**, 488
Editorial (1972). *Lancet*, **2**, 69
Foltz EL & White LE (1962). Pain 'relief' by frontal cingulotomy. *J. Neurosurg.*, **19**, 89
Fulton JF (1951). Frontal lobotomy and affective behavior, p. 159. New York: W. W. Norton & Co.
Knight GC (1964). The orbital cortex as an objective in the surgical treatment of mental illness. *Brit. J. Surg.*, **51**, 114
Knight GC (1972). Bifrontal stereotaxic tractotomy in the substantia innominata. In: *Psychosurgery* (Eds Hitchcock, Laitinen & Vaernet), p. 267. Springfield, Ill.: Charles C. Thomas.
Laitinen LV & Vilkki J (1972). Stereotaxic ventral anterior cingulotomy in some psychological disorders. *Ibid.*, p. 242.
Le Beau J & Pecker J (1949). La topectomie péricalleuse antérieure dans certaines formes d'agitation psycho-motrice au cours de l'épilepsie et de l'arriération mentale. *Rev. neurol.*, **81**, 1039
Le Beau J (1952). The cingular and precingular areas in psychosurgery (agitated behavior, obsessive compulsive states, epilepsy). *Acta Psychiat. Neurol. Scand.*, **27**, 305
Le Beau J (1954). Anterior cingulectomy in man. *J. Neurosurg.*, **11**, 268
Lewin W (1961). Observations on selective leucotomy. *J. Neurol. Neurosurg. Psychiat.*, **24**, 37
Livingston KE (1953). Cingulate cortex isolation for the treatment of psychoses and psychoneuroses. *Res. Publ. Ass. nerv. ment. Dis.*, **31**, 374
Scoville WB (1949). Selective cortical undercutting as a means of modifying and studying frontal lobe function in man. *J. Neurosurg.*, **6**, 65
Tow PM & Lewin W (1953). Orbital leucotomy: isolation of the orbital cortex by open operation. *Lancet*, **2**, 644
Whitty CWM, Duffield JE, Tow PM & Cairns H (1952). Anterior cingulectomy in the treatment of mental disease. *Lancet*, **1**, 475

CHAPTER 10

Observations on the transcallosal emotional connections
L V LAITINEN & J VÍLKKI

INTRODUCTION

Between January 1969 and October 1971 we carried out bilateral stereotactic rostral cingulotomies on 46 psychiatric patients (Laitinen, Toivakka & Vilkki, 1973). As 42 of them were operated on under local anaesthesia, various electrophysiological investigations were possible during surgery. The surgical target lay in the rostralmost part of the cingulum, below and in front of the knee of the corpus callosum. An almost constant finding was that electrical stimulation of target area 1 with 6 Hz caused an evoked potential in the contralateral frontopolar scalp EEG (Figure 10.1).

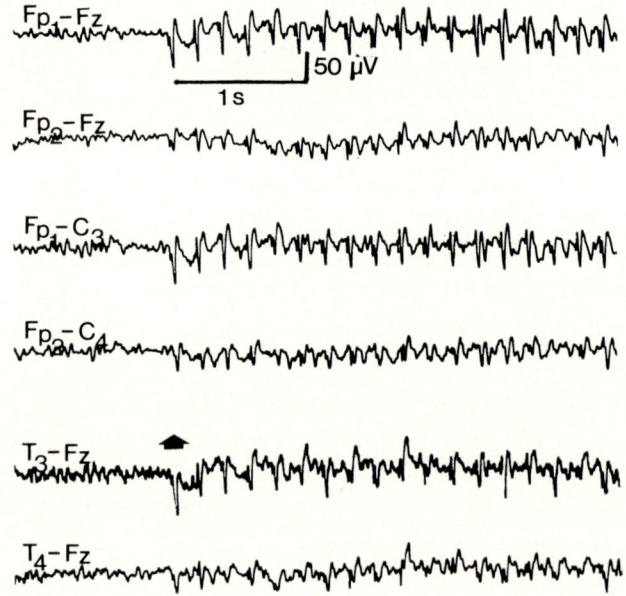

Figure 10.1 The evoked potentials in the left frontopolar derivations during bipolar stimulation of the right rostral cingulum (square waves, 6 Hz, 1 ms, 5 V). The arrow indicates the start of stimulation.

During one such operation an electrode was inserted into the rostral cingulum through the knee of the corpus callosum to investigate the transcallosal response. Electrical stimulation of the right side of the knee with 6 Hz caused a weak evoked potential in the contralateral frontopolar area. Subsequent stimulation with 60 Hz resulted in a sudden strong feeling of inner well-being and relaxation of the whole body of the patient, a 24-year-old girl suffering from schizophrenic anxiety. The response was reproduced several times; it was obtained from a limited area in the superficial layer of the knee. A lesion 6 × 6 mm in diameter was produced with high-frequency electrocoagulation; the centre of the lesion lay 6 mm from the midline. The electrode was then inserted into the left side of the genu, where electrical stimulation with 60 Hz again evoked the pleasant feeling, though less intensely than the right-sided coagulation. A similar lesion was produced on this side too. In addition to the callosal lesion, bilateral cingulotomy was carried out.

PRESENT SERIES

The clinical result of this operation, which we call anterior mesoloviotomy (Laitinen, 1972), was encouraging. Subsequently we have operated on 37 additional patients in the mesolovion. The clinical grouping of the patients is shown in Table 10.2. Anxiety and tension were the most dominant symptoms. The age of the patients varied from 21–58 y, with an average of 34 y. Duration of illness ranged from 2–27 y, with an average of 10 y.

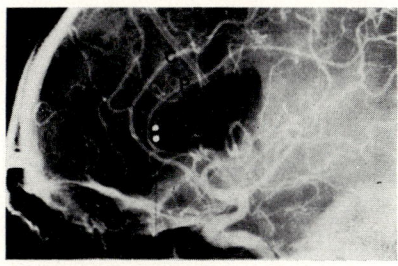

Figure 10.2 Combined air ventriculography and carotid arteriography to visualize the knee of the corpus callosum (white dots). The cingulum lies between the pericallosal (P) and callosomarginal (C) arteries.

METHODS

Laitinen's stereo-guide was used. For adequate localization of the knee of the corpus callosum, combined air ventriculography and carotid arteriography are necessary (Figures 10.2,3). The size, shape and site of the knee vary considerably from one patient to another. The target in the mesolovion lay 5–7 mm from the midline. The presumable size of the bilateral lesions ranged from 6 × 6 to 8 × 12 mm in diameter.

The pleasant response of well-being and relaxation to the high-frequency stimulation was obtained in most of those patients who suffered from primary anxiety, tension and fears. Those patients who suffered from depression or

Table 10.1 The pre- to postoperative changes in psychological test performances after anterior mesoloviotomy.

	Tests	Number of Cases	Direction of change	$P <$ *
Intelligence	Culture fair intelligence test†	20	Improvement	N.S.
Attention	Serial ordering of digits	17	Improvement	N.S.
Attention	Simple motor reaction time	20	No change	N.S.
Attention	Two-choice discrimination task	20	No change	N.S.
Psychomotor performance	Purdue pegboard (assembly)	19	Improvement	0·05
Imaginative capacity	Holtzman inkblot technique† (shortened form) number of rejections	25	Impairment	N.S.
Memory	Immediate recognition of inkblots†	24	Improvement	0·05
Memory	Delayed recognition of inkblots†	18	Improvement	0·05
Emotional state and attitudes	Eysenck personality inventory	18		
	'Neuroticism'		Improvement	0·05
	'Extraversion'		Decline	N.S.

* Two-tailed Wilcoxon matched-pairs signed-ranks test.
† Parallel tests were used in pre- and postoperative examinations.

obsessive-compulsive symptoms, even if accompanied by secondary anxiety, did not have any subjective sensation. Low-frequency stimulation with 3–6 Hz seldom caused subjective sensations. If they appeared they were of an unpleasant nature. It was surprising that no autonomic responses could be evoked by electrical stimulation of the knee of the corpus callosum.

One patient had an operative complication: there was excessive haemorrhage from the sagittal sinus at the burr hole margin. Bleeding could be stopped during surgery, but a sizeable blood clot was formed subdurally between the frontal lobes. This complication was presumably the cause of a marked mental slowing in this patient, who later made a good recovery.

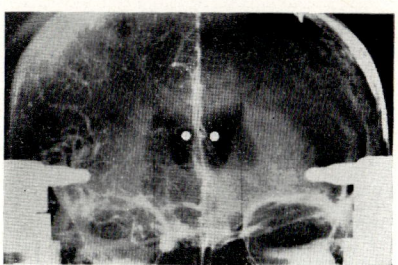

Figure 10.3 Anteroposterior view. The mesoloviotomy target lies 5–6 mm lateral to the midline, corresponding to the white dots.

PSYCHOLOGICAL EXAMINATIONS

The immediate effects of anterior mesoloviotomy on psychological test performances were assessed in those patients who performed adequately in preoperative tests (Table 10.1).

No pre- to postoperative average changes were seen in the tests of intelligence or attention. One patient had intraoperative subdural haemorrhage with postoperative confusion. Had this patient been excluded, there would have been a significant average improvement in the intelligence test performance ($P < 0.02$).

Imaginative capacity was assessed with a shortened form of the 'Holtzman Inkblot Technique'. The first 15 inkblots of a series of 45 were shown successively to the subject, and he was asked to say what they looked like or what they might represent. After our previous method, rostral cingulotomy, the number of inkblots about which the subject failed to report anything increased significantly ($P < 0.01$). Such a deficit was seen less frequently after mesoloviotomy.

Immediately after the 15 inkblots had been shown, a photograph of 45 inkblots was projected on the screen. The 15 inkblots which the subject had previously seen were randomly interspersed among the 30 new ones. The subject was asked to mark those 15 blots which he had seen earlier. After 1 hour all 45 inkblots were projected again on the screen but their mutual locations had been changed. The same procedure as above was repeated. Both immediate and delayed recognition improved after mesoloviotomy

In the Eysenck Personality Inventory a decline of 'neuroticism' was noticed. 'Extraversion' did not change.

In conclusion, psychological investigations indicate that anterior mesoloviotomy immediately improves the emotional state and possibly also some memory functions of the patients.

CLINICAL RESULTS

The short-term clinical results of 38 anterior mesoloviotomies are shown in Table 10.2. The new operation seemed to be effective against anxiety, tension and fears of neurotic, schizophrenic and epileptic origin. It was also powerful against schizophrenic catatonia. It was quite evident that anterior mesoloviotomy was absolutely ineffective against depression and obsessive-compulsive symptoms.

Table 10.2 The short-term results of 38 anterior mesoloviotomies. The follow-up time ranges from 1–12 months.

Diagnosis (ICD code)	Short-term results*					
	I	II	III	IV	V	Total
Schizophrenia (295.1,3,7,8,9)	4	10	2	1	—	17
Affective psychosis (296.2)	1	—	2	2	—	5
Anxiety neurosis (300.0)	2	3	3	2	—	10
Obsessive-compulsive neurosis (300.3)	—	—	—	1	—	1
Intractable pain and depression (304.3)	—	—	1	1	—	2
Erethic idiocy (315)	—	—	—	1	—	1
Temporal lobe epilepsy (345.3)	—	2	—	—	—	2
Total	7	15	8	8	—	38

* Improvement graded according to Pippard (1955): I Symptom free, II Much improved, III Improved, IV Not improved, V Worse.

DISCUSSION

Yakovlev & Locke (1961) and Yakovlev, Locke & Angevine Jr (1966) have shown that the core of the corpus callosum is formed of commissural fibres which unite the homotopic cortical areas of the two hemispheres. The superficial layers consist of the transcallosal cingulostriate fibres, which have their origin in the cingulum. Some run in the ventral lamina of the corpus callosum to the septum and to the contralateral stratum subcallosum and caudate nucleus. Others run in the dorsal lamina and perforate the commissural fibres in the contralateral hemisphere. Of these, some descend in the internal capsule, and others are distributed in the putamen and, according to Showers (1959), even in the pallidum, subthalamic area and substantia nigra.

We presume that in anxiety, tension and schizophrenic catatonia the interhemispheric cingulostriate fibres are hyperactive. These pathways may constitute the link between the emotional integrative system and its motor output.

Recently, an opinion was expressed (*Lancet*, 1972; Turner, 1972), that the callosal operation described here might be a sort of paramedian frontal lobotomy. Turner had made lesions in the frontal paramedian structures, 1 cm in front of the genu of the corpus callosum, and obtained good clinical results in the treatment of anxiety and aggressiveness. He therefore thought that mesoloviotomy interrupts the same anatomical pathways as his previous operation. This does not seem to be true: some years ago we carried out rostral cingulotomies (Laitinen, Toivakka & Vilkki, 1972) close to the callosal target, but definitely in the cingulum, medial to and presumably a little behind the target of Turner. The clinical results of cingulotomy and the psychological changes produced differed from those obtained with mesoloviotomy (Laitinen & Vilkki, 1973) and the responses of these two targets to electrical stimulation were quite different, and even opposite.

In Marchiafava-Bignami's disease the commissural fibres of the corpus callosum undergo demyelinization, which finally results in complete degeneration and cystic formation of the core of the corpus callosum (Castaigne, Buge, Canbier, Escourolle & Rancurel, 1971). The superficial layers, on the other hand, are perfectly preserved and so is the cingulum. The clinical symptoms of Marchiafava-Bignami's disease consist of mental deterioration, confusion, stupor, coma, muscular hypertonia, tremor, epileptic fits, etc., i.e. they are rather opposite to the effects of mesoloviotomy. This seems to be evidence that the beneficial effects of the anterior callosal lesions are due to interruption of the superficial fibres—we always aim at restricting the lesion to the anterior superficial layer of the genu. These fibres may, as Yakovlev's group (1961, 1966) has postulated, connect the cingulum with the corpus striatum of the contralateral hemisphere, or they may simply connect the two cinguli across the corpus callosum (Nauta, 1972). In some of our patients stimulation of the corpus callosum 6 mm lateral to the midline with low intensity caused relaxation of the ipsilateral side of the body and limbs, which seems to support the former theory.

Animal experimentation is still needed, however, to confirm our present hypothesis: in anxiety and tension the cingulostriate interhemispheric pathways are hyperactive and lesion to these pathways may result in relaxation and restoration of emotional well-being. So far there is no justification for a wider application of anterior mesoloviotomy until precise indications and limitations have been assessed.

ACKNOWLEDGEMENT

This study was aided by a grant to J. V. from Suomen Kulttuurirahasto.

REFERENCES

Castaigne P, Buge A, Cambier J, Escourolle R & Rancurel G (1971). La maladie de Marchiafava-Bignami: étude anatomclinique de dix observations. *Rev. neurol.*, **125**, 179

Laitinen LV (1972). Stereotactic lesions in the knee of the corpus callosum in the treatment of emotional disorders. *Lancet*, **1**, 472

Laitinen L, Toivakka E & Vilkki J (1972). Rostral cingulotomy for psychiatric disorders: electrophysiological, psychological and clinical findings. *Vopr. Neirokhir.* (in press)

Laitinen LV & Vilkki J (1973). Electrophysiological and psychological studies on the function of the rostral cingulum and the knee of the corpus callosum in man. *Psychiat. Fenn.* (in press)
Editorial (1972). Psychosurgery. *Lancet*, **2**, 69
Nauta WJH (1972). Personal communication.
Showers MJC (1959). The cingulate gyrus: additional motor area and cortical autonomic regulator. *J, comp. Neurol.*, **112**, 231
Turner E (1972). Stereotaxic lesions in the knee of the corpus callosum in the treatment of emotional disorders. *Lancet*, **1**, 755
Yakovlev PI & Locke S (1961). Corticocortical connections of the anterior cingulate gyrus, the cingulum, and the subcallosal bundle in monkey. *Arch. Neurol. Chicago*, **5**, 364
Yakovlev PI, Locke S & Angevine Jr JB (1966). The limbus of the cerebral hemisphere, limbic nuclei of the thalamus, and the cingulum bundle. In: *The Thalamus* (Eds Purpura and Yahr), p. 77. New York: Columbia University Press.

PART IV

ORBITO-FRONTAL INTERVENTIONS

CHAPTER 11

Anatomical placement of lesions in the ventromedial segment of the frontal lobe
RAYMOND L NEWCOMBE

INTRODUCTION

Lesions in the ventromedial segment of the frontal lobe for affective disorders, whether by open operation and cerebral incision or by stereotactic placement, depend for their position on an assumed degree of anatomical constancy of the target area in relation to the visible or radiological landmarks used. Physiological methods of localization in this area are of no proven clinical value. Topographical interpretation of the effect of such lesions therefore is limited by the degree of anatomical variation of the target area to the landmarks. This factor is more important than operative technique and instrumentation, provided the angle of approach determined by the point of entry into the brain is controlled and one of the more satisfactory methods of lesion production is employed.

In this study an analysis is attempted of the probable position of radiologically marked lesions in two operations, the bimedial rostral leucotomy (Greenblatt & Solomon, 1952; Falconer, 1954) and the stereotactic tractotomy of Knight (1964).

In the first operation the line of incision extends from the middle of the trephine opening, 2 cm in front of the coronal suture, to a position just anterior to the line of the sphenoidal ridge. The white matter is cut with a metal sucker for a width of about 2 cm subjacent to the grey matter medially and inferiorly. The incision skirts the front of the anterior horn, and therefore, should pass anterior to the head of the caudate nucleus in all cases. The lower end of the incision is marked with tantalum clips.

In the second operation the stereotactic lesion is produced by ^{90}Y implants. The site of the lesion was evolved from the approximate position of the posterior 2 cm of the orbital undercut operation. The target position is determined in the lateral x-ray by reference to the plane passing through the orbital roof laterally and the tuberculum sellae, and the plane perpendicular to the latter (Figure 11.1). Six yttrium seeds are placed on each side in the approximate position in relation to the skull shown in the figure. The dotted outlines represent the approximate area of β irradiation necrosis.

84 *Surgical Approaches in Psychiatry*

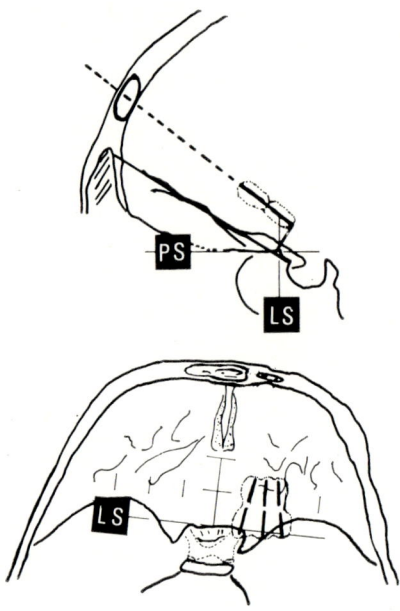

Figure 11.1 Diagram to show bony landmarks and approximate position of the yttrium lesion in stereotactic basofrontal tractotomy (Knight). PS, planum sphenoidale; LS, limbus sphenoidalis (anterior margin of sulcus chiasmaticus).

STEREOTACTIC TRACTOTOMY LESION

The position of the stereotactic tractotomy lesion of Knight within the brain has been described as being beneath the head of the caudate nucleus and lying in the substantia innominata. It is important to clear up a point of confusion regarding the latter term. The substantia innominata of Reichert appears to have been so called by an unknown student of Reichert's, who found that Reichert had not named the grey masses submerged in white matter in the area subjacent to the substantia perforata anterior, illustrated in his treatise of 1859–1861. The white matter of the substantia innominata merges with the white matter of the ventromedial segment of the frontal lobe in a thin strip above the olfactory hillock and the anterior margin of the anterior perforated substance. It is an area which fills the space between the anterior portions of the amygdaloid complex and the posterior boundary of the olfactory tubercle. The grey masses of this area are described in detail by Nauta & Haymaker (1969). Fibre systems are described by Miodonski (1967). The morphological features superficial to the substantia innominata are shown in Figure 11.2. The ventromedial segment of the frontal lobe is seen to be limited by the upturned posterior part of the gyrus rectus and the medial orbital gyrus.

The substantia innominata has alternatively been defined, in describing the site of ventromedial frontal lesions, as the area lying beneath the head of the caudate nucleus and overlying area 13 (Knight, 1964). This wider usage of the

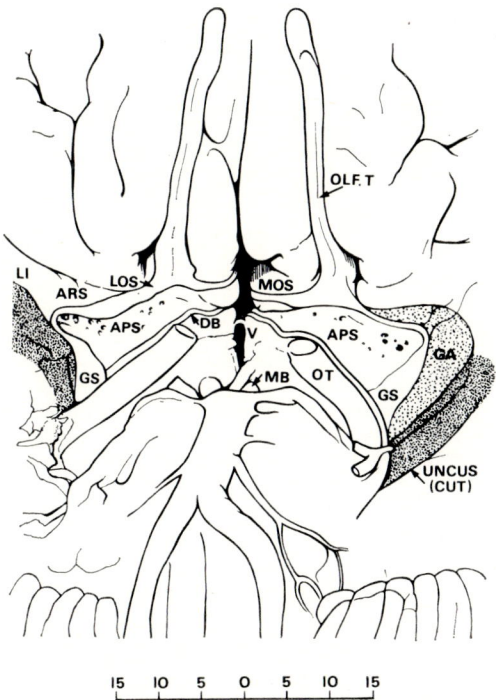

Figure 11.2 Anatomical feature of structures superficial to the substantia innominata (after Nauta). APS, anterior perforated substance; MOS and LOS, medial and lateral olfactory striae; DB, diagonal band of Broca; OT, optic tract; GS, gyrus semilunaris; GA, gyrus ambiens; MB, mammillary body; LI, limen insulae; ARS, anterior rhinal sulcus; OLF.T, olfactory tract.

term should be distinguished from the area known as the substantia innominata of Reichert.

In 25 patients who had a stereotactic tractotomy operation employing bony landmarks, the postoperative lateral x-rays were reviewed. The position of the yttrium seeds producing the lesions was measured in relation to the anterior commissure and the AC–PC line. The mean position at 10 mm from the midline is shown in Figure 11.3. The outlines were obtained by superimposition of 16 outlines of normal brains (van Buren & Maccubbin, 1962). It can be seen that the posterior limits of the mean lesion, and indeed the limit of the area defined by $2 \times$ S.D. of the co-ordinates, lie anterior to the upturned posterior part of the orbital cortex in all the representative normal brains. This makes it unlikely that the lesions in any of the 25 patients entered into the substantia innominata of Reichert, although they may well have influenced the cortical afferents and efferents passing through that area.

It can also be seen in Figure 11.3 that the posterior part of the lesion mean position, defined by the yttrium seeds, lies subjacent to the outlines of the head

86 Surgical Approaches in Psychiatry

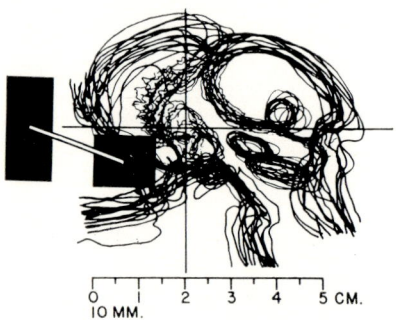

Figure 11.3 Mean position of stereotactic basofrontal tractotomy (Knight) in 25 patients, in relation to ventricular co-ordinates (white line). Horizontal line of the cross is the plane through the anterior and posterior commissures. The vertical reference plane passes through the anterior commissure. The outlines represent 16 superimposed sagittal sections at 10 mm from the midline (van Buren & Maccubbin, 1962). Rectangular shaded areas represent 2 × S.D. of co-ordinates of anterior and posterior limits of the lesions.

of the caudate nucleus and of the anterior horn of the lateral ventricle. Considering that the major yttrium lesion is about 5 mm in diameter, it is probable that some of these lesions involve the orbital segment of the head of the caudate nucleus, and lie near the anterior horn of the lateral ventricle. If the angle of insertion happened to be high, then the anteromedial part of the lesion might involve the tip of the anterior horn. A more extensive involvement of the thalamo-frontal radiation, which is concentrated in this area, might then occur. Since the angle of approach to the target area is determined in part by the height of the orbital roof at its highest point (about 30 mm from the midline) and in part by the placement of the burr hole just above the frontal air sinuses, the degree of involvement of the projection from the dorsomedial nucleus of the thalamus might be expected to vary from this cause (i.e. angle of approach) apart from any variation of the thalamo-frontal bundle in relation to the tip of the anterior horn.

PROXIMITY TO VENTRICLE AND CAUDATE NUCLEUS FROM BONY LANDMARKS
The 25 patients who had air studies, had their operations too recently for correlation of lesion position with clinical response. Therefore, one had to devise a method of estimation of lesion position from the plain postoperative x-rays. In any case it was likely that the bony landmarks were better indicators of the ventromedial segment of the frontal lobe than third ventricular co-ordinates (Newcombe, 1972). For this purpose the planum sphenoidale (PS) at the midline and the anterior margin of the sulcus chiasmaticus, or limbus sphenoidalis (LS) at the midline seemed to be the most appropriate landmarks, since the planum sphenoidale lies subjacent to the posteromedial tongue of the frontal lobe where it dips down into the olfactory groove. At about 1 cm from the midline the anterior horn and the caudate nucleus reach their lowest

point, and the more lateral degree of elevation of the orbital roof is unlikely to be relevant. In addition, the tuberculum sellae is very variable in contour and position, and lies further away from the relevant part of the brain. An analysis of the contours of the anterior fossa in 12 normal skulls, combined with the results of the variability study of 24 brains reported by Newcombe (1972), and the radiological data from the 25 patients who had air studies at the time of stereotactic tractotomy, resulted in the diagram shown in Figure 11.4. The details will be reported elsewhere. The probable range of the outlines of the ventral surface of the head of the caudate nucleus and of the external surface of the genu of the corpus callosum are shown in relation to the planum sphenoidale (PS) and the limbus sphenoidalis (LS). The diagram also gives an estimate of the lowest position of the tip of the anterior horn in the brains studies. There is a theoretical error of the position of structures in relation to the bony landmarks of plus or minus 4 mm but in practice the error would ap ear to be less.

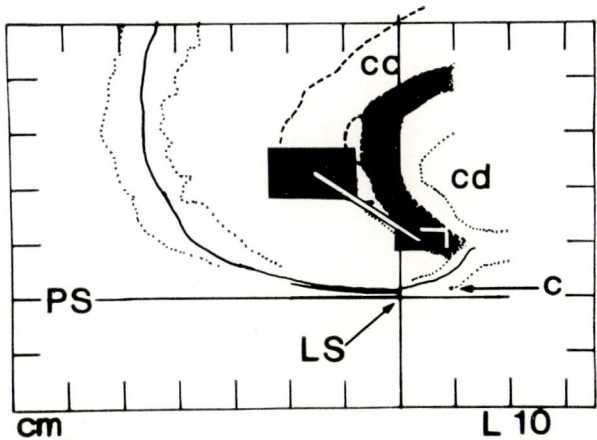

Figure 11.4 Mean lesion position of 25 patients treated by stereotactic basofrontal tractotomy (Knight) by reference to planum sphenoidale at the midline (PS) and limbus sphenoidalis (LS). Rectangular shaded areas 2 × S.D. of anterior and posterior co-ordinates of lesion limits. cd, range of outlines of ventral part of caudate nucleus in 24 normal brains; shaded area, 85% of observations; cc, range of outlines of corpus callosum near genu in the 24 brains; v, outline of lowest position of tip of anterior horn of lateral ventricle in any of the 24 brains.

To test the validity of the diagram as a means of estimating proximity to caudate nucleus and anterior horn, as well as anteroposterior placement, the brains of 8 patients who had had stereotactic tracotomy were used. An estimate of the degree of proximity to or probability of involvement of the caudate nucleus and the anterior horn by lesion was obtained by means of the diagram and the postoperative x-rays, with appropriate corrections for magnification. The estimates correlated well in seven of the eight instances with the independent assessment of Dr J A N Corsellis of the actual position of the

88 Surgical Approaches in Psychiatry

lesion. Also, the mean position of the yttrium seeds in the 25 patients who had had air studies, when defined by the bony co-ordinates PS and LS, is shown in Figure 11.4 and appears to correlate well with the findings demonstrated in Figure 11.3.

BIMEDIAL ROSTRAL LEUCOTOMY

Although the lesions in this operation are made under vision, their precise site is influenced by the position of the trephine holes, by the surgeon's estimate of the location of the sphenoidal ridge (itself a variable), by means of passage of a brain cannula, and by the fact that the anterior horn may not be visualized. The operation results in an incision just anterior to the tip of the horn, but if the ventricle is not encountered then no attempt is made to find it. These incisions always pass anterior to the head of the caudate nucleus, but if the

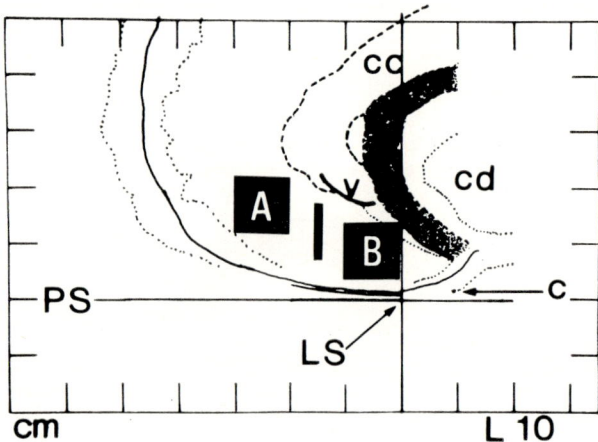

Figure 11.5 Analysis of bimedial leucotomy lesions, A, anterior group; I, intermediate placement; B, posterior group.

trephine holes happen to be suitably placed, and particularly if the surgeon is so inclined, the lesions may enter the posterior half of the ventromedial segment of the frontal lobe. By an ostensibly similar technique there is therefore a degree of scatter of the ventromedial segment involvement of the cuts in the anteroposterior direction. This offers an opportunity to test the theory that the more posteriorly placed lesions in the ventromedial segment are more effective.

From the Maudsley Hospital series of 54 patients reported by Post, Rees & Schurr (1968), 29 patients were selected and studied. In these, postoperative x-rays showing the lower end of the incision, marked by metal clips, were available, and there was less than 1 cm of separation of the clips on the two sides in the lateral film.

After appropriate corrections for x-ray magnification, the position of the most posterior marking clip in each patient was classified by its position in relation to the bony landmarks previously described. The distance in front of LS at 5 mm intervals of the most posterior marking clip of each patient was recorded. In 11 patients the posterior limit of the lesion lay within 1 cm of LS along the plane PS, and in 13 the posterior limit of the cut was at 20 mm in front of LS or more anterior. The 5 patients at the 15 mm interval are treated separately as an intermediate group to improve the separation of the anterior and posterior groups. Interpreted in terms of the diagram in Figure 11.5, the anterior group lies in general anterior to the genu of the corpus callosum in all instances, and the posterior group lies beneath the tip of the anterior horn and may extend in some cases beneath the head of the caudate nucleus. The position of the posterior group roughly corresponds to the position of the anterior half of the stereotactic tractotomy lesion.

CONCLUSIONS

It is not my purpose to consider the relative merits of the horizontal versus the vertical approach to the ventromedial frontal segment. The study shows that the lesion produced by stereotactic tractotomy lies somewhat further forward than may have been thought, since it does not involve the substantia innominata of Reichert except indirectly for example by fibre connections between the orbital cortex and the amygdaloid complex, or by interrupting frontal-hypothalamic pathways. The current surgical use of the term substantia innominata to describe subcaudate lesions, is to be distinguished from the original definition. In any case, it is clear that the substantia innominata of Reichert is not a suitable target for a stereotactic lesion because of the perforating vessels. In the placement of a lesion up to 15 mm from the midline in the posterior half of the ventromedial frontal segment, the lesion might be more centrally placed in the white matter if reference is made to the planum sphenoidale and the anterior horn of the lateral ventricle is outlined with air.

REFERENCES

Falconer MA (1954). The surgical treatment of mental disease. *Practioner*, **172**, 692
Greenblatt M & Solomon HC (1952). Survey of nine years of lobotomy investigations. *Brit. J. Psychiat.*, **109**, 262
Knight GC (1964). The orbital cortex as an objective in the surgical treatment of mental illness. The results of 450 cases of open operation and the development of the stereotactic approach. *Brit. J. Surg.*, **511**, 114
Miodonski R (1967). Myeloarachotectonics and connections of the substantia innominata in the dog brain. *Acta Biol. Warszawa*, **27**, 61
Nauta WJH & Haymaker W (1969). Hypothalamic nuclei and fiber connections. In: *The Hypothalamus* (Eds Haymaker, Anderson & Nauta.), p. 152. Springfield, Ill.: Charles C Thomas.
Newcombe R (1972). Landmarks for lesions of the substantia innominata. In: *Psychosurgery* (Eds Hitchcock, Laitinen & Vaernet), p. 289. Springfield, Ill.: Charles C Thomas.
Post R, Rees WL & Schurr PH (1968). An evaluation of bimedial leucotomy. *Brit. J. Psychiat.*, **114**, 1223
Reichert CB (1859–61). Der Bau des menschlichen Gehirns durch Abbildungen und mit erlauterndem Texte. Vol. 2 (1861), Tafel VI, Fig. 36, p. 162, Leipzig, Engelmann.
van Buren JM & Maccubbin DA (1962). An outline atlas of the basal ganglia. *J. Neurosurg.*, **19**, 811

CHAPTER 12

Neuropathological observations on yttrium implants and on undercutting in the orbito-frontal areas of the brain
J A N CORSELLIS & ALICE B JACK

MATERIAL

The brains of 11 patients have been examined in whom a bilateral orbital undercutting had been carried out. The observations have been compared with those made on the same number of patients in whom yttrium seeds had been implanted in the orbito-frontal areas of both hemispheres (Table 12.1).

All but one of the 22 patients had suffered from a depressive illness. It will be seen from the Table that the group with implants was older than the undercutting group, the mean age at operation and at death being about 13 years higher. Postoperative survival in the implanted group was shorter, with an average of 2 years, than in the undercutting group in which the average was 4 years. All the patients had died in one or other psychiatric hospital.

Table 12.1 Case material.

	Sex M	Sex F	Mean preoperative duration (y)	Mean age (y) at operation	Mean postoperative survival (y)	Mean age at death (y)
Orbital Undercut	4	7	7 (2–16)	54 (27–68)	4 (6/12–9)	58 (28–69)
Yttrium implant	4	7	12 (2–52)	68 (58–72)	2 (1/12–6)	70 (59–83)

ORBITAL UNDERCUTTING

The entry wounds in the cerebral cortex at the frontal poles were symmetrically placed; they measured approximately 2·0 cm horizontally and 0·5–1·0 cm vertically. Leptomeningeal thickening and cortical scarring was slight, and was localized to the edge of the wounds. Deep to the points of entry, the lesions fanned out posteriorly through the ventral half of the white matter of the prefrontal regions. Typical variations in the location and extent of the lesions are illustrated in Figures 12.1 and 12.2. Thus in the upper view of Figure 12.1, which is at an anterior coronal level, the lesion stretches across the full horizontal width of the white matter, deep to the orbital cortex. Posteriorly, in the lower view the lesion in the same hemisphere dies out between the anterior limits of the putamen and the posterior orbital cortex. These views may be contrasted with the upper half of Figure 12.2, in which the anterior part of the undercutting is smaller and is confined to the central part of the deep white matter. In the lower view it is seen to track back into the

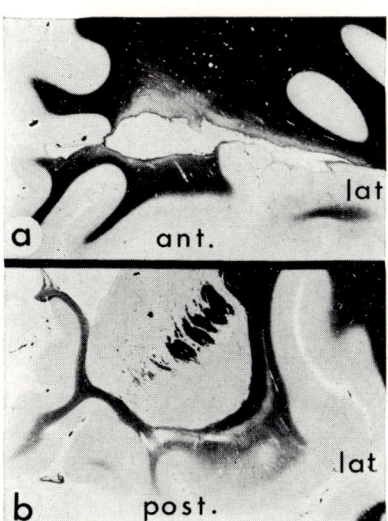 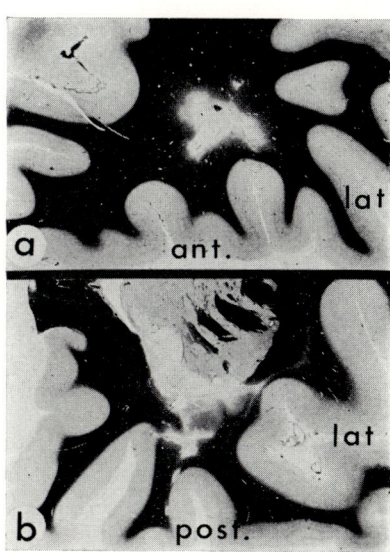

Figure 12.1 Coronally cut myelin-stained sections of orbital undercutting at anterior and posterior levels (R.H. 33/54, right hemisphere).

Figure 12.2 Similar views to those in Figure 12.1 showing less extensive operation with involvement in (b) of the corpus striatum (R.H. 61/60, left hemisphere).

ventral part of the corpus striatum which is therefore partially necrotic. This latter finding illustrates the commonest extension of the lesions, viz. in four of the 11 cases the striatum was entered on one side and in another four it was damaged bilaterally. Occasionally the orbital surface of the cortex was also perforated. In general, there was a tendency for the lesions to run more dorsally than intended, and in four instances the main lesion lay in the white matter, deep to the cingulate gyrus (Figure 12.3). The approximate extent in sagittal section, of the operation in ten of the 11 cases, is illustrated in Figure 12.4a. (In the 11th case the brain was exceptionally small, and on both sides the lesion had reached back to destroy most of the globus pallidus.)

YTTRIUM IMPLANTS
The entry marks ranged from minute and scarcely detectable puncture wounds to, in one case, a funnel-shaped defect which measured 2·0 cm in

diameter on both sides. The tracks of the inserting 'needles' penetrated the frontal cortex at varying dorsoventral levels along the surface of the frontal poles, but they tended to be more dorsally placed than the entry wounds in the orbital undercutting series.

Anteriorly, the lesions consisted of three parallel punched-out 'needle tracks', each 1–3 mm in diameter, which ran obliquely downwards and backwards through the central part of the frontal white matter towards the tip of

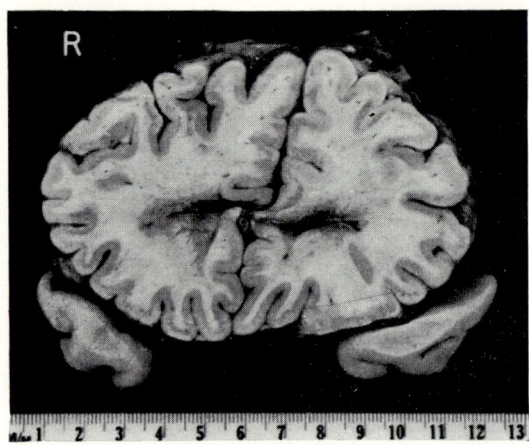

Figure 12.3 Coronal cut through fixed brain to illustrate undercutting which is at the level of the cingulate gyri (R.H. 138/67).

the anterior horn and below this to the head of the caudate nucleus. This course is illustrated in Figure 12.5a and b, the more anterior view (a) showing the lesions in the central white matter. In (b), at the posterior level, a grey ring or patch of necrotic tissue encircles the three implants on each side. The area is best shown in the left hemisphere. This may also be seen in Figure 12.6, which comes from myelin-stained sections of the same case as in the previous figure. The damage extends back into the head of the left caudate nucleus and into the ventral limits of the putamen. On the right side the three confluent rings of necrosis lie in the white matter between the tip of the anterior horn and the medial orbital cortex. The customary six implants on each side were usually placed symmetrically in the two hemispheres and, as seen in Figure 12.6, the tissue necrosis seldom extended more than a few millimetres into the surrounding tissue. In a few instances however, and, particularly in the elderly when cerebrovascular disease was present, the loss of myelin and the gliosis could be considerably more widespread, and in two cases, much of the cortical white matter of the prefrontal areas anterior to the implants was partially demyelinated. In five of the cases there was a small area of necrosis in the corpus striatum of one or both sides. The necrosis also tended to encroach on the deep surface of the posterior orbital cortex. The floor of the anterior horn was seen to have been entered on three occasions and an implant had travelled through the ventricles in two of them. In one of these patients a seed had migrated into the third ventricle and had led to an area of necrosis in the tuber cinereum. The angle of implantation and the approximate area of necrosis in ten of the 11 cases is shown diagrammatically in Figure 12.4b. (In the 11th case the necrotic areas were considerably larger, spreading into the globus pallidus and putamen of both sides.)

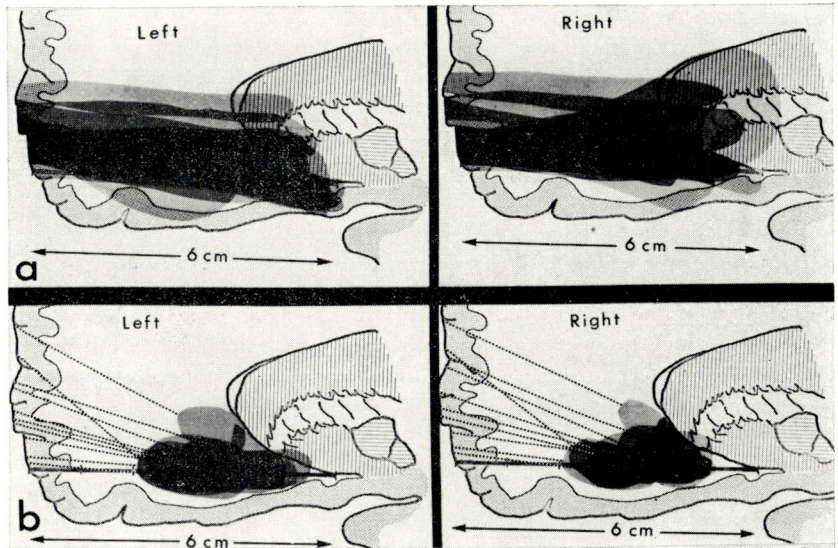

Figure 12.4 Diagrammatic representation of sagittal extent of undercutting in both hemispheres: a. orbital undercutting. b. yttrium implant.

This representation of the sagittal localization of the lesions in the two operations illustrates the main differences. Undercutting tends to destroy an extensive area of white, and even of grey matter, including cortex from the frontal pole back to, and often into the corpus striatum. The implants, on the other hand, are more accurately and more symmetrically placed, and they largely spare the anterior 2·0 cm of the frontal lobes. The area of necrosis around the implants however is usually centred anterior and ventral to the tip of the anterior horn, and it seldom runs more posteriorly than this. It therefore rarely involves the grey matter, which bridges across the most posterior limits of the region between the ventral surface of the corpus striatum and the overlying posterior orbital cortex. In other words, the region commonly affected lies for the most part anterior to that designated as the 'substantia innominata', since it is situated in the white matter anteroventral and ventral to the corpus striatum.

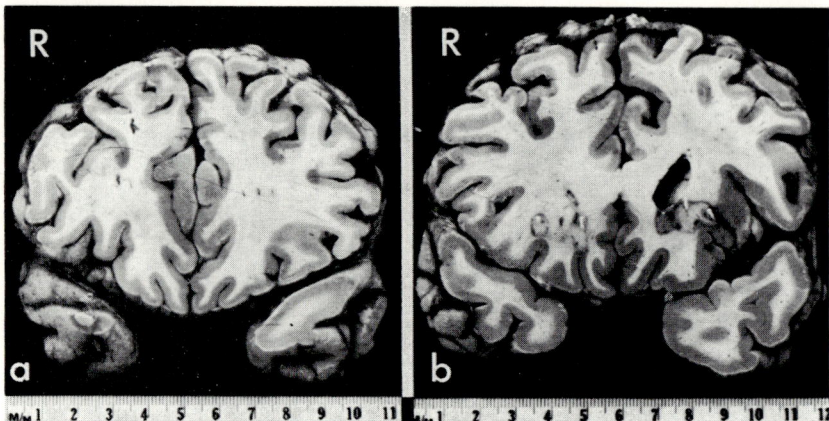

Figure 12.5 Anterior and posterior views of the brain with yttrium implant (R.H. 57/67).

SECONDARY DEGENERATION FOLLOWING ORBITAL UNDERCUTTING AND
YTTRIUM IMPLANTATION

Demyelination and gliosis was noticeably more severe in the ventral than in the dorsal part of the internal capsule (Figure 12.7). This fibre tract degeneration could be traced back into the thalamus and on to the dorsomedial nucleus. Within this nucleus, neuronal loss and astrocytic proliferation at anterior levels was most marked in the more dorsal and medial parts which underlie the magnocellular cap. This evidence of retrograde degeneration tended to move to the more medial edge of the nucleus (Figure 12.8) at more posterior levels, but it died out before the most caudal limits of the nucleus were reached.

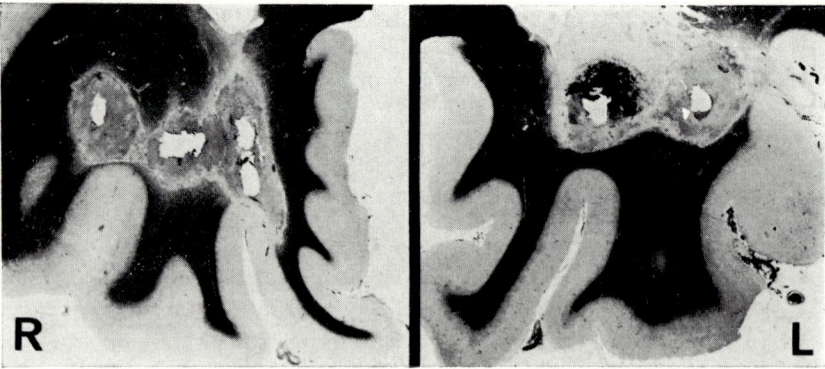

Figure 12.6 Close up view of myelin-stained sections from the case in the previous illustration. The direct involvement of the caudate nucleus by the implantation is seen on the left side.

Part IV—Orbito-frontal Interventions

The severity of the degeneration varied considerably from case to case, and in several, none could be identified with certainty. There was, moreover, the complicating factor of the age of death of these patients, for most were suffering from the effects of appreciable degeneration of the smaller cerebral vessels.

The cases help to confirm that the thalamo-cortical radiation to the orbital grey matter projects mainly from the medial part of the dorsomedial nucleus. It has not proved possible to assess the relative size of the radiation to the anterior as distinct from the posterior parts of the orbital cortex. The impression however was gained that the thalamic degeneration following yttrium implants tended to be less than that often seen in orbital undercutting. The intention is to pursue these anatomical studies further.

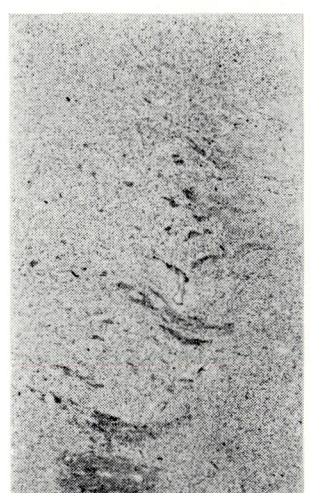
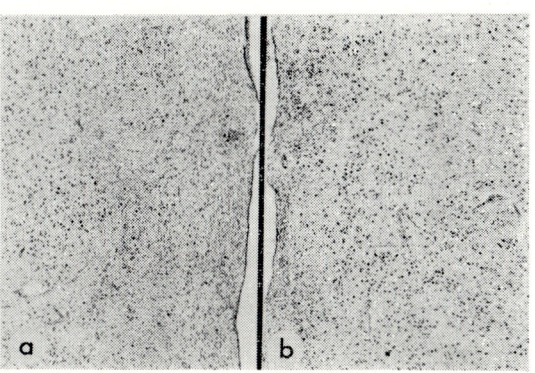

Figure 12.7 Left: Dense gliosis of the ventral bundles of the internal capsule at anterior striatal level.

Figure 12.8 Above: The anteromedial part of the dorsomedial nucleus of the thalamus on each side of the third ventricle. In a. the normal neuronal and glial picture is seen. In b. there is a marked loss of nerve cells and a noticeable glial increase.

CHAPTER 13

A review of patients with obsessional symptoms treated by psychosurgery
P K BRIDGES & E O GOKTEPE

INTRODUCTION

Although usually classified as neuroses, obsessional illnesses can carry a prognosis worse than almost any other psychiatric condition. The repetitive and apparently mechanical nature of obsessional symptoms tends to suggest to the neurosurgically naïve mind of the psychiatrist that psychosurgery must have a special therapeutic role in such illnesses, but there is probably only an element of truth in this.

It could be said that, with our present armamentarium of highly potent psychotropic drugs, and with other methods of psychiatric treatment now available, including other physical treatments, psychotherapy and behaviour therapy, some help can be given to all psychiatric patients except an unfortunate few with obsessional symptoms that seem to prove highly resistant to every available form of treatment. But not all patients with obsessional symptoms are so difficult to help, and in order to attempt to clarify our selection procedure we were led to review patients complaining primarily of obsessional symptoms who had been treated psychosurgically by Mr Geoffrey Knight. It was our aim to assess the results and to try to relate outcome after psychosurgery to factors which might have prognostic significance.

In a pilot study we extracted data from the review of Ström-Olsen & Carlisle (1971). We examined information they had obtained from patients who had presented obsessional symptoms and Table 13.1 shows the findings. In this series, patients of good outcome (Categories I and II) included about 50% of the sample. Of the remainder, five improved with persisting symptoms (III), eight were unchanged (IV) and one patient

Table 13.1 Obsessional patients from Dr Ström-Olsen's review.

Outcome	n	Mean age		Years between
		At onset	At operation	
I and II	14	30·86	44·64	13·78
III, IV, V	13	22·31	36·62	14·31

I Completely recovered, II improved—no treatment required but with slight residual symptoms, III improved, but still needing treatment—with persistent symptoms, IV unchanged, V worse.

became worse despite operation (V). It is apparent from the patients who did poorly that their illnesses began at a younger age on average than was the case with those who did well postoperatively. The years between onset and operation were about the same for the two groups.

PRESENT INVESTIGATION
It was then decided to review in more detail all patients with primary complaints of obsessional symptoms treated at least 3 years previously. This was a separate group from those mentioned above and the number involved this time was 28, but one could not be traced and three refused to co-operate. This left 24 patients, each of whom attended for a structured interview and brought with them a relative from whom a social history and assessment of the patient's progress was obtained. These 24 patients with primary obsessional complaints were compared to 24 control patients with primary complaints of depression, matched for sex and age. The depressed patients were also individually interviewed, as were their relatives, and the same data was collected. Of course, some of the primarily depressed patients also had secondary obsessional symptoms, and some of those presenting with obsessional symptoms complained of depression as well. All patients had a stereotactic tractotomy in the subcaudate region but several required two operations. This applied to six of the obsessional group and four depressed patients. The final improvement category after the second operation is included in the figures and there was at least 3 years between the second operation and the review.

Most of the additional operations consisted of a cortical undercut; these were carried out several years ago and this approach is now rarely used in this department. The best results from the second operation, in four cases, were obtained when there had been good improvement after the first one, but where symptoms had later reappeared and the second operation was then a subcaudate tractotomy. During the period covered by the study, stereotactic cingulate operations were coming into use, but they were not frequently performed at that time.

Table 13.2 Review of 24 obsessional patients with 24 depressed patients as controls.

	n	Mean age at interview	Outcome				
			I	II	III	IV	V
OBSESSIONAL GROUP							
Males	4	40·75	1	1	—	2	—
Females	20	42·80	7	7	6	—	—
All	24	42·41 ± 12·95	8	8	6	2	—
DEPRESSED GROUP							
Males	4	44·50	2	1	—	1	—
Females	20	46·85	4	10	5	1	—
All	24	46·46 ± 12·75	6	11	5	2	—

I recovered, no symptoms; II well, mild syptoms, little or no interference with daily life; III improved, significant symptoms remain which interfere with patient's life; IV unchanged; V worse.

At the time of the review all patients completed several psychological tests, intended to give further information about their current state. These results and other detailed findings will be published elsewhere (Bridges, Goktepe & Maratos, 1973).

Table 13.2 shows the composition of the two groups of patients with 24 in each. The usual five-point scale has been employed but with slight differences in definition to those given in Table 13.1. Function has been more emphasized than the need for treatment, because many patients, although managing well, continue to receive low doses of drugs such as diazepam and imipramine, which do not seem to be necessary. No patient in this series reported that they had become worse since the operation. Taking all grades of improvement together, 44 patients (92%) showed some improvement from the operations, but in the case of Category III this was slight and probably could not be confidently attributed to surgery. Therefore, those in Categories I and II are considered together as having a good outcome and those in Categories III and IV are grouped together as of poor outcome. In this case, 67% of the obsessional group clearly did well, as did 71% of the depressed group.

Table 13.3 Mean ages (years) at onset and at operation compared to clinical results.

	Outcome	
	I and II	III and IV
ONSET		
Obsessional group	28·75	22·00
Depressed group	28·06	33·00
OPERATION		
Obsessional group	38·50	35·25
Depressed group	39·76	43·86
TIME BETWEEN		
Obsessional group	9·75	13·25
Depressed group	11·70	10·86

Table 13.3 gives the mean age at onset and at operation for the two groups, and again it is apparent that obsessional patients with poor outcome had illnesses of earlier onset on average than those who did well. This is not so for the depressive group in which patients of poor outcome were rather older. The age at operation is similar for all groups, and the periods from onset to operation are between 10 and 13 years.

DISCUSSION

In psychiatry there are as yet no reliable objective means available for diagnosing patients accurately, and therefore, cases must be assessed solely on the basis of presenting symptoms. As a result of this, there is a tendency to group all patients with a given complaint into one diagnostic category, inevitably implying a unitary aetiology. An analogous situation would be the grouping of cases of oedema as one illness in the absence of knowing about cardiac, renal and other causes. The resulting confusion in assessing treatments empirically is obvious. One of the most important aspects of evaluating psychosurgery is to have uniform and reliable psychiatric diagnostic categories available, but this appears to remain an idealistic aim.

The present findings suggest that obsessional symptoms may be related to more than one aetiology. It may be that there is a true obsessional illness with an early onset in adolescence and a tendency to slow progression, as described by Pollitt (1957). This is likely to have a bad prognosis even with psychosurgery. In contrast, obsessional symptoms beginning later in life tend to respond better, and some of these are probably related essentially to depressive illnesses, although the depression may be latent in some cases.

Of course, age by itself is a relatively crude differentiating feature which appears to have some validity but which can be misleading. We recently operated on a girl of 24 years who became depressed after the birth of her child with increasing incapacity due to obsessional symptoms. She spent 6 months in hospital with little improvement despite electroplexy and other treatments. She was then discharged and for 6 months more she was completely housebound, cleaning the place incessantly and unable to look after her family without considerable support from others. Because she was so incapacitated, operation was carried out despite her young age and the relatively recent onset of symptoms, just over 2 years before. She proved to be one of the particularly satisfying cases in whom recovery was apparent a few days after a subcaudate tractotomy, and she returned home about 3 weeks later, remaining entirely well since. This was an early onset of obsessional symptoms probably based on a puerperal depressive illness.

Therefore, features other than age need to be sought and their relevance to prognosis established. Obviously an onset in pregnancy or in the puerperium may be important. Among the present 48 cases, no less than 14 (29%) began at this time. In the obsessional group there were eight, of whom six did well, and in the depressed group there were six related to childbirth, of whom all did well. Therefore, onset in relation to pregnancy appears to improve the prognosis considerably.

The relationship of symptoms may also be important. Among the 24 obsessional patients, ten complained of definite depression as a secondary symptom, and of these, eight did well. Among the depressed group six had significant obsessional symptoms as well, and three of these responded to operation. These findings are summarized in Table 13.4, from which it seems that the presence of depression appears to improve the prognosis.

Another feature which may help with prognosis is the type of onset. Of the 24 obsessional patients, 11 (46%) complained that the onset was sudden and 13 reported that their symptoms began gradually. Of the 11 with a sudden onset, 10 did well, but of the 13 with an insidious onset, only 7 (about 50%) did well. This is in contrast to the depressed patients among whom there were 9 who described a sudden onset and 5 (about 50%) did well, but of the 15 with an insidious onset, as many as 12 did well.

Table 13.4 Symptoms and outcome

Outcome	Obsessional group		Depressed group		
	Obsessions only	With depression	Depression only	With obsessions	Totals
I and II	7 (54%)	9 (82%)	14 (78%)	3 (50%)	33
III and IV	6	2	4	3	15
	13	11	18	6	48

From these findings it may be tentatively concluded that a relatively good prognosis may be expected in patients with primary obsessional symptoms after psychosurgery if the age of onset of the illness is near 30 years or older, if there is depression present, if the onset of the obsessional symptoms was sudden and, an especially good prognosis is associated with illnesses occurring in relation to pregnancy.

There is one further aspect which can only be mentioned briefly here. Obsessional symptoms are likely to remain as conditioned behaviour even when psychosurgery has perhaps reduced the abnormal emotional state associated with them. Therefore behaviour therapy after operation is often necessary in such cases. Behavioural treatment can be lengthy, and it may not be possible to arrange easily, but the possibility of residual symptoms which have become conditioned needs to be taken into account in follow-up assessments.

REFERENCES

Bridges PK, Goktepe EO & Maratos J. A (1973) comparative review of patients with obsessional neurosis and with depression treated by psychosurgery (*Brit. J. Psychiat.*, in press.

Pollitt J (1957). Natural history of obsessional states. *Brit. med. J.*, **1**, 194

Ström-Olsen R & Carlisle S (1971). Bi-frontal stereotactic tractotomy. *Brit. J. Psychiat.*, **118**, 141

CHAPTER 14

Additional stereotactic lesions in the cingulum following failed tractotomy in the subcaudate region
GEOFFREY KNIGHT

INTRODUCTION

A study of patients treated by stereotactic tractotomy reveals differences in response in certain subcategories which are significant in assessing results of operation in other areas of the brain. Modern thinking is leaning towards the view that anxiety is frequently not a primary state but the overt expression of an underlying depressive illness.

Our experience of over 600 lesions supports this. The subcaudate operation has been particularly successful in chronic depression, and those patients classified as anxiety states who have done best have been those in whom a depressive element can be detected. Obsessional illness also reveals a contrast between the better results obtained when obsessional illness is associated with depression as compared with pure obsessional neurosis of early onset, which always carries a worse prognosis.

The operation can be very successful in obsessional illness of the first category. A woman of 38 suffered from tension and anxiety since childhood. Following marriage to a sadist she developed multiple jerks and sweating, so severe that she had to change her clothes several times a day, and obsessional tidiness and depression. The effort to tidy her wardrobe was exhausting. She was unable to face meeting people. Strong suicidal impulses developed. Following operation 9 years ago she was immediately dramatically improved. Within 2 months the jerking, sweating, and suicidal impulses were gone; she was able to put things away in the wardrobe and forget all about abnormal tidiness. 'Formerly it had taken me ages to get away from it—I seemed to be glued to it.' She has maintained this complete cure.

Pure obsessional neurosis of early age onset is often difficult to influence by any measure, even the most elaborate open operation.

I have recently reviewed a woman of 43, who at 18 developed obsessions of contamination. Cortical undercutting in 1957, followed by cingulectomy in 1964, produced no improvement. In 1972 her hands are still almost raw from continuous washing.

PROBLEMS OF MULTIPLE LESIONS

In cases which failed to improve, we were at pains to discover if there was any point in making additional lesions in the cingulum. The formation of double lesions is confusing as it does not establish which focus is producing the benefit. For research purposes we feel that lesions should be formed consecutively at an appropriate interval to allow delayed recovery or for drugs or ECT to exert an enhanced effect after the operation. The majority of failures appear to be those of poor personality who are unsuitable for further operation. Among the relatively few in whom a second operation might be considered, the majority are cases of pure obsessional neurosis, although there are occasional cases of phobic anxiety or depression. There is evidence that tractotomy already exerts an influence on fibres coming from the amygdaloid region. Adolescent depression, associated with frequent self-mutilation, responds satisfactorily provided the operation is posterior enough to affect the fibres which pass to the temporal lobe. We therefore attempted to produce the equivalent of a superimposed cingulectomy, an operation which in our past experience gave good results in violent and aggressive patients and in some cases of obsessional neurosis. In cingulectomy the majority of area 24 is sucked out bilaterally to a depth of 1 cm which involves the subjacent cingulum bundle, the excision destroying fibres entering the cingulate cortex from the anterior nucleus of the thalamus through the anterior limb of the internal capsule, lesions extending 3 cm behind the ventricular tip being bound to pick these up.

TECHNIQUE OF CINGULOTOMY

Following a subcaudate operation, relays passing forwards from area 24 have already been interrupted. To produce an effect as far as possible equivalent to cingulectomy we used a linear lesion, which would interrupt afferent fibres to the cingulate cortex swinging medially above the head of the caudate nucleus and passing inwards through the internal capsule, as well as affecting the cingulum bundle itself and the medial parts of that bundle in particular. In the rat there is evidence of two relatively discrete systems in the cingulum. Medially situated fibres distributed to the cingulate cortex (fasciculus cinguli) are more numerous in the anterior parts. This would suggest that lesions in the medial part of the cingulum will have a greater effect upon the agranular cortex of area 24.

Two lines, each consisting of three radioactive seeds, are implanted, extending forwards from a point 3·5 cm behind the tip of the frontal horn, 7 mm above the roof of the ventricle, the lateral row 15 mm from the midline, and the medial row 10 mm from the midline. The lesion thus produced, extends from 6–15 mm lateral to the midline, which will bracket the cingulum bundle. This produces a strictly circumscribed lesion (Figure 14.1,2).

RESULTS

The results are determined by the clinical characteristic of the patient operated upon (Table 14.1). Seven patients have been treated. Operation

Part IV—Orbito-frontal interventions 103

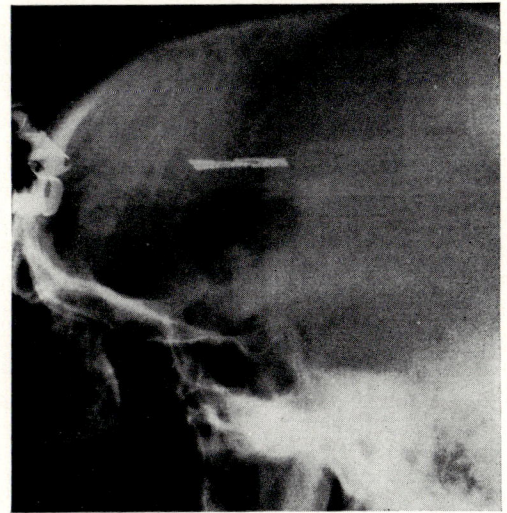

Figure 14.1 Lateral roentgenogram showing the radioactive seeds in the anterior cingulum.

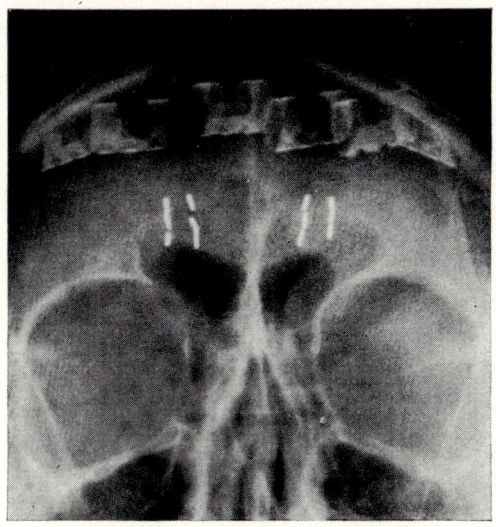

Figure 14.2 Anteroposterior view.

produced additional improvement in depressive illness or phobic anxiety, whereas no further influence was obtained in obsessional neurosis of early onset.

CASE REPORTS

Case 1—A nurse aged 30 developed phobic anxiety at the age of 17, with a fear of injuring herself with sharp objects. Depression with suicidal tendencies developed and her anxiety increased so that she had been unable to go out for 3 years. Stereotactic tractotomy was followed by relapse and re-emergence of severe tension and repetitive thoughts of self-destruction. Whenever she saw a sharp instrument, or bath in which she might drown herself, she felt that she could kill herself this way. It was this symptom that responded so well to a cingulate operation which was performed in March 1971. At first she insisted that her phobic anxiety was increased, and exhibited a good deal of hysterical behaviour, but after the administration of ECT, which had previously been ineffectual, she recovered completely.

Case 2—A woman aged 37, markedly depressed, with considerable anxiety for her personal relationships, developed obsessional guilt feelings concerning her father's death and mother's recent suicide. Stereotactic tractotomy relieved her basic depression but guilt feelings persisted. Following stereotactic cingulate operation in 1972 her preoccupations with her mother returned to some extent but were not so prominent and not so disturbing. She remained a very dependent type of woman and was liable to become slightly depressed if left alone. Therefore, she has subsequently required continuing psychiatric support.

Case 3—A somewhat similar case is that of a nurse aged 26 who, since the age of 15, has suffered from increasing depression requiring supportive psychotherapy and ECT with short-lasting effect. Stereotactic tractotomy in 1969 led to an initial improvement and for 6 months she was able to work as a children's nurse. However, she lost her position when she developed compulsive obsessions to hurt little children and compulsive violence against sexual organs, as a result of her original sexual traumata at the age of 10 when she was repeatedly assaulted. This led to the re-emergence of depression and suicidal thoughts. Bilateral cingulotomy has relieved her depression; she is more cheerful and more helpful, although it is too early as yet to observe the effect of surgery on obsessional features.

In only one of the five cases of obsessional neurosis did cingulotomy result in clinical improvement.

Case 4—A woman of 33 had been treated with ECT for obsessional compulsive neurosis while in her teens in New York. She became worse and worse, repeating everything she did over and over again, washing things unnecessarily. Stereotactic tractotomy in 1969 failed to produce any improvement, and the outlook was not regarded as promising. In July 1971 a cingulate operation at first produced little effect, but following concussion her symptoms abated entirely and have not as yet returned. With the exception of this one case which might perhaps be classified as a 'striking improvement', four other cases have failed entirely.

Case 5—A woman of 41 had, since the age of 18, obsessions of infection and a variety of other phobias and ritualisms. Following stereotactic tractotomy in 1970 her condition remained unaltered. She continued to have morbid thoughts of death and obsessional rituals, continuously imagining that she was near a cemetery and that God was going to strike her dead because of an unknown sin, and that she could not use her left hand properly because it was the wrong side. After bilateral cingulotomy in 1972 her condition remained unchanged, although she was objectively less tense.

Case 6—A woman of 30, who had suffered from obsessional phobias since the age of 17, subsequently developed depression and suicidal tendencies, being tortured by the thought that she might harm others if she did not perform certain rituals. She later developed bizarre thoughts of being strangled or bitten by snakes, but she was not apparently schizophrenic. Stereotactic tractotomy in 1971 produced an initial relief of her depression, but her obsessional thoughts remained largely unchanged. A cingulate operation in 1972 produced no improvement; in fact she felt her obsessions were more prominent.

Case 7—An Irish doctor aged 40, who had developed intense obsessional neurosis and washing obsessions, apparently arising at the age of 11 from the fear of threadworms, developed intense fears of contamination and tuberculosis which had haunted him ever since. Initially a bilateral cingulate operation was performed in 1971 without improvement, and a later subcaudate operation in the substantia produced no further effect.

Table 14.1 Results of cingulotomy following failed stereotactic tractotomy.

Case	Age years	Age of onset	Nature of illness	Previous operation	Cingulotomy	Result
M.S.	(30)	17	Phobic anxiety	1970	1971	Symptom free
J.W.	(41)	27	Depression Obsessional guilt feelings	1968	1972	Improved
J.P.	(26)	15	Depression Obsessional violence	1969	1972	Improved
L.N.	(33)	17	Obsessional cleanliness	1969	1971	Suddenly sympton free after concussion
V.B.	(41)	18	Obsessional ritualism	1970	1972	No improvement
V.R.	(30)	17	Obsessional rumination Depression	1971	1971	No improvement
J.P.	(40)	11	Obsessional neurosis	1971	1972	No improvement
J.Mc.	(32)	16	Obsessional rumination	1968	1969 Anterior cingulate	No improvement Social progress Able to work

Case 8—A woman of 32 had, since the age of 16, chronic obsessional neurosis with terrifying thoughts and preoccupations concerning people being cremated alive and babies being burnt. She felt that her thoughts were causing serious injury and death to others, and that she was in some way responsible for the deaths of innumerable infants. She was utterly without insight; she refused to be reassured and constantly repeated her fears to the same person. Stereotactic tractotomy in 1968 afforded no relief, and subsequent insertion of radioactive seeds into the anterior cingulate region had no additional benefit, although there was some social improvement in that she was now able to take a job as an audio typist, which directed her thoughts elsewhere for a portion of the day.

DISCUSSION

After unsuccessful tractotomy in the subcaudate area, additional cingulotomy can relieve extremely tense and depressed patients, but it does not appear to improve obsessional neurosis symptoms. Obsessional neurosis of early onset and without depression is notoriously difficult to eradicate by any means. One has seen cases in which four or five operations have been performed without effect, or until the last one results in a partial success by blunting the patient, who is subsequently less disturbed by persistent symptoms. Obsessional neurosis was sometimes improved by lower segment leucotomy because this produced a blunting of effect. I believe that there is still occasionally a justifiable indication for this operation to relieve patients of the real torture which persistent symptoms of this illness may inflict.

PART V

TEMPORAL LOBE

CHAPTER 15

Some properties of a lasting epileptogenic trace kindled by repeated electrical stimulation of the amygdala in mammals

GRAHAM V GODDARD & DAN C McINTYRE

INTRODUCTION
It is now well documented that repeated electrical stimulation of certain brain areas can lead to the progressive development of an epileptiform response to that stimulation (Goddard, 1967). When a brief burst of localized stimulation is delivered within the limbic system once each day at constant intensity, the response changes from little or no response initially, to local epileptiform after-discharge, progressively more prolonged, more intense and more widely propagating after-discharge, and, eventually, major behavioural convulsions. The effect has been called 'kindling' and has been observed in many animal experiments (Goddard, McIntyre & Leech, 1969; Racine, Okujava & Chipashvili, 1972).

Since the behavioural convulsions appear only after repetition of the stimulation, and cannot be induced in the naïve animal merely by raising the intensity of focal stimulation, the changes which underlie kindling appear to involve some reorganization of neural function, which requires time to complete. Furthermore, once these changes have occurred, they are shown to be relatively permanent. The major convulsion reappears upon the first or second stimulation even after many weeks in which stimulation has been omitted, and during which time the animal, both electrographically and behaviourally, appears to be relatively normal.

Control experiments have indicated that the change in brain function is not due to progressive destruction of neural tissue (Goddard, 1967), nor to gliosis, oedema, ionic poison, or any side-effects of net current flow (Goddard et al., 1969). The critical parameters of stimulation are a relatively high pulse frequency (25 Hz or more) and long intervals between the stimulation trials (at least 20 min, and optimally, 1 day). It seems to be likely that the effect is based on repeated tetanizing neuronal activation of a small but critical number of cells.

EPILEPTOGENIC LOCALIZATION IN THE BRAIN
Areas of the brain from which the kindling effect can be obtained most

readily are located within the limbic system, with the amygdala being the most responsive area. Much of the thalamus, brain stem and the more caudal structures of the extrapyramidal motor system are not responsive to the kindling procedures. When stimulating one of the responsive areas, however, the actual changes that take place are seen to be very widespread. Electrolytic destruction of the area around the electrode tip abolishes the convulsive response to stimulation through that electrode, but not if the intensity of stimulation is raised high enough to activate neurones on the periphery of that lesion. Thus, it is seen that, following kindling, the response can be triggered from neurones that had not received direct stimulation, but which had been synaptically activated during the kindling process.

Other studies (Burnham, 1971: Racine, 1969) have shown that kindling from a second electrode located in the limbic system, either ipsilateral or contralateral to the first electrode, will proceed more rapidly than would otherwise be expected if prior kindling had not been established from the first electrode. This facilitated transfer of the response to a second kindling site has been observed even after ablation of the original site of stimulation (Racine, 1972).

In the rat, repeated daily stimulation of the amygdala required approximately 15 trials before the appearance of bilateral forelimb clonus. Subsequent kindling from the contralateral amygdala required about half as many trials (50% savings). However, following six convulsions at one per day, triggered from this second electrode, an unexpected suppression of convulsions was observed when retesting the first electrode. Control animals which received rest intervals instead of kindling in the contralateral hemisphere, all showed retention of the kindling and responded with convulsions on the first retest trial. The animals which had received contralateral kindling required a mean of 5·1 daily trials before the convulsions were re-established at the first electrode

PHYSIOLOGICAL MECHANISM OF KINDLING

Figure 15.1 shows that the interference effect resulting from contralateral kindling spontaneously dissipated with time, and that within 2 weeks from the last contralaterally triggered convulsion, the original site of stimulation regained its power to trigger convulsions. Thus it would appear that the neural changes which underlie the kindling effect are actively maintained even though they may be suppressed temporarily by other convulsions.

It would be interesting to identify the nature of these lasting changes in brain function, i.e. to discover the anatomical or biochemical substrate of the kindled trace. This has not been done. Figure 15.2 is an electron micrograph of tissue taken from between 1 and 2 mm away from the electrode tip located in the rat amygdala. No structural abnormalities have been found to result from the kindling procedures. Studies are in progress to quantitatively and statistically analyse synaptic relationships in kindled and normal material, but no differences have yet been detected. Perhaps the changes are macromolecular and will not be structurally visible at the level of the electron

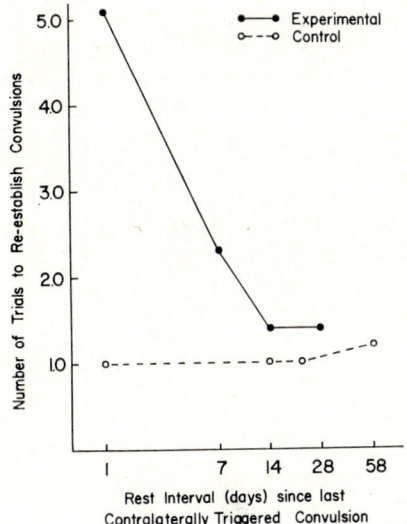

Figure 15.1 Spontaneous recovery of original focus of kindling as a function of time since the last convulsion triggered from the contralateral focus. Control animals did not receive contralateral stimulation and were permitted to rest for various intervals after the sixth behavioural convulsion triggered from the original (and only) focus.

microscope. Whatever their nature, however, it is clear that they are actively maintained for very long periods of time, and cannot be based on transient disturbances of homoeostatically controlled metabolism.

Electrophysiologically, the changes associated with kindling are not merely restricted to seizure activity. Racine, Gartner & Burnham (1972) have measured the amplitudes of evoked potentials in various structures of the brain, before and after kindling. The same electrode was used to deliver pulses to the amygdala for generating the evoked potentials and to deliver the repeated bursts of stimulation for generating the after-discharges and kindling. Two series of evoked potentials were recorded before kindling and two were recorded afterwards to ensure that the evoked potentials and changes in the potentials were stable. Significant changes in the late components of the potentials were observed in the ventromedial nucleus of the hypothalamus, preoptic area, hippocampus and frontal pole, following kindling from the amygdala. It is clear, therefore, that the new circuitry established by kindling can transmit synaptic activity more efficiently, not only in the seizure state, but also in the case of single pulse activation.

BEHAVIOURAL EFFECTS

Behavioural studies by McIntyre & Molino (1972) have demonstrated that the amygdala, following kindling, does not process normal physiological information in a normal fashion. They analysed the ability of several groups of rats to learn a conditioned emotional response. This consisted of pairing a warning

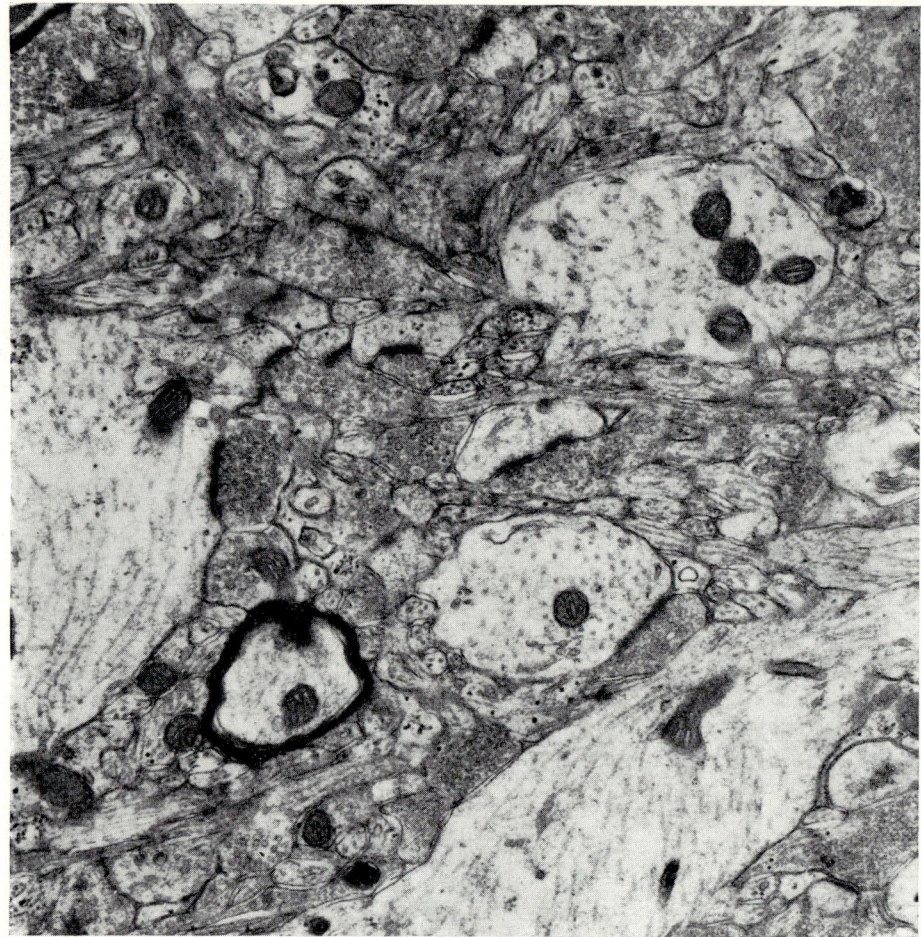

Figure 15.2 Electron micrograph of tissue taken from the amygdala of a kindled rat at a distance of 1 to 2 mm from the electrode tip.

tone with a foot shock when the animals were pressing a lever to obtain food. After several pairings, normal animals cease pressing the lever when the warning tone is presented, and the emotional response is quantified in terms of the number of lever presses during the tone as a ratio of the number of lever presses before the onset of tone. It is known that bilateral destruction of the amygdala severely retards the ability of rats to acquire this conditioned emotional response.

Previous work by McIntyre (1970) had shown that merely kindling by unilateral stimulation of the amygdala did not result in any lasting impairment of the rats' ability to learn a conditioned emotional response. However, McIntyre & Molino (1972) have demonstrated that when kindling is combined with a lesion of the contralateral amygdala, a lasting and severe impairment of the conditioned emotional response is observed. The control groups included: (1) normal animals, (2) bilateral electrodes in the amygdala without stimulation, (3) bilateral electrodes with a unilateral lesion of the amygdala, and (4) bilateral electrodes, unilateral lesion of the amygdala, and repeated daily stimulation of the contralateral amygdala with a 3 Hz alternating current that did not cause kindling. All of these groups learned the conditioned emotional response without significant impairment. The two experimental groups were severely retarded: (1) bilateral lesions of the amygdala, and (2) unilateral lesion of the amygdala combined with kindling of the contralateral amygdala using a 60 Hz alternating current (Table 15.1). The animals were not tested on the conditioned emotional response task until 3 weeks after the last stimulation trial, so it is unlikely that the deficit was caused by abnormal inter-ictal activity within the amygdala. Walters (1970) has shown that abnormal spike activity disappears within 2 or 3 days after the last convulsion. Therefore, it is clear that, accompanying the lasting changes in disposition to have convulsions and alterations of evoked potentials, kindled animals show lasting changes in those behaviour patterns that are normally controlled by the structure selected for kindling. The behavioural changes may not be apparent if the contralateral structure remains intact.

Table 15.1 Disruption of the ability to learn a conditioned emotional response 3 weeks after kindling. The animals were either bilaterally amygdalotomized or amygdalotomized on one side and stimulated on the other.

	Mean CER acquisition score	P-value compared to controls
Controls	0·822	—
Bilateral lesions	8·065	<0.001
Unilateral lesion + kindled focus	7·171	<0.001

In all of the above studies, the interval between each stimulation trial was relatively long, usually 24 h. It has been shown (Goddard *et al.*, 1969) that short intervals, or continuous stimulation, does not usually lead to convulsions. Some form of fatigue or habituation intervenes before the kindling process is complete. Similarly, animals that had been kindled previously did not continue having convulsions when stimulated continuously, but ceased responding after a few hours. Other studies (Essig, Groce & Williamson, 1961) have shown transient elevations of convulsion thresholds following stimulation. In all cases, however, when the animals were stimulated again at a rate of one trial per day, the convulsions reappeared.

Delgado, Rivera & Mir (1971) have recently shown a similar effect in monkeys. Thousands of stimulation trials were delivered through electrodes in the amygdala, using short intervals between each trial. Early in the experiment, epileptiform after-discharges developed and became more widespread, but later the stimulation ceased to evoke these responses.

It would not be correct to conclude that no lasting changes in brain function result from massed-trial stimulation, merely because the responses disappear during the course of the massed-trial series. It is possible that when the brain recovers from fatigue or habituation, after the end of the series, lasting changes similar to those associated with kindling, will be observed. This possibility has not received adequate investigation.

DISCUSSION

The studies reviewed here have several implications for the practice of psychosurgery and clinical applications of stimulation through depth electrodes. It is clear that repeated stimulation, especially in the temporal lobe, is likely to result in the development of seizure activity and, eventually, clinical convulsions. Convulsions are not likely to continue, however, since none of the experimental animals in the studies reported have been observed to develop spontaneous convulsions. Sometimes in kindled animals, repeated stimulations resulted in status epilepticus.

The expected therapeutic or diagnostic value of depth stimulation must be evaluated against the undesirable side-effects of kindling. To stimulate within the temporal lobe and to avoid kindling, is probably not possible unless very low pulse frequencies (3 Hz) are used. Unfortunately, these low frequencies have little value in most applications. If higher frequencies are used, and kindling or partial kindling results, the seizure activity or convulsions can be expected to cease when the stimulation is discontinued. The underlying changes and concomitant side-effects, however, cannot be expected to dissipate with time.

The most common clinical application of direct stimulation of the amygdala is for identification of an epileptic focus and selection of a site for subsequent ablation. Both hemispheres are often examined in this situation. In this particular application, therefore, it is important to recognize that any lasting behaviour changes which result from kindling of the 'normal' hemisphere are likely to be magnified when the contralateral ablation is made. Thus, the hemisphere for intended surgery should be identified as quickly as possible, and stimulation of the contralateral hemisphere held to a minimum.

It is possible that in extreme cases, bilateral stimulation (and kindling) will result in lasting personality changes that are therapeutically desirable. However, very little is known about these behavioural effects, and, at the moment, the probability of an undesirable result should be considered to be at least as high as the probability of a desirable result.

ACKNOWLEDGEMENT

This study was supported by the National Research Council of Canada.

REFERENCES

Burnham WM (1971). *Epileptogenic Modification of the Rat Forebrain by Direct and Trans-synaptic Stimulation.* Doctoral Dissertation, McGill University, Montreal.

Delgado JMR, Rivera ML & Mir D (1971). Repeated stimulation of amygdala in awake monkeys. *Brain Res.*, **27**, 111

Essig CF, Groce ME & Williamson EL (1961). Reversible elevation of electroconvulsive threshold and occurrence of spontaneous convulsions upon repeated electrical stimulation of the cat brain. *Exp. Neurol.*, **4**, 37

Goddard GV (1967). Development of epileptic seizures through brain stimulation at low intensity. *Nature*, **214**, 1020

Goddard GV (1972). Long-term alteration following amygdaloid stimulation. In: *The Neurobiology of the Amygdala*, (Ed Eleftheriou), **2**, 581. New York: Plenum.

Goddard GV, McIntyre DC & Leech CK (1969). A permanent change in brain function resulting from daily electrical stimulation. *Exp. Neurol.*, **25**, 295

McIntyre DC (1970). Differential amnestic effect of cortical vs. amygdaloid elicited convulsions in rats. *Physiol. Behav.*, **5**, 747

McIntyre DC & Molino A (1972). Amygdala lesions and CER learning: long-term effect of kindling. *Physiol. Behav.*, **47**, 1055.

Racine RJ (1969). *The Modification of Afterdischarge and Convulsive Behaviour in the Rat by Electrical Stimulation.* Doctoral Dissertation, McGill University, Montreal.

Racine RJ (1972). Modification of seizure activity by electrical stimulation: II. Motor seizure. *Electroenceph. clin. Neurophysiol.*, **32**, 281

Racine RJ, Gartner J & Burnham WM (1972). Epileptiform activity and neural plasticity in limbic structures. *Brani Res.*, **46**, 262

Racine RJ, Okujava V & Chipashvili S (1972). Modification of seizure activity by electrical stimulation: III. Mechanisms. *Electroenceph. clin. Neurophysiol.*, **32**, 295

DISCUSSION OF CHAPTER 15 BY O J ANDY

In discussing Dr Goddard's presentation, I would like to propose the concept that involvement of the septo-hippocampal system is necessary for generalization of an amygdaloid after-discharge. As will be noted from Figure 15.3,

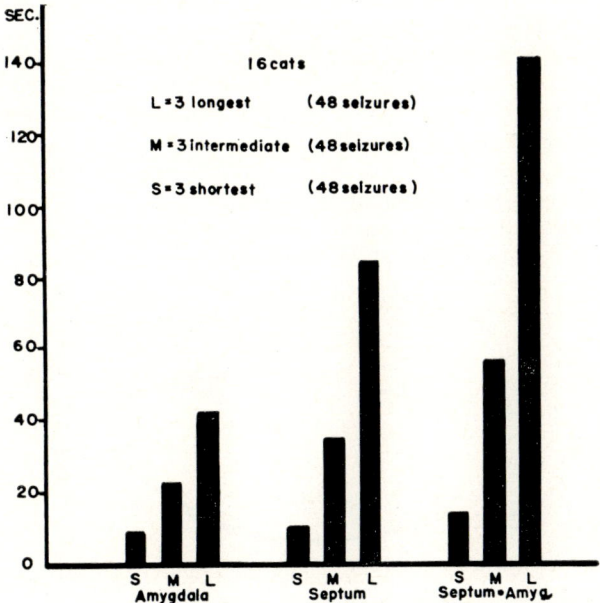

Figure 15.3 Average seizure duration in septum and amgydala.

116 *Surgical Approaches in Psychiatry*

repeated amygdaloid discharge durations are shorter than repeated septum discharge durations. Furthermore, repeated amygdala after-discharges over a period of time maintain an almost fixed seizure duration in relation to time (Figure 15.4, bottom line). In contrast, repeated discharges elicited from the

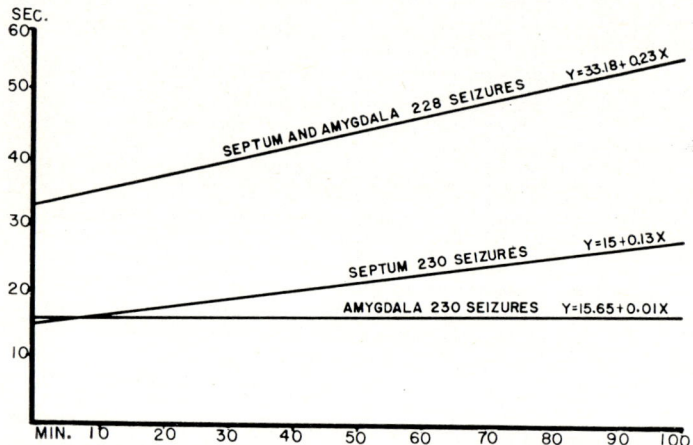

Figure 15.4 Repeated seizure durations in relation to time (septum, amygdala and septum plus amygdala).

septum alone or from a combination of the septum and amygdala, the discharge progressively increases in time (Figure 15.4, middle and upper lines, respectively). Note that the combined septum and amygdala discharge durations increase at a much faster rate with the combined stimulations than with either one alone. This facilitation is thought predominantly due to the septum. This is further supported by the observation that the amygdala tends to exert inhibitory effects upon septum after-discharge durations.

The increased duration resulting from septo-hippocampal participation occurs through a mechanism of reciprocal inhibitions (Figure 15.5), in which

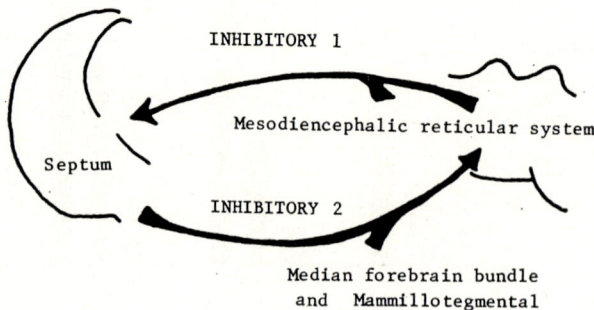

Figure 15.5 Modulation of septum after-discharge durations.

the septo-hippocampal propagated discharge inhibits, at the brain-stem level, a pre-existing reticular inhibitory input to the limbic system. This concept is supported by the observation that within the mesodiencephalic reticular system, stimulation will inhibit and ablation will facilitate the prolongation of limbic after-discharges. Furthermore, following mesodiencephalic lesions, self-sustained neocortical discharges result from septal stimulation but not from amygdala stimulation. Finally, the resulting gliosis demonstrated by the authors, tends to potentiate the seizure process and thus would further facilitate development of generalized seizures through septo-hippocampal involvement. The ipsilateral facial movement during the amygdaloid discharge is a result of the characteristic ipsilateral brain-stem propagation of amygdaloid discharges while the opposite amygdala is passively involved and in a state of hyperexcitability.

CHAPTER 16

Epileptic ammonshorn sclerosis and schizophrenia: negative correlation
TURNER McLARDY

CLINICO-PATHOLOGICAL OBSERVATIONS

In the 476 consecutive autopsy brains investigated neuropathologically at a 1,000-bed USA state general mental hospital during 1965–1970, not one of the 18 brains displaying ammonshorn sclerosis (AHS) of the classical temporal lobe epilepsy (TLE) type (i.e. affecting CA4 and CA3 as well as CA1) came from a patient with a recorded history of schizophrenic illness (beyond transient paranoid delusions in one chronic alcoholic). The macroscopically shrunken and histologically gliosed appearance in 16 of the 18 was consistent with the AHS having been present since childhood. Seizures in childhood featured in the clinical records of only five, but early-life medical histories are notoriously inadequate for state mental hospital patients, who are often paupers and admitted as adults. Nine of these 18 were admitted at over the age of 60, another six at over 40. Five were diagnosed primarily as epileptics, five as chronic alcoholics, seven as cerebrovascular accidents (CVA), and one as a post-traumatic state. The two showing unshrunken ungliosed AHS were CVA cases. A postadmission history of seizures was present in 15 of the 18.

Of the 476 patients concerned, 96,* i.e. approximately one-fifth, had reportedly suffered a serious schizophrenic illness, a feature almost certainly seldom missed in the medical history of state hospital patients, even when admitted for chronic alcoholism or CVA. Other things being equal, therefore, one would have expected three or four instances of schizophrenic illness among the 18 AHS cases. There were none. No 'unequal thing' could be found in the selection criteria for admission to hospital, or for autopsy (42% of total deaths), to explain the negative correlation ($p<0.05$).

In another five instances of shrunken gliosed AHS from pre-1965 material, where full statistics were not available, there were likewise no clinical histories of schizophrenic illness.

In all 23 cases the 'resistant sector' CA2 (McLardy, 1969) was spared to a greater or lesser degree, and the uncal CA3 transition zone of cells towards amygdala was incompletely sclerosed. The granular cells of gyrus dentatus were 100% sclerosed in three cases.

* Two of these 96 gave a case-record history of earlier TLE, but neither of them showed AHS.

DISCUSSION

Purely clinical reports of a negative correlation between schizophrenia and epilepsy in general, constituted one of the main bases for seizure-therapies for schizophrenia, begun in the 1930s (Meduna, 1938). A 'notable absence of chronic psychoses' in TLE operates, whose biopsy displayed AHS, was reported by Falconer (1968). None of the seven paranoid psychotics from a group of over 500 adult mental defectives, investigated by Reid (1972), suffered from epilepsy. Such considerations, together with the clinico-pathological observations reported above, provoke the hypothesis that abnormal neuronal circuit activity caused by childhood AHS tends to prevent development of schizophrenic illness. At first sight this might seem contradictory to Slater, Beard & Glithero's (1963) delineation of a subset of schizophrenic illnesses developing in apparent causal sequence to TLE. In their series of 69 cases, five of the 11 biopsied were found to manifest AHS. Detailed neuropathology is not however given. It may be that all five differed from my 23, in that they had complete sclerosis of either CA2 or the uncal CA3 transition into amygdala, or both. Again, they may have had 100% sclerosis of the granular cells of gyrus dentatus. In June of this year I came upon the first instance, in 8 years at Boston State Hospital, of a patient with a history of TLE (since aet 2), developing serious schizophrenic illness (at aet 22). She died at the age of 54 from breast-cancer metastases. Her left hippocampus showed classical epileptic sclerosis with sparing of CA2 and much of the uncus. The granular cells of gyrus dentatus, however, were 100% faded, i.e. there was probably no mossy-fibre-system input to pyramidal neurons of the hippocampus.

The more detailed hypothesis becomes, therefore: abnormal circuitry activity due to incomplete sclerosis of neurones of, or directly synapsing with, the hippocampal mossy-fibre system, promotes TLE and inhibits any proclivity towards schizophrenia, whereas the completion of such sclerosis, (on the average, 14 years after the first seizure), tends to stop the TLE, and release any proclivity towards schizophrenia. My three cases with 100% sclerosis in gyrus dentatus presumably had no such proclivity.

CONCLUSIONS

If the foregoing deductions prove valid, e.g. after rescrutiny of the hippocampal neuropathology in Slater et al.'s (1963) and Falconer's (1968) materials, then (1) they may constitute a contraindication to operative removal of ammonshorn tissue, for instance to prevent pre-TLE scholastic deficits (Funk & Meyerhoff, 1969), in children with a schizophrenic parent, (2) such children might be testable for schizophrenic proclivity during blocking of conduction in the mossy-fibre system, transiently, by an intraventricular injection of saline 33% saturated with H_2S (McLardy, unpublished), and (3) the preventive value might be explored of, for instance, an inset stimulating electrode in one ammonshorn, simulating TLE abnormal activity in children of schizophrenic parents—especially those who showed up positively in the H_2S test.

ACKNOWLEDGEMENTS

This work was partly supported by US Public Health Service Grant 2-ROI 09755-02 COM from the National Institute of Neurological Diseases and Stroke. For histological aid I am beholden to John Carpenter, Madelon Winston and Marvin Mitchell.

REFERENCES

Falconer MA (1968). Surgical treatment of drug-resistant epilepsy due to mesial temporal sclerosis. *Arch. Neurol. Chicago*, **19**, 353

Funk S & Meyerhoff H (1969). Children with seizure disorders in school. *Off. Gesundh. Dienst.*, **31**, 430

McLardy T (1969). Ammonshorn pathology and epileptic dyscontrol. *Nature*, **221**, 877

Meduna L (1938). General discussion of the cardiazol therapy. *Amer. J. Psychiat.* Suppl., **94**, 40

Reid AH (1972). Psychoses in adult mental defectives: II. Schizophrenic and paranoid psychoses. *Brit. J. Psychiat.*, **120**, 213

Slater E, Beard AW & Glithero E (1963). The schizophrenia-like psychoses of epilepsy. *Brit. J. Psychiat.*, **109**, 95

CHAPTER 17

Pathological substrates in temporal lobe epilepsy with psychoses
MURRAY A FALCONER

PATHOLOGICAL SUBSTRATES

At the Second International Conference on Psychosurgery held in Copenhagen in 1970, I reviewed the pathological substrates found at operation in patients who had been submitted to unilateral temporal lobectomy for drug-resistant epilepsy in two personal series, each consisting of 100 consecutive patients. The lesions could be divided into the following four subgroups:

(1) *Mesial temporal sclerosis*. This was found in just over half of the cases. The lesion is a sclerotic process which affects particularly the hippocampus, amygdala and uncus. It is an acquired rather than an inherited lesion, resulting not from birth trauma, but usually from an asphyxial episode occurring in early infancy, such as a prolonged febrile convulsion. The nerve-cell damage thus sustained, leads to a sclerotic process which 'ripens' into an epileptogenic lesion. It is the most common single cause of intractable habitual epilepsy arising in the first decade of life. It is also the most common single lesion found at autopsy in the brains of chronic epileptics, and when present, is unilateral in 80% of cases. In my experience it is frequently associated with aggression as well as with epilepsy. Following operation, the best results, not only with regard to relief of epilepsy, but also with regard to improvement in social adaptation, occur whenever this lesion is encountered.

(2) *Hamartomas (small cryptic tumours)*. These occur in 20–25% of neurosurgical material. Most are of filial origin, and are situated in or close to the amygdala and parahippocampal regions. They should be regarded as developmental abnormalities. Only a third of them develop their habitual epilepsy within the first decade of life.

(3) *Scars and infarcts*. These are found in only 10% of cases. We often cannot tell whether infarcts and traumatic scars are responsible for the epilepsy or the result of it. The occasional scar due to an old cerebral abscess is clearly causal to the epilepsy. Patients with these lesions usually have late onset of epilepsy.

(4) *Non-specific lesions*. Often they take the form of gliosis but without definite neuronal abnormalities. These occur in 20–25% of cases. This group tends to have late onset of epilepsy, and, although some of them are benefited, the results of surgery on the whole are the poorest of any group.

(5) *Cortical dysplasia.* This is a rare lesion, akin to tuberose sclerosis but with important histological differences, and without the stigmata of this condition. We have so far only reported five instances of this lesion affecting the temporal lobes, but some of them were benefited.

RESULTS OF SURGERY

The results of surgery clearly relate to the presence of definite lesions. The best results are found in cases of mesial temporal sclerosis. Thus in our second series of patients, operated on and followed up for 2–10 years, more than 50% of cases with mesial temporal sclerosis became completely seizure-free following unilateral temporal lobectomy, compared with only 33% in the other pathological groups. Their epilepsy was appreciably improved in 45 of the 47 patients with mesial temporal sclerosis. Similarly good results in social adaptation were usually seen whenever mesial temporal sclerosis was the pathological substrate. Episodic aggression is particularly liable to occur in young epileptics with mesial temporal sclerosis, and Taylor (1969) showed that when overt aggression is relieved by operation, it results in a return to normality and is not just a matter of 'taming'.

PSYCHOSIS AND TEMPORAL LOBE EPILEPSY

Today, however, I want to discuss the relationship between psychosis and temporal lobe epilepsy, for our experience seems to indicate that the nature of the psychosis may be related to the pathology. Thus in our series there were 23 patients who had had a psychosis at some period of their epileptic illness. In 12 of these the psychosis, usually schizophrenia, was present before operation and continued to persist afterwards, even though the epilepsy had usually disappeared. Yet not one of these 12 cases had mesial temporal sclerosis. About half of them had hamartomas, the others non-specific lesions. In the remaining 11 patients who had had a psychotic illness either before or after operation, but not a continuing psychosis, we encountered episodic confusional psychoses, paranoid psychoses, even severe depressive states. Seven of these 11 patients had mesial temporal sclerosis.

In 1963 Slater, Beard & Glithero reported on 69 epileptic patients who had also developed a psychotic illness—an association which they thought was greater than could occur by chance alone. Among the points which they raised were, that the epilepsy usually antedated the psychosis by a long interval, which in their material was a mean of 14 years. Often at the onset of the psychosis the fits would change pattern, but not constantly so. Whenever this psychosis took on a schizophrenic-like pattern, there were often paranoid ideas which might become systematized, with ideas of reference, auditory hallucinations of a menacing kind, and a frank thought disorder with the use of condensed words and inconsequential sentences. There were however some points of difference of a qualitative rather than a quantitative kind. Thus religiose colouring of the paranoid ideas was common, while the effect tended to remain warm and appropriate, and there was no deterioration to the hebephrenic type of schizophrenia. Slater and his colleagues tried to correlate these psychoses with many of the symptomatic features of the epilepsy and its past medicinal treatment, but they made no attempt to correlate the epilepsy and the psychosis with the pathological substrate. Eleven of their patients have been operated on, seven of them by myself.

We therefore have brought up to date the follow-up of 12 patients with psychosis and temporal lobe epilepsy, submitted to unilateral temporal lobectomy and reported by Serafetinides and myself in 1962. These patients were all taken from our first series of 100 consecutive patients, and they are arranged in chronological order. Follow-up now extends for 12–18 years. Seven of the patients were male and five female. The laterality of the lesion was evenly represented between the right and left hemispheres. Three types of psychosis were recognized, acute confusional psychosis, psychosis with a strongly paranoid basis, and a schizophrenic-like psychosis. The psychiatric label allocated to each patient was made by Serafetinides, and subsequently confirmed by Slater and his colleagues (Slater et al., 1963).

In five cases the underlying substrate was mesial temporal sclerosis, while in four others it was hamartoma. In two it was non-specific, and in one it was a cortical infarct. These figures indicate a disproportionate number of hamartomas, compared with the 10% incidence of these lesions in the series as a whole.

All the patients had psychomotor seizures, and six had grand mal attacks as well. Except in the one case with a cortical infarct where the psychosis preceded the epilepsy, in the others the epilepsy antedated the psychosis, usually by many years. The epilepsy in most of the patients has been greatly improved since operation, and in many cases their psychosis also. There were three patients diagnosed as schizophrenic-like, and all three were improved with regard to their epilepsy, two becoming fit free and the third almost so. In all three the schizophrenic state still persists 18, 13 and 12 years later, but is much less florid. As regards the pathological substrate, two had hamartomas of the amygdala, and only one mesial temporal sclerosis. This last patient has recovered sufficiently to lead an independent working life, but has a slightly withdrawn personality. In the remaining nine cases the diagnosis was usually either acute confusional psychosis or paranoid psychosis, and the lesions encountered included mesial temporal sclerosis and hamartomas, as well as non-specific lesions, in approximately equal proportions.

RELIGIOUS CONVERSIONS

Incidentally, Dewhurst & Beard (1970) recently reported six patients who, against a background of temporal lobe epilepsy, had experienced sudden religious conversions. Two of their patients had been operated on by myself, and both had mesial temporal sclerosis as the pathological finding. In both, the epilepsy had been late in onset, although in one there had been a history of four grand mal seizures at the age of 4 years. In both, the psychosis took the form of an acute confusional state, and in one (Case 10) the conversion experienced did not occur until 14 years later, 4 years before operation. In the other it occurred shortly after the onset of epilepsy and 12 years before operation. Both patients were still psychotic at the time of operation, but subsequently both made good recoveries. Follow-ups are now 16 and 12 years respectively.

CONCLUSIONS

From these data it would seem that a psychotic illness can sometimes complicate temporal lobe epilepsy, and that somehow the form it takes is related to the pathological substrate. Thus, hamartomas have a disproportionately high incidence compared with mesial temporal sclerosis, particularly when the psychosis resembles schizophrenia. Episodic confusional states, as well as paranoid psychotic states, can also occur with mesial temporal sclerosis. These latter psychotic states may disappear, if, as often happens after operation, the epilepsy is relieved. However, if the psychosis is a schizophrenic one, it tends to persist, although in a less florid form and even though the epilepsy completely disappears. The precise relationship between schizophrenic-like psychoses and temporal lobe epilepsy on the one hand, and hamartomas of the temporal lobe on the other, remains a mystery.

REFERENCES

Dewhurst K & Beard AW (1970). Sudden religious conversions in temporal lobe epilepsy. *Brit. J. Psychiat.*, **117**, 497

Serafetinides EA & Falconer MA (1962). The effects of temporal lobectomy in epileptic patients with psychosis. *J. ment. Sci.*, **108**, 586

Slater E, Beard AW & Glithero E (1963). The schizophrenic-like psychoses of epilepsy. *J. ment. Sci.*, **109**, 95

Taylor DC (1969). Aggression and epilepsy. *J. psychosom. Res.*, **13**, 229

CHAPTER 18

The results of stereotactic treatment of the aggressive syndrome
P NÁDVORNÍK, J POGÁDY & M ŠRAMKA

INTRODUCTION
We were interested, above all, in the value of stereotactic treatment for the various forms of continuous, chronically current, serious aggressivity or erethism with or without mental retardation, when all contemporary methods of treatment, including psychotropic drugs, had proved unsuccessful.

PATIENTS AND METHODS
The number of patients and the review of the stereotactic targets are shown in Table 18.1.

The unilateral operations were in most cases combined with surgery in other structures (Diemath & Nievoll, 1971).

The mentally retarded patients were examined and assessed by an experienced psychiatrist before and after surgery, the others by a psychologist and a psychiatrist who, after collaboration, recommended the patients for surgery. The stereotactic procedure was performed by our neurosurgical team with the aid of Riechert's apparatus, after consideration of the clinical picture and the election of the target of choice.

A rating scale was created to describe the behaviour of the patients.

Experience of the value of the stereotactic treatment of the aggressive syndrome was acquired from 43 patients with mental retardation, psychopathy, epilepsy and schizophrenia. The surgery was carried out in the thalamus, the amygdalo-hippocampal complex or the posterior hypothalamus.

In treating epileptics we combined posterior hypothalamotomy with surgery in the amygdalo-hippocampal complex on the side on which the deep electrodes revealed epileptic activity. In one case the epileptic seizures disappeared totally.

Posterior hypothalamotomy was performed bilaterally as recommended by Sano, who introduced this method (Sano, 1962). Only in one case did we have to interrupt surgery after a one-sided procedure because of haemorrhage. The bleeding started after removal of the electrode from the site of the coagulation. Perhaps the coagulated nervous tissue somehow became attached to the surface of the electrode tip, the temperature of which was raised to above 80 °C, and some vessels were torn off. The blood penetrated into the third ventricle and caused deep unconsciousness. The patient was immediately operated on in the classical manner and the clots were removed. The passage through the ventricular system was freed and the patient was saved.

At the present time we use an electrode of which the surface temperature is controlled by a thermistor. During 30 s of high-frequency coagulation it destroys about 30 mm^3 of the tissue. The lesion is small in comparison with the destruction in the nucleus amygdalae or the thalamus. The

Table 18.1 Clinical diagnosis and surgical targets in 43 patients operated on stereotactically for aggressive behaviour.

Diagnosis	No. of patients	Surgical target	Bilateral	Left	Right
Idiocy	11	Dorsomedial thalamus	2	—	1
		Anterior thalamus	2	1	1
		Amygdala	1	2	—
		Amygdala and left putamen	1	—	—
		Posterior hypothalamus	1	—	—
Imbecility	17	Dorsomedial thalamus	1	3	1
		Anterior thalamus	7	—	—
		Amygdala	3	—	—
		Amygdala and left Hippocampus	1	—	—
		Posterior hypothalamus	1	—	—
Debility	5	Dorsomedial thalamus	2	—	—
		Amygdala	1	1	1
Psychopathy	5	Posterior hypothalamus	5	—	—
Epilepsy	3	Posterior hypothalamus	1	—	—
		Posterior hypothalamus and both amygdalas and both hippocampus	1	—	—
		Posterior hypothalamus and both amygdalas and both hippocampi	1	—	—
Schizophrenia	2	Posterior hypothalamus	1	—	—
		Posterior hypothalamus and left Dorsomedial thalamus	—	—	1
Total	43		31	7	5

mammilothalamicus fasciculus should be left intact, because damage may be followed by temporary disorientation. We have seen this in one of our patients.

For the visualization of the brain structures we use air, insufflated at the time when the stereotactic device is fixed on the head of the patient. The electrodes for recording the spontaneous potentials of the deep structures and for their stimulation are introduced before the coagulation electrode itself.

Their position is repeatedly monitored by means of roentgen pictures. Simultaneous recording of ECG during stimulation of the posterior hypothalamus shows us any acceleration of the heart action.

DISCUSSION

In the group of idiots, the most effective of the structures in which surgery was carried out to diminish aggressive or erethic behaviour was, in our experience, the posterior hypothalamus. Stereotaxy in the thalamus or in the amygdalo-hippocampal complex did not make the patient calm. Similar results were obtained in the group of imbeciles.

It seems to us that symmetrical, bilateral operations are more effective if performed at a single session. We obtained this experience in the debility group, in which reduction of aggressive behaviour was effective after bilateral dorsomedial thalamotomy performed simultaneously rather than successively. Bilateral thalamotomy was effective in some patients of the debility group. (Nádvornik, Bureš, Komias, Libus & Němeček, 1967).

But surgery to the thalamus has undesirable side-effects. It tends to impair the activity of the patient, his mood and sometimes his interest in his work. It is the behaviour prompted by the better side of their characters that is lost in these patients. It was for this reason that we abandoned thalamotomy. (Poblete, 1970).

Nor does surgery to the nucleus amygdalae alone seem to us to be effective or indicated. This procedure was carried out mainly in cases where the patient had epilepsy currently or in his past history. The procedure in the nucleus amygdala and particularly stimulation of the structures of the gyrus hippocampus is sometimes dangerous. In one case the outcome was fatal, owing to a refractory reflexive status epilepticus, which appeared immediately after surgery. Nevertheless, in some cases the combination of amygdalectomy with hippocampectomy is very useful in the treatment of epilepsy.

In other patients without mental retardation we performed the basic surgery in the posterior hypothalamus and only exceptionally combined this with a lesion in the amygdala or thalamus.

It proved that after posterior hypothalamotomy the patient is rid of his aggressive behaviour, in most cases without impairment of the desirable side of his personality.

Stereotactic treatment of aggressive behaviour affects the functional mechanism of mental activity, about which too little is known in detail. A new level of regulation of behaviour is achieved, which is more acceptable to the patient and to society. Pharmacological treatment is a synergist of psychostereotaxis. The technical performance of surgery is easier to achieve than perfect evaluation of the effects on the behaviour of the patients.

According to standard evaluation of the behaviour before and after surgery, posterior hypothalamotomy seemed to give the best results.

REFERENCES

Diemath HE & Nievoll A (1971). Effects of combined lesions in the dorsomedial thalamic nucleus and in the contralateral amygdala on erethic behaviour. A follow-up study. Collection of abstracts. *Internat. Symposium on Stereoencephalotomy,* Bratislava.

Nádvorník P, Bureš O, Komias V, Libus J & Němeček S (1967). Zmeny psychiky po stereotaktických operacích u eretických oligofreniků. *Čs. psychiatrie,* **62,** 79

Poblete M (1970). Stereotaxic thalamotomy (lamella medialis) in aggressive psychiatric patients. *Confin. neurol.,* **32,** 326

Sano K (1962). Sedative neurosurgery: with special reference to posteromedial hypothalamotomy. *Neurologia, med.-chir. Tokyo,* **4,** 112

CHAPTER 19

Which is the better amygdala target, the medial or lateral nuclei? *(For behaviour problems and paroxysm in epileptics)*
H NARABAYASHI & F SHIMA

INTRODUCTION

The number of patients subjected to stereotactic amygdaloid surgery has been increasing continuously but slowly during the 14 years since the first trial by myself in 1958. The average number of cases has been ten a year, including both adult and child cases, but no operated brain is yet available for post mortem study.

Our observations in these 14 years have indicated the following findings. (1) Severe behaviour problems, such as violence, uncontrollable explosive behaviour, unsteadiness of mood or poor concentration span, are very favourably, sometimes dramatically, influenced or improved when the symptoms are based on the epileptic aetiology in the wide sense. (2) Further, in about two-thirds of these emotionally greatly improved cases, the clinical seizures, especially those of grand mal type, and EEG paroxysms are diminished. Focal seizures are influenced less. The effects on the epileptic seizure or paroxysm mostly parallel those on behaviour problems. (3) Thirdly, in the greatly improved cases, the threshold for barbiturate anaesthesia often falls, usually to about half the preoperative dosage level. (4) No psychological, intellectual or automatic side-effects have appeared even after bilateral lesions, in either postoperative or follow-up studies up to 14 years.

The amygdala is a big nucleus, composed of numerous subnuclei, and was named the 'olfactory thalamus' by McLean. The question on which attention is now focused is which subnuclei within the amygdala are better as the target of surgery aimed at influencing behavioural disorders and at the same time diminishing the epileptic paroxysmal phenomena. Apart from neuro-anatomic analysis, the functions of the subnuclei of the amygdala are not well studied or understood, in contrast to the detailed knowledge of the thalamic subnuclei, such VL, Vim and VPL. This short paper discusses whether the medial nuclear group or the lateral group is the more important for emotional and behavioural function in the light of our clinical experience.

PATIENTS AND METHODS

Cases 61 to 127 are discussed here. Ten non-epileptic cases were excluded from the study and another ten cases were lost owing to change of address of the family, sometimes overseas, or to insufficient observation at follow-up. Of a total of 47 cases, all with definite epileptic aetiology, 20 were operated on unilaterally and the others bilaterally. The location of the surgical lesion in each case, i.e. the position of the tip of the electrode, is measured on the x-ray films about its lateral distance from the midline. For the sake of convenience, the border between the medial nuclear group and the lateral nuclear is arbitrarily estimated in the adult Japanese brain as about 20 mm from the midline, although the actual situation is not so simple, as will be pointed out later. Individual differences due to age and size of the brain were also considered. The lateral distance of the lateral extreme of the brain from the midline is measured on the film and the ratio of this distance to the adult mean value is estimated in each case. This ratio is used to estimate the lateral distance of the nucleus in each child case. Parallax on the film is also calculated and excluded. In lateral view, the location of the nucleus is calculated in relation to the tip of the temporal horn mostly by air study, and the insertion needle is moved down from the frontal burr hole in a slightly posteromedial direction. In addition to the roentgenological measurement, physiological devices, such as injury discharges and localized spontaneous spikings from the amygdala as well as olfactorily evoked discharges from the nucleus, were routinely used to verify the exact insertion of the needle in the amygdala. For details of these techniques, reference should be made to our previous publications. (Narabayashi, 1970, 1972; Narabayashi & Mizutani, 1970; Narabayashi, Nagao. Saito, Yoshida & Naghata, 1963).

RESULTS
The effect on behavioural or emotional abnormalities was classified as follows. (A), the best grade, means sufficient improvement in the patient's emotional status to enable him to return to his previous or adequate environment, such as his job or school life. (B) also means great improvement but still insufficient to allow him to resume his previous occupation. Although most of these patients stay at home, they cause much less trouble to the family. (C) means that improvement is slight as compared with (A) and (B), and in (D) behaviour is not influenced or is worse. Category (A″) is the remarkably improved and benefited cases, which cannot be considered abnormal or pathological at all after surgery in any intellectual, emotional or social respect. These normalized A″ cases work as able members of the community, and may occupy fully responsible positions in a company or factory, or be pleasant pupils at school.

On EEG and clinical epileptic seizures, grade (a) denotes the marked abolition of paroxysmal phenomena such as diffuse or localized spike discharges or slow-wave paroxysms, as well as complete diminution of clinical seizures even without medication. (b) denotes similar improvement but of less marked degree. (c) is a slight diminution of epileptic features in both EEG and clinical aspects. (d) is unchanged. (a″) is the extraordinarily improved or almost completely normalized cases in both EEG and clinical seizures.

Part V—Temporal Lobe

Table 19.1 List of 47 cases showing the site of the lesions in terms of their distance from the midline, and the grade of clinical effects on the behavioural abnormality and on the EEG paroxysms. L = Left-sided lesion; R = Right-sided lesion; B = Bilateral lesion.

			Distance of lesions from midline			Effect of lesion on	
Case no.	Age (y)	Sex	15 mm	20 mm	25 mm	Behavioural abnormality	Clinical seizures and EEG paroxysms
61, M.N.	6	m	L			A	a
65, K.Y.	12	m		B		B–C	a
66, H.K.	18	m		L		B–C	c
67, H.N.	41	m		L		B	d
70, Y.O.	12	f	L			C	d
71, N.M.	13	m	R			A	a
73, S.S.	33	m		L		A	a
74, K.U.	5	m		B		B	a
75, M.C.	10	m	R			A″	a″
76, S.H.	5	f	L			A″	a″
82, H.T.	11	m		L		A	b–c
84, M.F.	8	m		L		B	d
85, M.I.	5	f	R			B	a
86, H.K.	6	m	R			A	b
89, H.Y.	7	m		L		B–C	a′
90, H.M.	5	f	R			B–C	d
91, T.M.	5	m	R			A	a
92, Y.T.	10	m		B		A″	a
93, T.S.	5	m	B			C	d
94, T.S.	8	m	B			A″	a″
95, C.S.	7	f		R		C	d
97, S.S.	8	m	B			A″	a
98, S.S.	6	m	B			B–C	a
99, N.I.	13	f		B		B	a
100, K.T.	13	m	B			A	a
101, Y.A.	5	f	L			A	
102, K.N.	8	m	L	R		B–C	
103, T.N.	13	m		L	R	B–C	
104, N.I.	5	f		B		C	b
105, S.Y.	9	m	L	R		B	c
107, T.O.	6	f	R	L		C	c
109, K.S.	18	m		B		B	a
110, K.N.	38	m	L	R		A	b
111, M.S.	6	m	B			C	d
112, K.S.	34	m	L			A	a
113, M.K.	5	m		L		A″	b
115, T.N.	6	m		B		B	d
117, H.M.	7	m	L	R		A″	d
118, K.O.	6	f		B		B	c
119, Y.H.	5	m		B		B	c
121, S.K.	21	m	B			A″	a

Table 19.1—*continued*

			\multicolumn{3}{c}{Distance of lesions from midline}	\multicolumn{2}{c}{Effect of lesion on}

			15 mm	20 mm	25 mm	Behavioural abnormality	Clinical seizures and EEG paroxysms
122, K.K.	6	f		B		A	b
123, K.A.	8	m		B		B–C	a
124, M.K.	8	m		B		A″	b
125, I.I.	18	m		B		A″	a
126, K.Y.	24	m		B		A″	b
127, M.F.	24	f		B		A″	a

In Table 19.1 a description of each case is given, showing the site of the lesion, and the effects on both behavioural and epileptic features. Our impression from observations in a previous series of cases indicated that the calming effects of this procedure and the effects on the epileptic paroxysmal symptoms are parallel in most of the cases, as previously described (Narabayashi & Mizutani, 1970). It was also our experience that a lesion located a little more medially had a better effect and therefore, in most of the cases in this table, the targets of the surgical lesions were in the area 18–20 mm lateral of the midline. Table 19.2 is a summary of the same cases arranged according to the laterality of the lesion.

In most of the twelve dramatically influenced patients, i.e. those of (A″) grade, the lesions are all distributed in this intermedian area, bilaterally in nine and unilaterally in three, except in one case, in which the lesion was more medial (case 117). In the much less improved or unaffected patients (C grade) the lesions were distributed more laterally. As shown in Table 20.2, in the greatly improved group (including both A and A″) the lesion was produced in relatively medial areas, especially in the area 17·5–20 mm from the midline, but also more medially, whereas of the less improved or unaffected patients a higher proportion had more laterally located lesions. From these observations it seems that to achieve the calming effects aimed at, the relatively medially and not extremely medically located lesion is preferable than the lateral one. Similar observations were also made on the effects on epileptic and paroxysmal symptoms, which were formerly described and interpreted as being mostly parallel to improvement in the behavioural or emotional sphere (Narabayashi & Mizutani, 1970; Narabayashi *et al.*, 1963).

DISCUSSION

In practice, differentiation of the medial from the lateral group is not difficult, when physiological study is supplemented by an exact x-ray study visualizing the temporal horn. Depth recording of the discharges evoked from the amygdaloid nucleus by olfactory stimulation is sometimes quite useful for such

Table 19.2 Summary of 47 cases classified by the grade of effects.

Behavioural abnormality in 47 patients Grade of effect	Effects of amygdalotomy on Laterality of lesions (mm)		
	medial 15–17·5	medial 17·5–20	lateral 20
A″–A	Case no. 91 93 98	Case no. 61 101 71 110 74 112 75 113 76 117 82 121 86 122 92 124 94 125 97 126 99 127 100	Case no. 73
No. of patients	3	23	1
B or B–C	Case no. 90 102 105	Case no. 85 109 115 118 123	Case no. 65 66 67 84 89 103 119
No. of patients	3	5	7
C	Case no. 70 111		Case no. 95 104 107
No. of patients	2		3

identification. The medial nucleus receives the direct inflow from the olfactory system through the lateral olfactory tract and the potentials evoked in this nucleus are quite large, sharp and spiky. In the lateral group they are blunt and smaller.

Morphological classification of the subdivision of the amygdaloid nucleus, which has been based mainly on Nissl stain, is very diverse and different in animal species and even in the opinions of the individual investigators. Taking the most commonly accepted division, corticomedial nuclei and basolateral nuclei, the above-mentioned effective area seems to be part of the corticomedial group, especially of its lateral part, and seems to be very close to and perhaps to involve the stria terminalis, which mainly projects into the hypothalamus. However, the possibility of involvement of the basal nucleus in such a lesion still remains.

Hall & Genesen-Jensen (1971) have given a beautiful histochemical demonstration that, in the brain of the guinea-pig the medial nuclear group is monoaminergic in nature and the lateral group cholinergic. The stria terminalis shows the highest concentration of monoamine oxidase, which receives its impulse mainly from the medial nuclear group, but to some extent from the basal nucleus.

Amygdalotomy for epileptic behavioural disorder is therefore assumed to be effective when it succeeds in eliminating the area involving the stria terminalis, which is characterized by strong projection to the hypothalamus and by its high content of monoamine oxidase.

REFERENCES

Hall E & Genesen-Jensen FA (1971). Distribution of acetylcholinesterase and monoamine oxidase in the amygdala of the guinea pig. *Z. Zellforsch.*, **120**, 204

Narabayashi H (1970). Long term results of stereotaxic amygdalotomy. *Advances in Neurological Sciences*, **14**, 169 (Japanese).

Narabayshi H (1972). Stereotaxic Amygdalotomy. The Neurobiology of the amygdala. In: *Advances in Behavioral Biology* (Ed Basil E. Eleftheriou), **2**, 459. New York: Plenum.

Narabayashi H & Mizutani T (1970). Epileptic seizures and the stereotaxic amygdalotomy. *Confin. neurol.*, **32**, 289

Narabayashi H, Nagao T, Saito Y, Yoshida M & Nagahata M (1963). Stereotaxic amygdalotomy for behavior disorders. *Arch. Neurol. Chicago*, **9**, 1

CHAPTER 20

Fundus striae terminalis, an optional target in sedative stereotactic surgery

J A BURZACO

INTRODUCTION

The two prevailing therapeutic targets in sedative neurosurgery are the amygdala (Narabayashi & Uno, 1966) and posterior medial hypothalamus (Sano, 1962). It seems that between these two structures a complex, subcortical system mediates the regulation of affective and aggressive reactions.

Fernandez-Molina & Hunsperger (1959, 1962) found that the aggressive reactions produced by stimulation of the dorsomedial part of the amygdala were abolished by destruction of the stria terminalis at the level of its fundus. Since then, many contradictory reports have appeared (Hilton & Zbrozyna, 1963; Hunsperger & Bucher, 1967) but without sufficient evidence to justify a definitive conclusion.

METHODS

We used Leksell's stereotactic method. Under general anaesthesia, air ventriculography was done to visualize the reference points: the walls of the third ventricle and the anterior and posterior commissures. The ventricular border of the anterior commissure was used as the centre of the three-dimensional system. The lesion was aimed at the precommissural and commissural components of the fundus striae terminalis. The co-ordinates were as follows: $x = 3$ mm rostral to the posterior border of the anterior commissure; $y = 0$ mm, on the intercommissural line and $z = 5$–6 mm lateral to the wall of the third ventricle. The bare tips of the electrodes were 6 mm long and the interelectrode distance was 4–5 mm.

The angles of introduction of the electrodes were: $\alpha = 15$ degrees, $\beta = 30$ degrees and $\gamma = 30$–45 degrees.

The lesions were produced with bipolar RF current, raising the temperature to 60–65 °C. The presumed size of the lesions was 60–75 mm^3.

The surgical procedure did not present any special difficulties, except in patients with a dilated ventricular system; when one of the electrodes might enter the lateral ventricle. We checked this possibility by slowly withdrawing the electrodes 6 mm dorsally, after the stylets had been removed. If the tip of the electrode is within the ventricle, a few drops of CSF will come out. In such a case we reduced the value of the γ angle to 15–30 degrees or moved the target 1–2 mm laterally.

RESULTS

Between May 1966 and December 1971 a unilateral stereotactic lesion was made to the fundus striae terminalis in 13 patients (Burzaco & Gutierrez, 1968). All patients were referred for surgical treatment through a psychiatric department, neurological, neuroroentgenological, EEG and psychological routine examinations had been performed.

The surgical procedure was well tolerated and the postoperative course was uneventful. Transient pyrexia up to 38·5 °C for 4–6 days was observed in about a third of the cases. Increased food intake was seen in five patients for 1–2 weeks. In one patient this hyperphagia persisted for 3 months producing a total weight increase of 20 kg.

There were two patients who had suffered from temporal lobe epilepsy. The epileptic fits had been infrequent but they had presented with severe behavioural disturbances. In both of them the fundus of the stria terminalis ipsilateral to the epileptic focus was coagulated. Two years after the operation both patients were practically free (grades I–II) from behavioural disturbances. A reduction in the number of seizures was also observed.

In the remaining 11 patients contralateral amygdalotomy was performed, in addition to the lesion in the fundus striae terminalis. Three of them were adults with normal IQs in whom a severe psychopathic personality and aggressive behaviour had put them in conflict with the law and they were facing the risk of long-term confinement. The postoperative improvement in behaviour was remarkable (grade I) and the aggressive outbursts completely disappeared. Eight patients had a low IQ (50 or less). They were restless, compulsive, destructive and aggressive. Their ages ranged from 10–25 years. Postoperatively, five of them could be discharged (grades I and II). Three improved (grade III) but not sufficiently to return to family life.

CONCLUSIONS

The present study shows that small stereotactic lesions in the fundus region of the stria terminalis may suppress violent aggressive behaviour in selected patients. This area may be chosen as the surgical target in the following cases:

(1) when bilateral lesions are considered necessary and amygdalotomy or posteromedial hypothalamotomy is to be done on the contralateral side,

(2) after unsuccessful amygdalotomy or hypothalamotomy, or

(3) in cases of temporal lobe epilepsy where the focus is clearly or possibly bilateral.

REFERENCES

Burzaco JA & Gutierrez D (1968). Trastorno de conducta postencefalitico (su tratamiento por cirugia esterotaxica). *Arch. de Neurobiol.*, **31**, 69

Fernandez-Molina A & Hunsperger RW (1959). Central representation of affective reactions in forebrain and brain stem; Electrical stimulation of amygdala, stria terminalis and adjacent structures. *J. Physiol. (London)*, **145**, 251

Fernandez-Molina A & Hunsperger RW (1962). Organization of the subcortical system governing defence and flight reactions in the cat. *J. Physiol. (London)*, **160**, 200

Hilton SM & Zbrozyna AW (1963). Amygdaloid region for defence reactions and its efferent pathway to the brainstem. *J. Physiol. (London)*, **165**, 160

Hunsperger RW & Bucher VM (1967). Affective behaviour produced by electrical stimulation in the forebrain and brainstem of the cat. In: *Structure and Function of the Limbic System* (Eds Adey and Tokizane), *Progr. Brain Res.*, **27**, 103. Amsterdam: Elsevier Publishing Co.

Narabayashi H & Uno M (1966). Long range results of stereotaxic amygdalotomy for behavior disorders. *Confin. neurol.*, **27**, 168

Sano K (1962). Sedative neurosurgery. *Neurologia, med.-chir.*, **4**, 112

CHAPTER 21

Long-term assessment of stereotactic amygdalotomy for aggressive behaviour
J SIEGFRIED & A BEN-SHMUEL

Stereotactic psychosurgery, involving selective localized lesions, presents a promising approach to the problem of the functional role of deep structures of the brain and their relationship to behavioural symptoms. In the treatment of aggressive behaviour stereotactic amygdalotomy has become widespread in the last few years. A marked or relatively satisfactory calmness in patients has been reported as a result. However, an objective assessment, and particularly, a long-term assessment of the results is often insufficient. This is due to the fact that the neurosurgeon himself is not able to judge the results of his operation, since he only sees the patients just before and shortly after the operation. Too often we are dependent on poorly trained and frequently rotating personnel in the psychiatric clinics to evaluate the effectiveness of our treatment. The same problem presents itself in the decision to undertake a surgical approach. For this reason, we have tried to follow a scheme of investigation which would permit us to judge the efficiency of the operation more objectively.

METHODS
To determine whether surgery is indicated, a very thorough examination is necessary, and even then, it is only decided on after repeated attempts at conservative treatment have failed. To obtain sufficient information, we have constructed a detailed questionnaire which is carefully filled out by the head of the psychiatric clinic. In addition to a history and diagnosis, we need a detailed knowledge of the psychiatric and physical state of the patient to evaluate objectively the results of our procedure. The preoperative examination includes details about the state of consciousness, orientation, memory, intelligence, thinking capacity, compulsive behaviour, delusionate idea, hallucinations, affectivity, contact, drives, and, of major importance, an exact analysis of the patient's aggressiveness. We undertake annually a postoperative examination of the patient, and this paper reports the results of the first of these.

The stereotactic amygdalotomy was performed with the stereotactic frame of Riechert. Two small burr holes of 2 mm diameter were made in front of the coronal suture. After stereotactic puncture of the frontal horn, ventriculography with Dimer-X was performed. About 1·5 cc of Dimer-X was injected, with the patient lying supine. Then, in the sitting position x-ray examinations were made. A good visualization of the temporal horn is thus obtained. An electrode was then inserted into the amygdala at a point situated about 3 mm in front of the temporal horn and 7 mm above the horizontal line drawn from its inferior edge. The electrode is situated at 20–23 mm lateral to the midline. By use of a side electrode, multiple high frequency coagulations were made. Two-thirds of the amygdala was thereby presumably destroyed.

RESULTS

Bilateral stereotactic amygdalotomy was made on a series of eight patients.

CASE REPORTS

Case 1 involves a 60-year-old woman, who became ill for the first time 43 years ago, and has been hospitalized practically continuously. She suffers from a catatonic schizophrenia. Clinically she demonstrates an affective obliteration, depersonalization, a compulsion to speak, an excessive need to eat, stereotypes (in speech and in repeated movements of the head). She frequently falls into a deep schizophrenic state of excitement, screams and believes she is dead. At such times she is very aggressive. Before surgery she received a long-term daily therapy of 200 mg Melleril-Retard, 25 mg Largactil/tid, 6 mg Haloperidol. She often received a large number of other medications also. A year after her bilateral amygdalotomy, the patient still believes she is dead, but says so less often. The periods of excitement have decreased in number. Contact has improved. However, hardly any of the stereotypes have changed. When we visited the patient, she was receiving 200 mg Nozinan. She was again able to be integrated with the other patients. No new manifestations were observed.

Case 2 is a 26-year-old male, who suffers from erethic idiocy and exhibits a serious state of excitement and aggression, suicidal tendencies, stereotypes with hour-long rubbing movements of his feet on the bed frame or on the linen until he bleeds or seriously wounds himself. After the bilateral amygdalotomy the patient showed no signs of improvement. However, a year later an additional stereotactic coagulation of the dorsomedial thalamus resulted in a definite improvement in his condition. He is now easier to manage. Although the aggressive periods still occur, they have become less frequent. No new sensations have appeared.

Case 3 involves a 24-year-old female, who suffers from a chronic catatonic hebephrenia. The patient lives in an autistic world of illusions (she believes she is pregnant and that her child is in danger of being eaten), serious aggressiveness towards her surroundings, negativity and an absence of contact. She uses only yes and no answers. She stereotypes by rocking to and fro in bed and by grimacing. After bilateral amygdalotomy the patient showed a distinctly improved affectual approachability. The aggressions are still present, but they manifest themselves less frequently. One particular dramatic improvement can be observed. As reported, preoperatively she offered only yes or no answers. She was unapproachable and screamed constantly. Now depressive moods clearly began to appear. The patient actually began to express her dissatisfactions, to complain of homesickness and to exhibit fear. In short, she opened her soul, as the psychiatrists say.

Case 4 is a 51-year-old female chronic paranoid patient with a persecution complex, optic and auditive hallucinations, and states of excitement and aggressiveness, which appear every few days. After surgery the patient was relatively quiet for 10 months. Lately however, she had to be isolated again. The states of excitement appear every 3 or 4 weeks, so that on the whole the patient can be seen to have improved. The hallucinations also appear to have decreased.

Case 5 involves a 17-year-old male, who suffers from imbecility following cerebral birth trauma. Clinically, he exhibits states of excitement and aggressiveness in the form of biting and scratching. The surgery resulted in a marked improvement after only 3 months. Whereas before he would only bite at himself he now only bites and scratches at others.

Case 6 involves a 16-year-old female, who suffers from erethic idiocy. She exhibits very severe states of excitement and aggressiveness and a serious tendency to self-destruction. After bilateral stereotactic amygdalotomy the patient showed no signs of improvement. An additional bilateral dorsomedial thalamotomy kept the patient very subdued for 4 months. Then she committed a tentative suicide, became aggressive again and died suddenly of an unknown factor.

Case 7 is a 21-year-old female with previous debility, who suffers from a paranoid-hallucinogenic schizophrenia with severest hallucinations and insane actions. Her IQ (after HAWIE) is 72%. In May 1970 we performed a bilateral amygdalotomy. A few days after this procedure the condition of the patient deteriorated. Whereas before the operation she often criticized the nursing staff with lewd remarks, shortly afterwards she remained reserved. Three to four weeks after the procedure, however, her behaviour reverted back to its previous condition. She began tattering several sets of bed linen a day. These acts of destruction came out of the blue. After 5-6 weeks stereotypic behaviour became evident. The patient stroked her forehead with her right hand continually, and extended and flexed her fingers in rapid succession, so that her thumb moved repeatedly between her fingers. At this time consciousness was also distorted. Hallucinations increased. In addition, she displayed a marked tendency towards autistic and perverse lines of thought. She wanted to marry off the ward doctor to the ward sister at any cost and to become their child. She emptied her meals on the ground, claiming that the floor told her it was hungry. She sat down on a very small clay elephant in order to ride it, and then proceeded to drink her own urine because it was wonderfully warm, etc. Most tormenting for the patient herself were nightly hallucinations. In them she saw men and machines coming through the window towards her. She saw knives closing in on her from the walls and cutting off her head. It rolled on the ground and blood flowed from it. The patient claimed to have heard voices, which commanded her to destroy. Since the operation the patient has been continuously soiled with her urine and stool, and has even begun to eat the stool. She displayed increasing signs of dementia in the form of defective orientation, loss of long- and short-term memory, word-finding difficulties and tendencies towards perseveration. Subjectively, the patient declared she lost her sense of awareness. She would not allow herself to be properly examined. Thereupon, we performed a bilateral electrical coagulation of the dorsomedial thalamic nuclei with practically no results, so that in May 1971, we performed a bilateral prefrontal leucotomy. A year later the nursing staff reported that the patient was in the same state as before the bilateral amygdalotomy.

Case 8 involves a 24-year-old female, who suffers from catatonia with sudden aggressiveness and suicidal tendencies. After bilateral stereotactic amygdalotomy her condition improved so much that she was allowed home 8 months later.

CONCLUSIONS

In our series of eight patients, the complete absence of aggressive behaviour one year after bilateral amygdalotomy can be confirmed in only one case. A reasonable improvement is shown in four others. However, it can be said with certainty that the first results are encouraging. One must not forget that we operated only on cases which were resistant to all conservative therapy. Therefore, the limited success we obtained with bilateral amygdalotomy—a relatively risk-free procedure—is all the more significant. In the course of our postoperative investigations, we asked all staff members of psychiatric clinics the following question: With the knowledge of our results, would you recommend the continuation of our procedure? The answer was a unanimous yes. The clinic personnel face great difficulties daily while caring for these patients. Thus, they value even the slightest chance of improvement. With the exception of Case 7, we found no significant postoperative side-effects after a year. This detailed study of a series of eight patients shows that bilateral stereotactic amygdalotomy is in some cases a useful treatment for aggressive behaviour.

CHAPTER 22

Observations on the development of an assessment scheme for amygdalotomy

E R HITCHCOCK, G W ASHCROFT,
V M CAIRNS & L G MURRAY

INTRODUCTION

It is obvious that psychosurgery has become the focus of growing attention and increasing scrutiny. Recent adverse criticism can be refuted only by objective evidence of the results of psychosurgical procedures. Early assessments of psychosurgery were admirable surveys and analyses including both operative, psychological and psychiatric data (Partridge, 1950; Petrie, 1952). It is unfortunate that subsequent studies have not been so detailed nor so objective. A complete assessment of any psychosurgical procedure can only be made with information about psychiatric, psychological and surgical events; and to be relevant each must be related to the other so that the surgical procedure is only carried out on patients who have had complete preoperative assessments, thus enabling comparison to be made with postoperative results of similar cases earlier in the series. Similarly, the effects of psychosurgical lesions on psychological and psychiatric performances on testing must be related to an exact siting of the target and the extent of the surgical ablation.

The type of patient likely to be referred for psychosurgery, especially those referred for the treatment of aggression, is particularly resistant to most conventional methods of assessment. Psychological testing is extremely difficult since the absence of co-operation and motivation is usually a contributory reason for referral.

This necessitates the use of objective measurements of patient behaviour which make no demands on the patient's co-operation and can provide quantitative assessments even in the most unco-operative patient.

At the last conference we reported on a pilot study assessing patients submitted to amygdalotomy (Hitchcock, Ashcroft, Cairns & Murray, 1972). We have adhered as closely as possible to the assessment scheme described, with pre- and postoperative psychological and psychiatric assessment, including a one-month pre- and postoperative period of inpatient psychiatric hospitalization in the ward of the Brain Metabolism Unit.

In this paper we present some of our findings during the development of a comprehensive scheme of assessment. The first few patients in the series were treated with only sketchy pre- and postoperative assessments. More recent follow-up studies of some of these early cases have utilized the more comprehensive assessment procedures now available. We wish to report our results to date for all our cases.

We will also mention briefly some of the more recent extensions as the amygdalotomy project has developed from an isolated surgical project into a multidisciplinary team approach, with benefit to all participants.

PATIENTS

Our attempts to evaluate the effectiveness of amygdalotomy in a group of 17 patients over the past 5 years with increasingly detailed pre- and postoperative assessments of behaviour have emphasized the complexity of factors contributing to behaviour and the difficulty of evaluating the degree of change produced by surgical intervention.

All patients were referred from either neurologists or psychiatrists. Unfortunately, because of his association with the project our assessing

14 AMYGDALOTOMY CASES

	Pre - op	Post - op
At Home	10	9
Hospitalised	4	5
Total	14	14

OCCUPATION

		Pre - op	Post - op
Open Employment	Regular	2	2
	Occasional	2	3
Sheltered Occupation		2	4
No Occupational Activity		8	5
Total		14	14

Figure 22.1 Domicile and occupation.

psychiatrist is unable to refer patients personally in that such a referral would obviously influence his assessment and possibly his staff's ratings. A number of patients referred have come from other sources therefore, largely from neurologists, although over the past few years there has been an increasing referral from a large neighbouring mental hospital. This expansion of the project has been most interesting and we have been able to have discussions and exploration of views of clinicians who are not themselves directly involved in the project but who have referred patients for amygdalotomy. Although at first such participation and discussion was treated with some reserve since it might influence assessment and control studies, in practice it increased the accuracy of assessment by permitting a longer period of pre- and postoperative observation, so that we are now in many cases able to have an assessment in the referring hospital, an immediate preoperative assessment of one month in the special unit, an assessment during admission for the surgical procedures, and a postoperative assessment in the special unit, after which the patient returns to the referring hospital. A strong history of aggression was obtained in all cases. Many of these patients in whom the prime reason for referral was that of aggression, had associated personality disorders.

As far as occupational activity is concerned, three patients previously incapable of any form of occupational activity are now either employed or attending industrial therapy units (Figure 22.1).

The ages of the patients ranged from 8–44 years. Intellectual level was low in the majority of cases (Figure 22.2).

There were twelve males to five females, a male predominance of more than 2 : 1, and in keeping with other series. This high incidence of male aggressivity is interesting although relevant only to the selected patients and it does not necessarily bear a relationship to the population as a whole. Thirteen of the 17 patients were epileptics and in one case there was a past history of a mild epilepsy.

One patient had episodic impulsive automatic behaviour which might be regarded as epileptic phenomena but on no occasion was any epileptic activity demonstrated by electroencephalography nor was there any past history of epilepsy, although there was a family history of temporal epilepsy in a sibling. The association between impulsive behaviour and epileptic phenomena is an unresolved problem and further study has yet to be made in these cases.

NEUROSURGICAL STUDIES

Although the opportunity for chronic electrode studies rarely arose, such investigations were done whenever possible and when the indications appeared correct for the patient's management. The value of chronic electrode studies is difficult to assess and our own experience in this project has been limited. We have inserted electrodes into the amygdala, and in five patients, into the hippocampus bilaterally.

When the patients were admitted to the neurosurgical wards they were investigated by routine neurosurgical investigations such as straight skull

Part V—Temporal Lobe 145

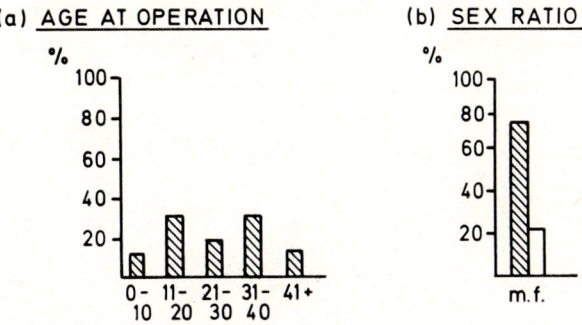

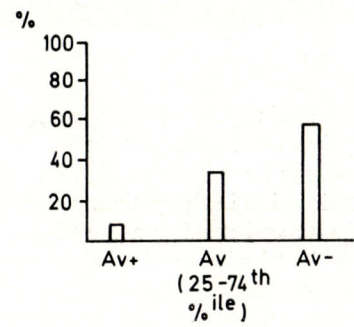

Figure 22.2 Age distribution, sex ratio and preoperative intellectual level.

x-ray, cerebral isotope scan and air encephalography. Although no tumours or other space-occupying lesions were revealed in any of the patients, in a few cases it was helpful in indicating ventricular enlargement and temporal lobe distortion.

The early approaches to the amygdala were transfrontal, the electrode traversing other parts of the brain than the temporal lobe. Although the possible damage must be small, to eliminate any possibility of damage to such structures influencing the assessment of patients, the direct transtemporal approach has been used for all but the first two or three cases. A further advantage of this approach has been a shorter brain track and an opportunity to record and stimulate en route to the amygdala. The first few cases were treated using the Leksell stereotactic system but the direct temporal approach was not possible with this instrument. Therefore, all other cases were treated

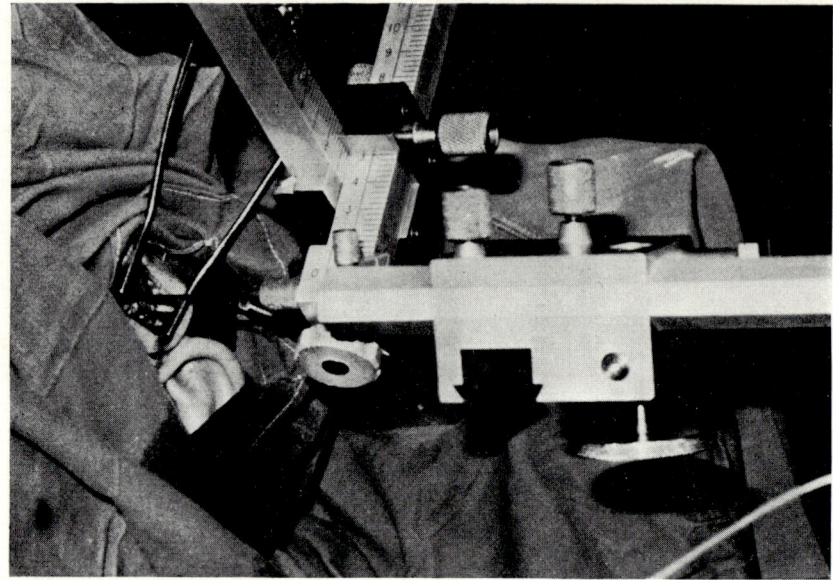

Figure 22.3 Transtemporal insertion of electrode using the direct attachment.

using a different stereotactic system (Hitchcock), which permitted the transtemporal approach (Figure 22.3, 4).

A total of 19 operations have been carried out. In one case no lesion was made owing to a deterioration in the patient's condition following application of the stereotactic frame and making a burr hole. This patient will not be analysed here. One patient had contralateral amygdalotomy 3 years after the first lesion. Two patients had unilateral lesions only and the remaining 14 had bilateral one-stage operations. In one of them surgery was too recent for any follow-up data to be included.

Whenever possible, procedures were performed without premedication under local anaesthesia. Nine patients were operated on under local anaesthesia and one was anaesthetized for the preliminary stereotactic procedure and when the probe was inserted the patient was allowed to waken up. The remaining eight patients had bilateral amygdalotomy performed under general anaesthesia because of their aggressive behaviour, and were considered too disturbed to undergo the procedure under local anaesthesia. Even those who were considered suitable for local anaesthesia often behaved violently during stimulation of temporal lobe structures, disturbing the sterile environment and trying to tear the stereotactic instrument from their heads. Five of the 17 patients showed extreme restlessness and disturbed behaviour during the procedures. As aids to checking the accuracy of electrode placement, steel ball markers were usually inserted at the sites of the lesions for subsequent radiological verification. Although in the postoperation period some patients were so disturbed that they removed their dressings and fingered their

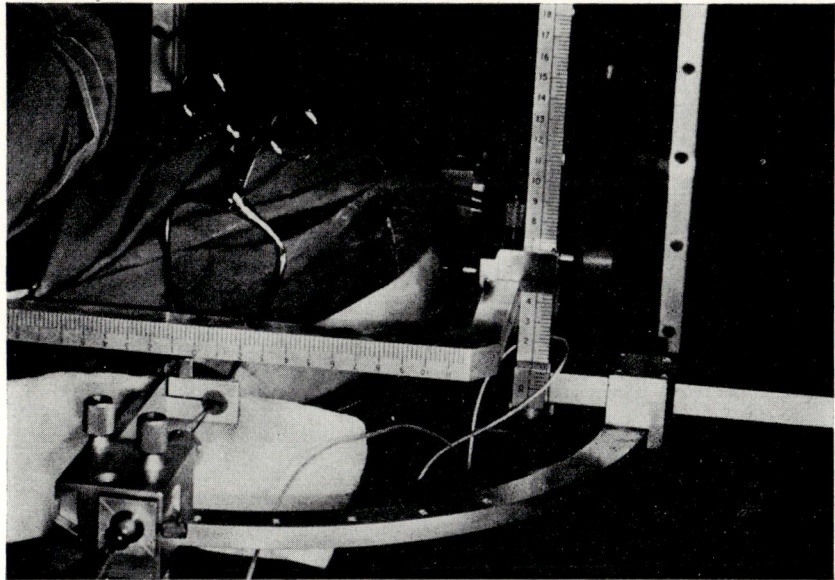

Figure 22.4 Transtemporal insertion of electrode using the quadrant arc.

wounds, postoperative infections were minimal and no serious infection arose.

BIOCHEMICAL AND PHYSIOLOGICAL STUDIES
Because of the close association of the amygdala with the hypothalamus and its influence on the endocrine system it is hardly surprising that hormonal disturbances were manifest postoperatively in some patients, the most impressive being a patient who developed acute and severe gynaecomastia. The project has broadened therefore to include a biochemical study performing hormonal assay, examining the continuous urinary testosterone excretion pre- and postoperatively. Although originally it was hoped to include all patients in this particular study, the variation in urinary excretion in females was such that this test was considered unreliable, and at the present time the estimations have been done on male patients only.

Biochemical analyses in the pre- and postoperative periods have been confined to CSF concentrations of amines. The amygdala is rich in 5HT and if this contributes to the 5HIAA metabolite levels of CSF one could expect to see changes in the CSF concentration of 5HIAA postoperatively.

Because bilateral amygdalotomy in primates is said to alter the facility to habituate neural responses to repeated external stimuli, a standard habituation method has been developed by the special unit to determine the habituation of the skin conductance response to repeated auditory stimuli. The habituation of other arousal responses such as skin vasoconstriction, heart rate changes and blocking of alpha EEG rhythm are also recorded routinely, but measurement and interpretation of these results present problems and analysis has been difficult. Despite the association of all members of the team and an attempt to control the medication, the difficulties of management of these patients in terms of their aggression and/or epilepsy are such that many of these studies have been spoiled by the sedative effects of medication or non-standardized drug regimes pre- and postoperatively.

PSYCHIATRIC AND PSYCHOLOGICAL STUDIES

Over the years our experience has shown that control situations are almost impossible to achieve, may be undesirable, and in themselves by producing a stress situation, affect assessment ratings. Eventually by discussion and experience a compromise situation has been reached where a known environment is used for pre- and postoperative assessment and where medication is stabilized as much as possible.

The psychiatric assessment comprises preliminary outpatient interview by a consultant psychiatrist, and the patient is then admitted for a month's inpatient preoperative assessment in the special unit at a time dictated by the operation date previously arranged. The admission to the special unit enables a fuller psychiatric assessment in the relatively controlled setting. The patient is continuously rated by trained nursing staff with the Hargreaves Nursing Rating Scale (28 behavioural items) (Hargreaves, 1968), providing daily ratings during the immediate pre- and postoperative inpatient psychiatric observation. However, it has not been applicable to all cases, and we have found that The Adaptive Behaviour Scale (Nihira, Foster, Shellhaas & Leland, 1969) enables a more general assessment to be made by a wider range of raters, is much less time-consuming, and is useful in obtaining information about the patients living at home. Neither of these scales is ideal for every case in our series, but we have very few instances where the scales were not felt to provide the relevant information. The Hargreaves scale was designed for use with acute psychiatric cases. The Adaptive Behaviour Scale was designed for use with institutionalized retardates. However, within the standardization population level of intelligence was not a significant factor in relation to degree of maladaptive behaviour. Our cases include a large proportion at the lower end of the intellectual scale. We have now made use of the scale in 11 cases, obtaining pre- and postoperative ratings in eight cases, and postoperative ratings only, in three cases. Relatives have sometimes been asked to complete ratings, either as the sole means of assessment available or in addition to ratings made by staff in hospital and industrial therapy units (Figures 22.5,6).

The data for violent and destructive behaviour indicate that of the four male cases on whom pre- and postoperative ratings were made, three showed a substantial drop (two to zero). Postoperatively one of these has a follow-up of 5 years. One of these four with a moderately high preoperative level showed no substantial improvement. Of the four female cases (all were preoperatively more violent than 90% of an equivalent population) only one showed marked improvement. This is the only female case living at home and is also the one

Part V—Temporal Lobe   149

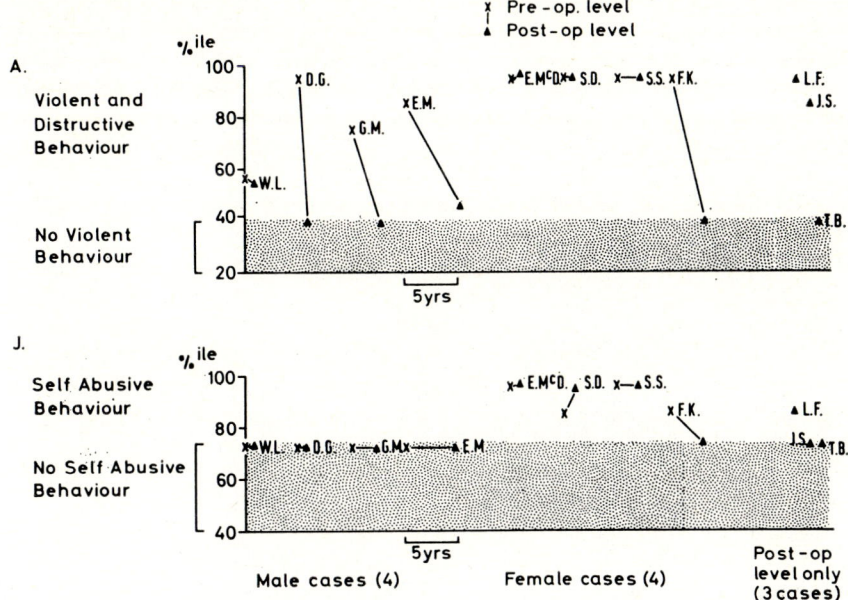

Figure 22.5 Adaptive behaviour scale.

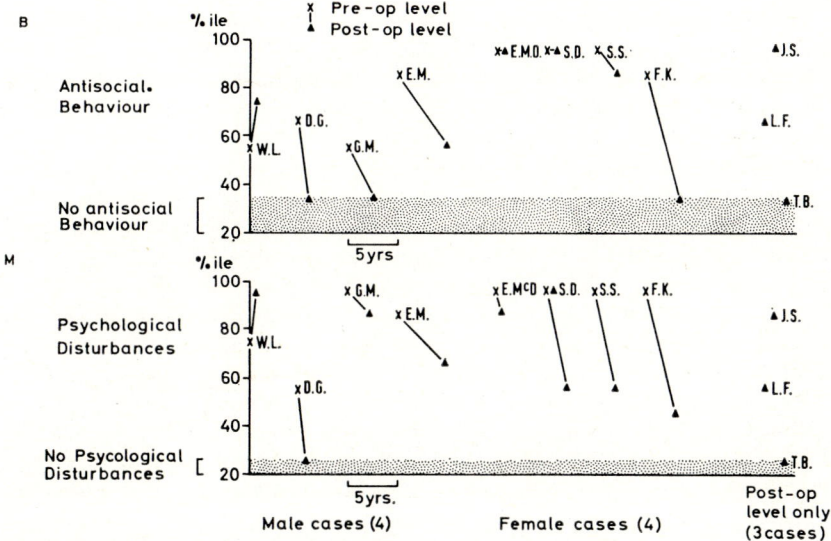

Figure 22.6 Adaptive behaviour scale.

with the longest follow-up (3 years). Four patients showed zero violent and destructive behaviour at the time of the most recent follow-up but five showed a postoperative level of violence higher than 80% of the population.

It is of interest that all four females but only one of the seven males showed any self-abusive behaviour. This behaviour was modified in only one patient postoperatively (the female who also showed a substantial drop in violent behaviour). The cases showing self-abusive behaviour pre- or postoperatively were the cases who also showed the highest level of violent behaviour postoperatively. Antisocial behaviour follows a similar pattern to that noted for violent behaviour, except in one male case where there was a postoperative increase. A range of behaviour such as reaction to frustration, mood changes and hypochondrical tendencies are covered in the area labelled psychological disturbances. All cases showed some degree of such disturbance preoperatively and nine cases postoperatively. Six cases showed a decrease (improvement) postoperatively, one an increase in level and one no real change. Three of the four cases showing greatest overall improvement could be described as having adolescent problems preoperatively and in the fourth there was a change in domestic circumstances.

At the 2nd International Conference on Psychosurgery in Copenhagen, Ursin (unpublished discussion) emphasized the fact that the most objective assessments of behaviour were obtained when the patient's behaviour in a standard situation was observed. This encouraged us to continue the efforts we had already been making to devise such situations. While it is too early to be able to report on pre- and postoperative changes in behaviour in these situations, we would like to mention three such measures which we are now using.

The first is a task designed to provide a measure of tolerance of frustration. The patient is required to draw around a number of different designs by looking at the mirror image of the paper on which he is drawing. The results are quantified in terms of the length of time spent on the task and the number of items attempted.

The second is a tracking task using a pursuit rotor. The patient has a number of trial runs at different speeds. He is then encouraged to adjust the speed himself (providing a measure of choice of level of difficulty). Next, the speed is fixed at a moderate rate, and the buzzer (providing feedback) switched off. A series of false 'success' readings are given, followed by a series of 'failure' readings. This is alternated for dominant/non-dominant hand and for several different patterns and provides a differential measure of the patient's persistence when succeeding and failing.

The Third method is a modification of the Gibson Spiral Maze (Gibson, 1965) in which the patient is required to trace a path through this circular maze, using his non-dominant hand. The test is administered under three conditions. First, the patient is left alone to complete the task; then the patient is stressed every 15 s to increase his speed; and lastly, the patient is stressed every 15 s to increase his accuracy. Variation in time taken and number of errors provide a measure of reaction to a mildly stressful situation.

Part V—Temporal Lobe   151

The aim of these three techniques is to put the patient in mildly frustrating or stressful situations. It was not considered desirable to create situations of a severely stressful nature as it was felt that this would have immediate repercussions in terms of patient management, and would also be likely to preclude any further co-operation in future testing. Hence the variable in the first two techniques is the time spent prior to the patient's decision to terminate the task. It is emphasized to the patient, both before and at fixed intervals during the task, that *he* decides when to stop.

Preliminary results indicate that there is a relationship between levels obtained on the Adaptive Behaviour Scale and other ratings and performance on tasks of a frustrating nature. Much further work is required in terms of obtaining normative data before the value of these techniques is established.

Where possible standard methods of personality assessment are also used. However, most personality questionnaires are of limited application in view of the low intellectual level of many patients.

RESULTS OF AMYGDALOTOMY
The 16 Personality Factor Questionnaire (Cattell, Eber & Tatsuoka, 1970)

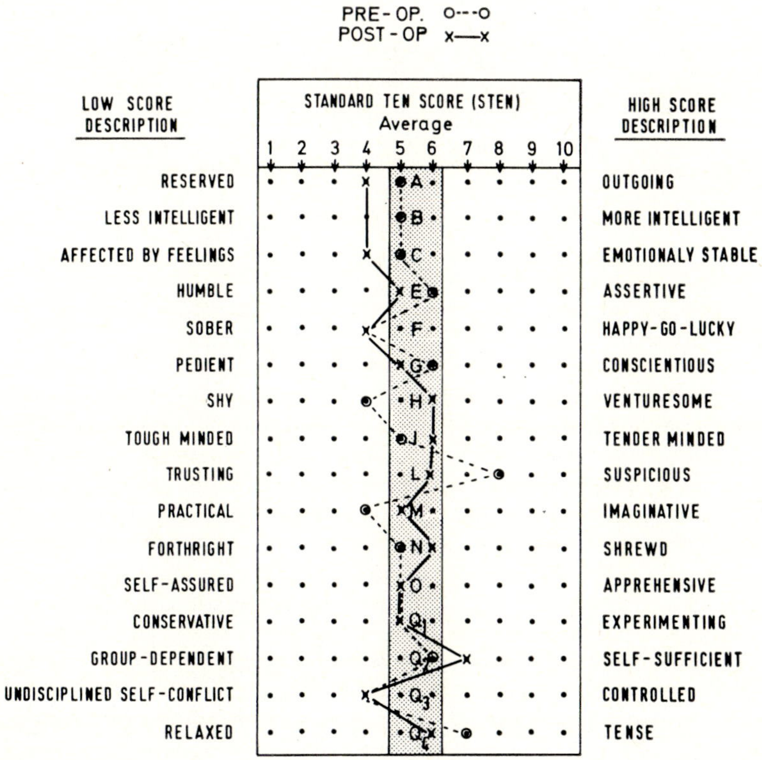

Figure 22.7 Sixteen personality factor test profile (five amygdalotomy cases).

revealed very few changes postoperatively. The majority of pre- and postoperative scores were within the average band. The most extreme preoperative score was on the factor of suspiciousness. Postoperative score was average. The only other change noticed was a decrease in shyness (Figure 22.7).

On the Hostility and Direction of Hostility Questionnaire (Caine, Foulds & Hope, 1967), the most notable feature was the very high total hostility (both pre- and postoperatively). Scores were more than two standard deviations above the normal mean and one standard deviation above the mean score for Personality Disorders. While there was no real change in total level postoperatively, there was a slight increase in intropunitiveness (Figure 22.8).

	Mean total score		Direction	
			(+ scores are intropunitive)	
Amygdalotomies	Pre	Post	Pre	Post
5 cases, Pre & Post-op scores	26.8	25.4	+1	+5.8
4 cases, post-op scores only	24.7		+1	
Normative Data				
Normal controls	13		+0.5	
Personality disorder	18		+1.4	

Figure 22.8 Hostility and direction of hostility questionnaire.

We continue to use all the tests previously documented (Hitchcock et al., 1972) in the assessment of cognitive function (Figure 22.9).

Amygdalotomy did not cause any significant changes in performance on tests of general intellectual function and short-term memory. We were also looking in more detail at memory function and learning, since an alteration in certain learning processes follows amygdalotomy (Andersen, 1972) and some of our patients, or their relatives, reported specific types of memory impairment. Previously we had concentrated on tests of short-term memory function on which deficits were not being detected.

We have therefore supplemented our battery by the inclusion of a further subtest from Williams Memory Scale (Williams, 1968—a test of non-verbal learning (the Rey-Davis pegboard test).

There may be an association between an impairment in face recognition following right temporal lobectomy and the type of deficit reported by some of our patients postoperatively, and we now also include a modification of a face recognition test, with the patient being required to select, from 24 photographs of faces, the 12 which he saw 1½ minutes previously.

COMPARISON OF PRE- AND POST-OPERATIVE TEST RESULTS

Raven's Progressive Matrices			
Mean change in score	No. +	No. -	No. same
+3.5	10	2	0

Mill Hill Vocabulary Scale			
Mean change in score	No. +	No. -	No. same
+1.7	6	4	2

Graham Kendall Memory for Designs			
Mean change in score	No. +	No. -	No. same
+0.7	7	4	1

Sentence Repetition		
No. +	No. -.	No. same
2	3	8

Figure 22.9 Cognitive function.

DISCUSSION

The potential value of these areas of study is debatable. On the basis of our experience of dealing with a selected group of patients submitted to a bilateral discrete psychosurgical procedure attempting to modify one aspect of behaviour, we would suggest that all psychosurgical studies should include a full psychiatric and psychological assessment, and that follow-up should be of at least 2 years. Whilst it is appreciated that the immediate effects of operation may be a valuable indication of suitable targets, only long-term follow-up with formal assessments can provide an adequate evaluation of the results of particular procedures.

The surgical procedure of amygdalotomy is relatively simple, and, although we have had no pathological verification, radiological technique is so good that target location was accurate. The amount of destruction necessary for a good result, however, is less well known. Some of our lesions have been small, and no attempt has been made to destroy the whole amygdala. The surgical target lay in the most medial part of the amygdala. Complications have been small and largely related to immediate postoperative difficulties of management. However, in one patient, as the result of an injury sustained during the removal of an indwelling electrode inserted via the transfrontal approach, a severe right hemiplegia was produced, which resulted in a considerable disability in one arm. The original lesions were small because of the fear of complications, but later on we tended to make larger lesions in an attempt to destroy a major part of the medial nucleus of the amygdala. To date we have had no complications from these large lesions.

Preliminary assessments indicate that very few cognitive changes are detectable following bilateral amygdalotomy. In several recent cases subtle memory deficits have been noted, both clinically and on tests, but they have been transitory and only detected in the first three postoperative months.

Throughout this study a major problem has been the care of violent patients in situations other than psychiatric hospitals. The introduction of such patients into a neurosurgical ward results in disruption and difficulties which may well influence nursing and medical staff assessment. It continues to be difficult to make relatives and attendants aware of the possible results of surgery, which in this particular series has been the apparently modest aim of reducing aggressive behaviour. Because these patients usually have associated personality disorders, and because, either as a result of their behaviour or associated with their behaviour, their social and domestic circumstances are invariably disturbed, it is important that the surgeon establish at a very early interview, the hopes of relatives and attendants of the outcome of successful surgery. It is our experience that unless the aim of surgery, in this case the elimination or reduction of aggression, is clearly stated, patient, relatives and attendants may be disappointed when their other multitudinous problems remain.

Our sample is small, and because all our assessment techniques were not available throughout the study, firm conclusions cannot be drawn. Our short-term results, however, in cases followed up for less than one year, are less impressive than many other published studies (Narabayashi, Nagao, Saito, Yoshida & Nagahata, 1963; Heimburger, Whitlock & Kalsbeck, 1966).

Long-term assessments are more relevant and the longer the follow-up the more reliable the assessment. However, during such long-term observation variables other than the surgical procedure itself result in behavioural changes, and it is important that such long-term evaluation consider also the effects of maturation, domestic changes, occupational status and other factors. It is also difficult to determine how far changes in social factors were caused by or resulted in changes of behavioural pattern.

A study of a matched control group of patients with aggressive behaviour not referred for surgery would be extremely valuable, and it is hoped to include this in the next part of our research.

Bearing in mind the above limitations, it may, nevertheless, be useful to indicate such trends as have emerged. Being male, having a mental age of more than 6-year level, living at home and with the aggressive behaviour confined mainly to the home situation, would appear to offer a greater chance of improvement postoperatively. The importance of adequate rehabilitation facilities, prolonged postoperative psychiatric support and good communications between all those involved in management, cannot be overstressed.

ACKNOWLEDGEMENTS

We wish to express our appreciation of the support provided by the Mac-Robert Trust and our thanks to the Research Secretary, Mrs E. Cumptsey.

REFERENCES

Andersen R (1972). Differences in the course of learning as measured by various memory tasks after amygdalotomy in men. In: *Psychosurgery* (Eds Hitchcock, Laitinen & Vaernet), p. 177. Springfield, Ill.: Charles C Thomas.

Caine TM, Foulds GA & Hope K (1967). *Manual of the Hostility and Direction of Hostility Questionnaire*. London: University of London Press Ltd.

Cattell RB, Eber HW & Tatsuoka M (1970). *Handbook for the Sixteen Personality Factor Questionnaire (16 P.F.)*. Champaign, Ill.: Institute for Personality and Ability Testing.

Gibson HB (1965). *Manual of the Gibson Spiral Maze*. London: University of London Press Ltd.

Hargreaves WA (1968). Systematic nursing observation of psychopathology. *Arch. gen. Psychiat.*, **18**, 518

Heimburger R, Whitlock CC & Kalsbeck JE (1966). Stereotaxic amygdalotomy for epilepsy with aggressive behavior. *J.A.M.A.*, **198**, 741

Hitchcock ER, Ashcroft GW, Cairns VM & Murray LG (1972). Preoperative and post-operative assessment and management of psychosurgical patients. In: *Psychosurgery* (Eds Hitchcock, Laitinen & Vaernet), p. 164. Springfield, Ill.: Charles C Thomas.

Narabayashi H, Nagao T, Saito Y, Yoshida M & Nagahata M (1963). Stereotaxic amygdalotomy for behavior disorders. *Arch. Neurol. Chicago*, **9**, 11

Nihira K, Foster R, Shellhaas M & Leland H (1969). *Adaptive Behavior Scales: Manual*. Washington DC: American Association on Mental Deficiency.

Partridge M (1950). *Prefrontal Leucotomy*. Oxford: Blackwell.

Petrie A (1952). *Personality and the Frontal Lobes*. London: Routledge & Kegan Paul Ltd.

Williams M (1968). The measurement of memory in clinical practice. *Brit. J. soc. clin. Psychol.*, **7**, 19

PART VI

MISCELLANEOUS AND MULTIPLE LESIONS

CHAPTER 23

Stereotactic anterior capsulotomy in anxiety and obsessive-compulsive states
T BINGLEY, L LEKSELL,
B A MEYERSON & G RYLANDER

INTRODUCTION

In the search for a safe and accurate alternative to various types of open prefrontal leucotomies a stereotactic procedure has been developed, bilateral anterior capsulotomy, which aims at destruction of the anterior part of the internal capsule. Investigations by Meyer & Beck (1954) formed the functional and anatomical background for the choice of this particular target. On pathoanatomical material from an extensive series of patients who had undergone open leucotomy, they showed that the optimal clinical results had been achieved when the lesion included the fibres within the internal capsule. According to the same authors, it is within this anterior part of the internal capsule that the prefrontal-thalamic pathways are funnelled to form a discrete, well-defined fibre tract. Figure 23.1 shows a brain section made in the coronal plane about halfway between the tip of the frontal horn and the anterior commissure. The internal capsule occupies the space between the head of the caudate nucleus and the putamen. Two electrodes, 6 mm apart and with tips exposed 10 mm, have been placed over the internal capsule to demonstrate that in this particular coronal plane a fairly small lesion may effectively interrupt most of the fibre tracts passing through the anterior part of the internal capsule.

During the 1950s, when the method of stereotactic anterior capsulotomy was first introduced, an initial series of 116 patients with various psychiatric disorders was operated upon and an attempt was made to divide all fibres in the anterior capsule. However, in these operations there were considerable variations both in the localization and in the size of the lesions in the internal capsule. Surgically the technique was found to be very safe. This group of patients comprised cases of schizophrenia, depression and obsessional and anxiety neurosis. In a follow-up study covering 2–6 years Herner (1961) found that the obsessional group benefited most.

On the basis of these experiences, bilateral anterior capsulotomy has been performed on a group of 17 patients with a definite diagnosis of obsessive-compulsive neurosis. In the present study the stereotactic technique and the target co-ordinates as well as the size of the lesions were the same in all the patients. Standardization of the operative technique seemed necessary to

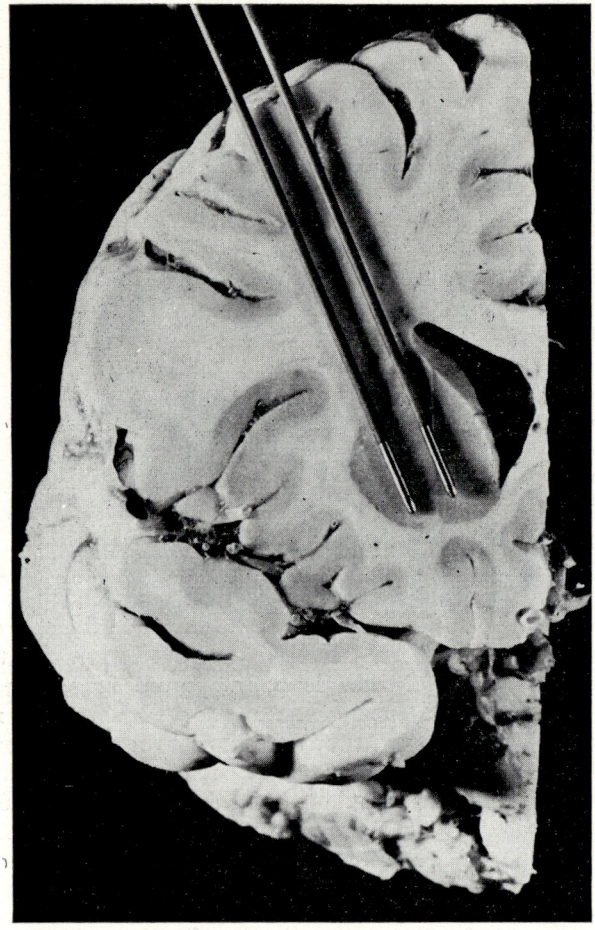

Figure 23.1 Coronal section of the brain exposing the anterior part of the internal capsule located between two lesioning electrodes 6 mm apart.

permit reappraisal of anterior capsulotomy as a routine technique for the treatment of severe obsessive-compulsive neurosis.

TECHNIQUE AND MATERIAL

Localization is based on an operation programme with preselected co-ordinates, the reference points being the tip of the frontal horn, the anterior commissure and the midline, which were visualized with pneumoencephalography (for further details see Leksell, 1971). The co-ordinates were: $x = 17$ mm anterior (to C.A.); $y = 0$ mm (relative to CA.–C.P. line); $z = 20$mm from mid-line. Bipolar RF lesions measuring about 20 mm in height and 8mm in width were produced. The relation of the target area to the

Part VI—Miscellaneous and Multiple Lesions 161

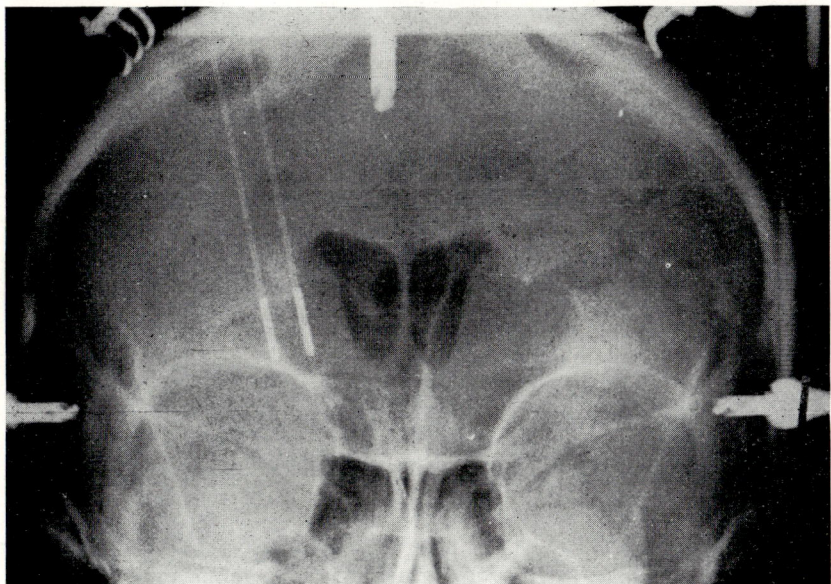

Figure 23.2 Intraoperative roentgenogram with lesioning electrodes in one side. Target area lies 20 mm from the midline.

ventricular system as well as the angle of the electrodes appears from x-ray depicted in Figure 23.2. The operative procedure was carried out under local anaesthesia alone and it was thus possible to communicate with the patient. Electrical intracerebral stimulation with varying frequencies was generally performed.

There were ten men and seven women of ages from 22–53 years, with a mean age of around 40. All the patients were suffering from severe states of obsessive-compulsion with accompanying anxiety. Care was taken to choose patients with a good basic personality, which was considered important for successful postoperative rehabilitation. Most of the patients were totally or greatly incapacitated although a few were just able to carry on with their work but on the verge of breaking down. All had been in mental hospitals several times and had been given every available kind of psychiatric treatment. They had thus all had intensive supportive psychotherapy, group psychotherapy, behavioural therapy or, in a couple of cases, psychoanalysis. In addition, all patients had had intensive treatment with psychotropic drugs. Four patients had previously undergone 'psychosurgical' operations; standard lobotomy had been performed in one patient and superior undercutting in two. These three patients had experienced temporary relief from their symptoms after their first operation, but had then relapsed. The fourth patient had had an anterior cingulotomy one year earlier, performed by ourselves but without effect.

Table 23.1 shows the duration of illness. The duration ranged from 3·5–32 years, with a mean of 15 years. This shows that the series consists of patients with a very long history of suffering and disability, in whom very long persistent therapeutic efforts had failed.

Table 23.1 Duration of illness

Duration in years	Number of cases
2–5	3
6–10	4
11–15	2
16–20	3
over 20	5
	Total 17

RESULTS

Immediate effects
Electrical intracerebral stimulation during the operation did not elicit subjective psychic or sensory-motor effects in any case. To assess the immediate effects of the lesion on memory, concentration and orientation the patient was questioned during the operation. None of the patients experienced any effect after the first lesion was made, regardless of whether this was in the dominant or the non-dominant hemisphere. After the second lesion on the other side, however, some but not all patients reported a feeling of relief from anxiety and tension. In addition, in some cases, after the production of the second lesion, there was mild confusion and slight disturbance of memory.

During the first 2–4 days after operation about half of the patients became moderately confused and disorientated. These symptoms invariably disappeared within a few days. Transient hemiparesis developed a few days after the operation in two patients, one of whom also had two epileptic fits. In both cases angiography revealed a unilateral subcortical expanding lesion, presumably due to venous intracerebral bleeding caused by insertion of the electrodes. These two patients recovered spontaneously within a week and there were no residual neurological symptoms at the time of discharge. All the patients showed a marked decrease in initiative during the first or second postoperative week, but this symptom gradually disappeared with time and with the aid of psychotherapy and reactivation.

Follow-up results
Table 23.2 shows the length of time that the patients have been observed since the operation. The first patient in the series was operated on in December 1970 and the last in May 1972. The mean period of observation is about 8 months. In addition to the clinical psychiatric examination, psychometric tests were given to the majority of the patients before and after the operation. There was no indication, judging from these results, that the operation had caused any intellectual deterioration. This fact was confirmed by the patients themselves as well as by close relatives.

Apart from the transient postoperative loss of initiative, no serious personality changes were observed. In two cases, however, there appeared to be a mild tendency to inactivity which is still present several months after the operation. In some patients there was a slight reduction of 'inhibition' in social behaviour. However, this was considered a change for the better by

Table 23.2 Length of follow-up

Months	Number of cases
10–19	5
5–9	7
2–4	5
	Total 17

themselves and their relatives, as before the operation they had been handicapped by shyness and great difficulty in making contact with other people. They claimed that they were in a better mental state than ever before and this was confirmed by their relatives.

Table 23.3 shows the results of the operation as classified in four different groups:

(a) Free from the symptoms that led to the operation.
(b) Much improved, some symptoms remaining but considerably alleviated.
(c) Slightly improved, most symptoms remaining but alleviated.
(d) Unchanged or worse.

Table 23.3 Short-term effects of capsulotomy

Effect of operation	Number of cases
(a) Free from symptoms	9
(b) Much improved	3
(c) Slightly improved	4
(d) Unchanged	1
	Total 17

As seen, 12 patients (9 + 3) out of 17 benefited considerably by the operation, i.e. so far the operation has been successful in about 70% of our series of 17 patients. It should be stressed that the follow-up period for several of the patients is too short to permit a final evaluation of the result. It is our experience that the final outcome of the operation is largely determined by the degree of intensive postoperative rehabilitation provided for an adequately long period of time.

On the basis of these early results it is felt that bilateral anterior capsulotomy can be regarded as a safe and effective method for the treatment of severe and chronic states of obsession and compulsion accompanied with anxiety. Work is now in progress to find out whether it is possible to achieve the same therapeutic results with an even smaller lesion, on the assumption that in the anterior capsule the fibres originating from the frontal convexity are separate from those coming from the orbital cortex.

REFERENCES

Herner T (1961). Treatment of mental disorders with frontal stereotaxic thermo-lesions. *Acta Psychiat. Neurol. Scand.*, Suppl., **36**, 36

Leksell L (1971). *Stereotaxis and Radiosurgery.* Springfield, Ill.: Charles C Thomas.

Meyer A & Beck E (1954). *Prefrontal Leucotomy and Related Operations: Anatomical Aspects of Success and Failure.* Edinburgh and London: Oliver and Boyd.

CHAPTER 24

Technique and assessment of limbic leucotomy
DESMOND KELLY, ALAN RICHARDSON & NITA MITCHELL-HEGGS

INTRODUCTION
There are two important limbic circuits which appear to be concerned with emotion. (a) *The medial limbic circuit* of Livingston & Escobar (1973), which was originally described by Papez (1937), passes from the septum via the cingulum bundle in the cingulate gyrus to hippocampus, and via fornix to mamillary body, via mamillo-thalamic tract to anterior thalamus, and finally via anterior thalamic radiations to cingulum bundle (Figure 24.1). Meyer, McElhaney, Martin & McGraw (1973) stimulated the medial limbic circuit in the anterior cingulate region and obtained affective responses and physiological changes in conscious patients. Subsequently anterior cingulotomy resulted in significant overall improvement in a variety of psychiatric disorders. Ballantine, Cassidy, Flanagan & Marino (1967) and Brown & Lighthill (1968) also obtained good results with cingulotomy, and Lewin (1961)

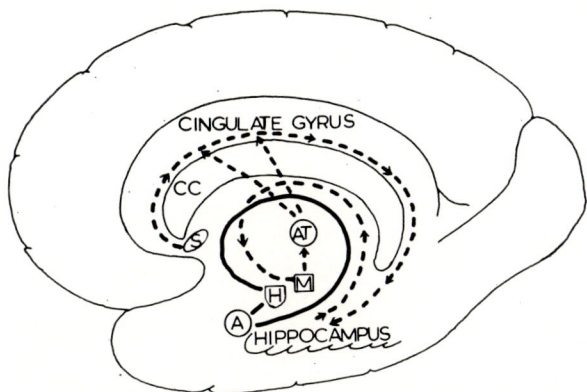

Figure 24.1 **The Papez circuit** (broken line) passes via the cingulum bundle, in the cingulate gyrus, from septum (S) to hippocampus, and via fornix to mammillary body (M), via anterior thalamic radiations to cingulum bundle.
The defence reaction circuit (solid line) passes from hypothalamus (H) via stria terminalis to amygdala, and via amygdalo-fugal pathway to hypothalamus.

Surgical Approaches in Psychiatry

considered that the beneficial results of cingulectomy in obsessional neurosis were due to interruption of the 'reverberating' Papez circuit. (b) *The defence reaction circuit* passes from hypothalamus via stria terminalis to amygdala, and via the amygdalo-fugal pathway back to hypothalamus (Figure 24.1). Electrical stimulation of this circuit leads to the defence reaction in animals and acute anxiety has been obtained from stimulation of the hypothalamus and amygdala in conscious patients. Several workers have made lesions in this circuit: in the posteromedial hypothalamus (Sano, 1966), amygdala (Balasubramaniam & Ramamurthi, 1968) and stria terminalis (Burzaco, 1973) with clinical improvement in severely disturbed patients.

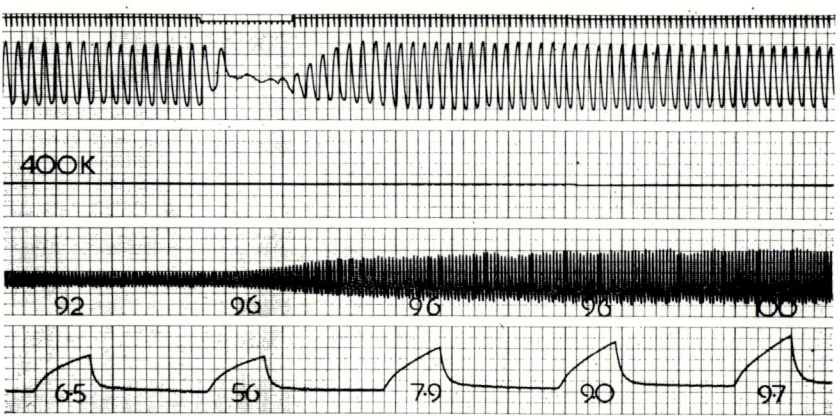

Figure 24.2 Polygraph recording during stimulation of the lower medial quadrant of the frontal lobe with 8 V, showing marked decrease in amplitude of respiration. There is increased physiological arousal following stimulation as evidenced by changes in heart rate and forearm blood flow.
Channel 1 time trace in seconds, line depressed during stimulation
Channel 2 respiration
Channel 3 skin resistance in kΩ
Channel 4 finger pulse with heart rate in beats per minute
Channel 5 forearm blood flow in ml/100 ml/min.

The frontal cortex both monitors and modulates limbic mechanisms (Nauta, 1971), and the object of limbic leucotomy is to interrupt some fronto-limbic connections, and in addition to make lesions in one of the main limbic circuits, in the anterior cingulate gyrus (Figures 24.5, 6).

Target location is in part determined by physiological responses obtained from electrical stimulation, since this may indicate functional pathways which mediate patterns of pathological behaviour (Figure 24.2). We have found autonomic changes from stimulation of the lower medial quadrant of the frontal lobe under general anaesthesia, but the area of responsiveness is usually very small, and one may pass from maximum to nil response over a distance of 4 mm. Respiratory changes are most marked, and a short period of apnea is usual (Figure 24.2). We have found similar physiological responses from other parts of the limbic circuits described, namely the anterior cingulate area (Figure 24.3) and amygdala (Kelly, 1972, Figure 2.44). This evidence, and that of others, suggests that there are functional emotional pathways associated with autonomic activity running through these parts of the brain (Kelly, Richardson & Mitchell-Heggs, 1973).

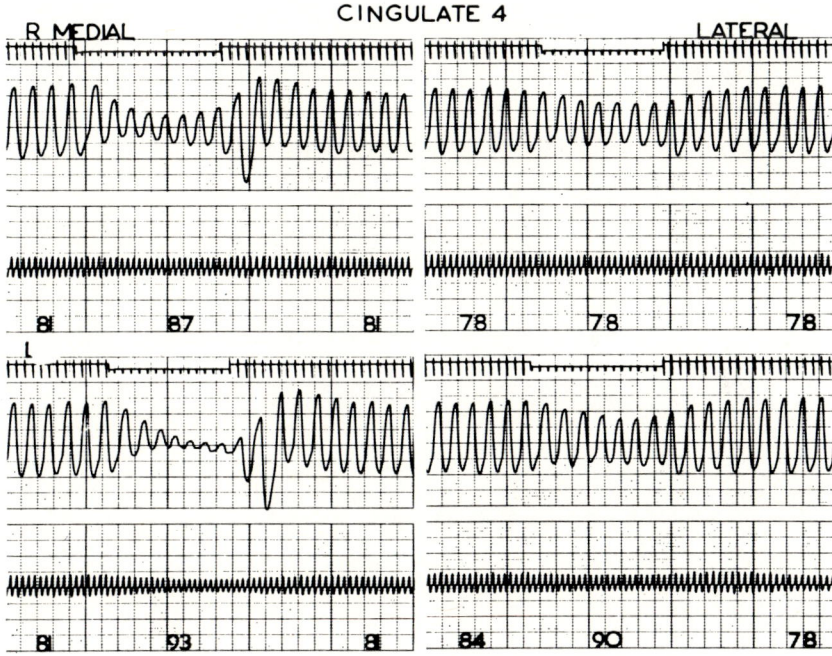

Figure 24.3 Polygraph tracings during stimulation of anterior cingulate gyrus under general anaesthesia (Site 1: Figure 24.5, lateral roentgenogram; Figure 24.6, anteroposterior view). The right and left medial and lateral targets were stimulated with 8 V showing changes in respiration and heart rate.

PRE- AND POSTOPERATIVE ASSESSMENT

Clinical, psychometric and physiological evaluations (Kelly, 1972) have been made before, and 6 weeks and 1 year postoperatively. The preliminary results on 40 patients examined 6 weeks after limbic leucotomy are summarized here (Kelly, Richardson, Mitchell-Heggs, Greenup, Chen & Hafner, 1973). The psychometric ratings were not completed on 4 patients because of language difficulties, and one patient was too ill to be tested (Table 24.1). There was a significant reduction in neuroticism, but no change in the extraversion score on the Maudsley Personality Inventory. Depression was significantly reduced on the Beck and Hamilton scales and on the Middlesex Hospital Questionnaire (MHQ). Anxiety was significantly reduced on the

168 *Surgical Approaches in Psychiatry*

Taylor, Hamilton and MHQ scales (free-floating anxiety and phobic anxiety). The somatic anxiety and obsessional scores on the MHQ were also decreased significantly.

Physiological arousal was also assessed preoperatively and 6 weeks after leucotomy and showed a significant reduction in 'basal' forearm blood flow

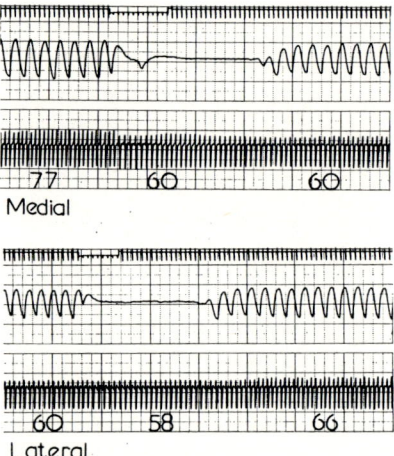

Figure 24.4 Polygraph tracings showing changes in respiration during stimulation of medial and lateral target sites of the amygdala.

Table 24.1 Psychometric mean values before and after limbic leucotomy ($N = 35$).

		Pre	Post	p
MPI	Neuroticism	30·8	23·1	0·001
	Extraversion	12·9	14·2	NS
Depression	Beck	26·4	18·7	0·001
	Hamilton	21·5	10·5	0·001
Anxiety	Taylor	31·9	24·1	0·001
	Hamilton	22·2	12·3	0·001
MHQ	Anxiety	11·6	10·0	0·01
	Phobic	7·1	5·7	0·01
	Obsessional	11·3	10·2	0·05
	Somatic	8·2	5·5	0·001
	Depressive	10·6	7·9	0·001
	Hysteric	5·3	4·7	NS

heart rate and blood pressure (Table 24.2). Anxiety was rated on a 10-point scale with 'zero' representing no anxiety and '10' maximum anxiety. The observer-rating on this scale fell significantly, but the self-rating, although it decreased appreciably, failed to reach the 0·05 level of significance. There was a significant decrease in the observer and self-ratings of depression on a similar 10-point scale

Table 24.2 Basal mean physiological and psychological ratings before and after limbic leucotomy ($N = 37$).

	Pre	Post	p
Forearm blood flow	3·9	2·8	0·01
Heart rate	86·5	77·9	0·001
Systolic bp	126·5	118·7	0·01
Diastolic bp	82·8	76·6	0·05
Anxiety observer rating	4·7	3·2	0·001
Self rating	4·8	3·8	NS
Depression observer rating	4·6	3·8	0·05
Self rating	5·5	4·3	0·05

The numbers of patients in each diagnostic category are shown in Table 24.3. There were 17 patients suffering from obsessional neurosis, 5 with depression, 9 with chronic anxiety and 6 with schizophrenia. There were single patients suffering from depersonalization, anorexia nervosa, and personality disorder with severe phobic anxiety. The patients' mean duration of symptoms was 11 years and their mean number of hospital admissions was 4·5. All but 4 had received at least one course of ECT, 24 had undergone one or more courses of modified narcosis, combined with ECT and antidepressants, and 27 had received formal psychotherapy or psychoanalysis. Eleven patients had previously made determined suicidal attempts and 9 had undergone previous psychosurgery of a more extensive type.

Table 24.3 Clinical ratings 6 weeks after limbic leucotomy.

	N	I	II	III	IV	V	% of total improved
Obsessional neurosis	17*****	1	6	6	4	0	76
Depression	5*	1	1	2	1	0	80
Chronic anxiety	9**	1	1	3	4	0	55
Schizophrenia	6*	0	1	3	2	0	66
Depersonalization	1	0	0	0	1	0	—
Anorexia nervosa	1	0	0	1	0	0	—
Personality disorder	1	0	0	0	1	0	—
Total	40	3	9	15	13	0	67

* Previous operation

The patients were rated (Table 25.3) as I Symptom free, II Much improved, III Improved, IV Unchanged and V Worse (Pippard, 1955). The overall improvement was 67% (I, II, III). The results were rewarding in obsessional neurosis (76%), which is a particularly difficult illness to treat, as evidenced by the fact that 5 had undergone previous psychosurgery without appreciable benefit. These patients had primary obsessional neurosis with an early age of onset, and long intractable illnesses. Mean age of onset was 21 y; 10 patients of the 17 had an onset of illness before the age of 20. The affective component of their obsessional illnesses was not marked. This group of patients is generally considered to carry a poor prognosis, even with psychosurgery. With stereotactic tractotomy those who were recovered or much improved were significantly older when their symptoms appeared (mean age 31 y) compared with those who remained unchanged (mean age 20 y) (Bridges & Goktepe, 1973). The small number of depressives did well, but the patients with anxiety neurosis had a less favourable early outcome than obtained with rostral (McKissock, 1959) and modified prefrontal leucotomy (Jackson, 1954).

One of the main advantages of the multidisciplinary approach to assessment is that the effect of different operations on target symptoms can be compared (Kelly, Richardson, Mitchell-Heggs, Greenup, Chen & Hafner, 1973). Global ratings alone are too crude for this purpose. An indication of the type and severity of the preoperative psychiatric status can be obtained by examining the psychometric profiles of different groups of patients.

Table 25.4 Wechsler Adult Intelligence Scale before and 6 weeks after limbic leucotomy ($N = 30$).

IQ	Pre	Post	Difference	p
Verbal	107·7	108·3	+0·6	NS
Performance	98·3	102·2	+3·9	0·01
Full scale	103·9	106·0	+2·1	0·05

The Wechsler Adult Intelligence Scale was also administered to the patients before and 6 weeks after limbic leucotomy (Table 24.4). The performance and full-scale IQ *increased* significantly, and on none of the subtests was there a significant decrease in the postoperative score. The significant increase may well be due to a practice effect—but there is no evidence that the operation produces intellectual impairment.

SURGICAL TECHNIQUE

The stereotactic method employs the Leksell instrument, as this represents a satisfactory compromise between complex instruments and complicated and therefore less accurate calculations. In its unmodified form the technique precludes obtaining lateral x-rays with the probe in position; changing from one target site to another is time-consuming and the angles of approach are limited.

The ventricular system and major subarachnoid cisterns are outlined with air and x-rays taken in anteroposterior and lateral projections, with the patient supine. Carefully controlled general anaesthesia is used throughout the procedure.

Target zones for the medial quadrant are mapped between vertical lines 1 cm anterior to the base of the clinoid process and 1 cm posterior to the tip of the frontal horn. They are 1 cm above the anterior fossa floor and 6 and 14 mm from the midline (Figures 24.5,6). Further lesions may be made 5 mm above these. The target zones for the cingulate lesions are on a vertical line from the base of the anterior clinoid process, 5 mm above the ventricle and a

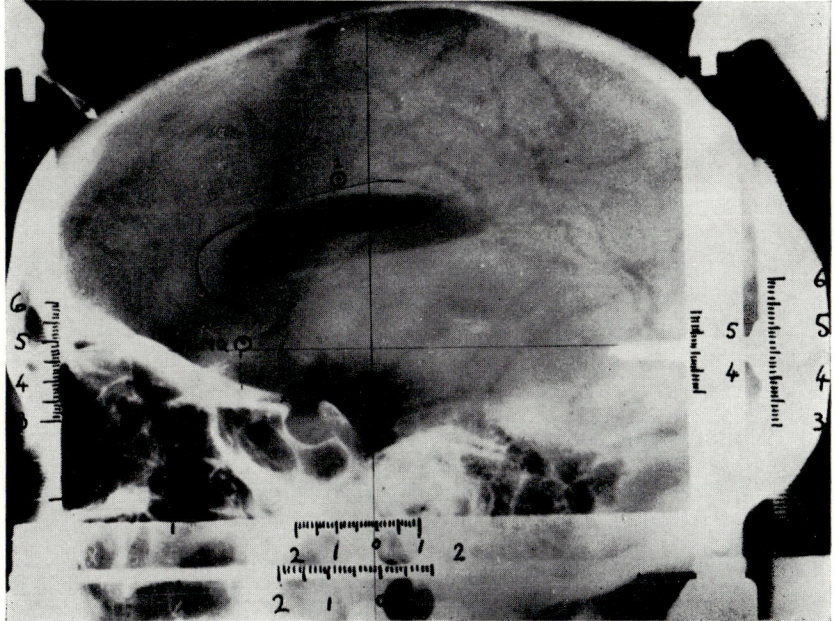

Figure 24.5 Lateral air ventriculogram showing the lesion sites 1 and 2 in the anterior cingulum and LMQ in the lower medial quadrant.

variable distance from the midline, according to the size of the ventricles. One lesion site is at the lateral extremity of the ventricular border and the second is 8 mm medial to this. The posterior cingulate lesions are mapped 15 mm posterior to these and are usually 3 cm posterior to the tip of the frontal horn. Stimulation is then performed in the target zones using 60 Hz at 8 V. Physiological change indicates an active zone. The objective is to identify physiologically active zones and to interrupt the pathways by making suitable lesions.

The lesions are produced by a cryogenic probe, with a freezing tip 3 mm in diameter and 4 mm in length. Experimental studies have shown that reducing the tip temperature to −70 °C for 5 minutes and then allowing slow rewarming produces a lesion 7–8 mm in diameter. The lesion is avascular; the temperature gradient is high, so that the margins of partial tissue damage is minimal. The tissues do not adhere to the probe tip once it is rewarmed. The probe is suitably rigid, so that it is not deviated from the target direction by its passage through the brain.

The cryogenic or 'freezing-probe' technique seems a safe and reliable lesion-making method and has been attended by no postoperative complications. If for any reason a further operation is necessary, it is a simple matter to repeat the procedure, knowing with some precision the situation and extent of the original lesions.

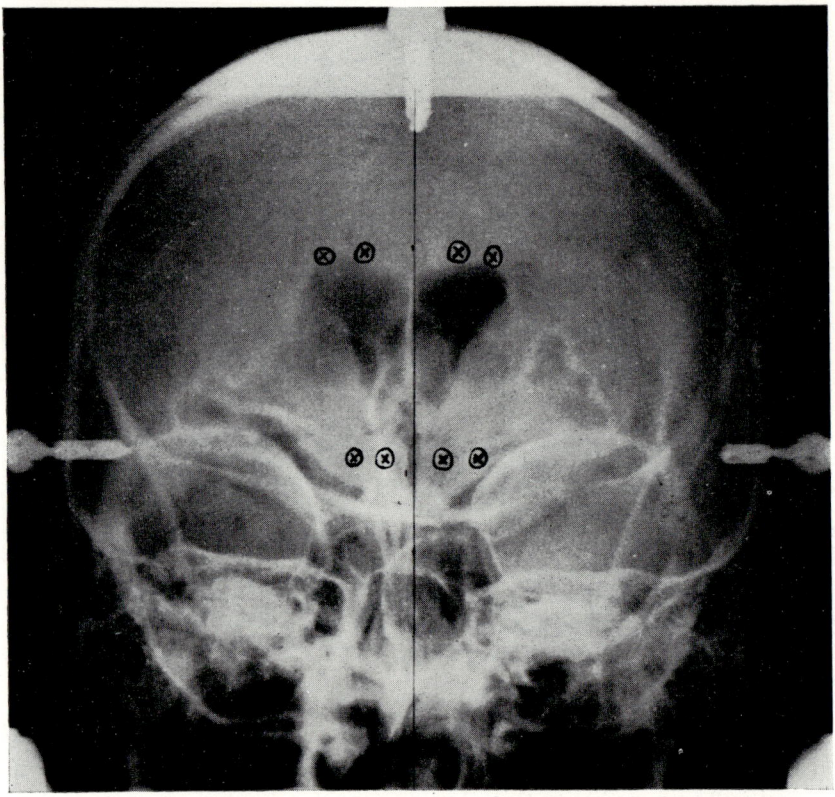

Figure 24.6 Anteroposterior air ventriculogram showing the cingulate lesion sites above the roof of the lateral ventricles and the sites of lower medial quadrant lesions in the frontobasal area.

In conclusion, we have used a well-established stereotactic technique which has a high degree of accuracy for lesion placement. The target zones we use are also well established, but we hope to increase the accuracy, or at least the symmetry of lesion placement by using electrical stimulation to monitor our anatomical landmarks. Finally, we use a cryogenic technique for lesion-making as we feel that this may contribute to the safety and accuracy of the procedure.

REFERENCES

Abrahams VC, Hilton SM & Zbrozyna A (1960). Active muscle vasodilatation produced by stimulation of the brain stem: its significance in the defence reaction. *J. Physiol. (London)*, **154**, 491

Balasumramaniam V & Ramamurthi B (1968). Stereotaxic amygdalotomy. *Proc. Austr. Assoc. Neurol.*, **5**, 277

Ballantine HT, Cassidy WL, Flanagan NB & Marino R (1967). Stereotactic anterior cingulotomy for neuropsychiatric illness and intractable pain. *J. Neurosurg.*, **26**, 488

Bridges PK & Goktepe EO (1973). A review of patients with obsessional symptoms treated by psychosurgery. In: *Surgical Approaches in Psychiatry* (Eds Laitinen and Livingston), Lancaster: Medical and Technical Publishing Co Ltd.

Brown MH & Lighthill JA (1968). Selective anterior cingulotomy: a psychosurgical evaluation. *J. Neurosurg.*, **29**, 513

Burzaco JA (1973). Fundus striae terminalis, an optional target in sedative stereotactic surgery. In: *Surgical Approaches in Psychiatry* (Eds Laitinen and Livingston), Lancaster: Medical and Technical Publishing Co Ltd.

Hilton SM & Zbrozyna AW (1963). Amygdaloid region for defence reactions and its efferent pathway to the brain stem. *J. Physiol. (London)*, **165**, 160

Jackson H (1954). Leucotomy: a recent development. *J. Ment. Sci.*, **100**, 62

Kelly D (1972). Physiological changes during operations on the limbic system in man. *Cond, Ref.* **7**, 127.

Kelly D (1972). Psychiatric diagnosis and the assessment of psychosurgery. *Bulletin Internat. Congr. Psychosurg.* **2**, 9.

Kelly D, Richardson A & Mitchell-Heggs N (1973). Stereotactic limbic leucotomy: neurophysiological aspects and operative technique. *Brit. J. Psychiat*. In press.

Kelly D, Richardson A, Mitchell-Heggs N, Greenup J, Chen C & Hafner RJ (1973). Stereotactic limbic leucotomy: a preliminary report on 40 patients. *Brit. J. Psychiat*. In press.

Lewin W (1961). Observations on selective leucotomy. *J. Neurol. Neurosurg. Psychiat.*, **24**, 37

Livingston KE & Escobar A (1973). Tentative limbic system models for certain patterns of psychiatric disorder. In: *Surgical Approaches in Psychiatry* (Eds Laitinen and Livingston), Lancaster: Medical and Technical Publishing Co Ltd.

McKissock W (1959). Discussion on psychosurgery. *Proc. Roy. Soc. Med.*, **52**, 206

Meyer G, McElhaney M, Martin W & McGraw CP (1973). Stereotactic cingulotomy. In: *Surgical Approaches in Psychiatry* (Eds Laitinen and Livingston), Lancaster: Medical and Technical Publishing Co Ltd.

Nauta WJH (1971). The problem of the frontal lobe: a reinterpretation. *J. Psychiat. Res.*, **8**, 167

Papez JW (1937). A proposed mechanism of emotion. *Arch. Neurol. Psychiat.*, **38**, 725

Pippard J (1955). Rostral leucotomy: a report on 240 cases personally followed up after $1\frac{1}{2}$ to 5 years. *J. Ment. Sci.*, **101**, 756

Sano K (1966). Sedative stereoencephalotomy, fornicotomy, upper mesencephalic reticulotomy and postero-medial hypothalamotomy. In: *Progress in Brain Research* (Eds Tokizane and Schadé). Amsterdam: Elsevier Publishing Co.

CHAPTER 25

Psychological changes after selective frontal surgery (especially cingulotomy*) and after stereotactic surgery of the basal ganglia

M CHOPPY, N ZIMBACCA & J LE BEAU

Observation of the postoperative behaviour of patients submitted to selective frontal psychosurgery led us to separate at least two main groups: the lateral 'convexity group' (area 9 and 10) exhibiting the classical frontal syndrome and the 'mesial group' (area 24 and 32).

Psychological studies developed with the help of the Maudsley School (Eysenck, 1952; Petrie, 1952) gave what is perhaps objective confirmation of the clinical observations: The main difference was found along the introversion–extraversion scale; while the patients of a 'convexity' group showed decreased introversion scores, the mesial group patients showed no change or some increase in introversion. The differences were less marked for the 'neuroticism' factor which generally decreased, and variable in other tests for differentiating psychotics from non-psychotics (Choppy, Le Beau & Petrie, 1955; Petrie & Le Beau, 1956).

More recently, in the course of an analysis of the results of cingulate surgery, we reported some psychological findings after cingulectomy and after cingulotomy. Today we present a tentative comparison of objective psychological assessments of two types of brain operations differing greatly from one another.

METHODS
Selective prefrontal psychosurgery
Surgery was always bilateral. Four main types of approaches were studied:

(*a*) resection or undercutting of areas 9 and 10 ('convexity' patients),
(*b*) resection or undercutting of areas 11, 13 and 14 ('orbital' patients),
(*c*) resection of areas 24 and 25 (cingulectomy) and
(*d*) mesial undercutting of areas 24, 25, and a variable part of 32 (cingulotomy).

*'Cingulotomy' in this paper means subcingulate leucotomy.

Pre- and postoperative studies of the (a), (b) and (c) patients were published in 1954 and 1956 by Le Beau and Petrie & Le Beau. The postoperative tests were performed 6–8 weeks after surgery. The results of earlier tests (average 2 weeks) are given here. The (d) group (cingulotomy) will be described in greater detail in this paper, which reports the results of tests performed, on the average, 5 weeks postoperatively.

Stereotactic surgery of the basal ganglia
These operations were always unilateral and were limited either to the pallidum or more frequently to the posterior thalamus. Thus we present three groups of patients (lesion in right pallidum, right thalamus or left thalamus) submitted to tests both preoperatively and 1–4 weeks after surgery.

CINGULOTOMY
Cingulotomy means section of cingulate white matter. This operation should

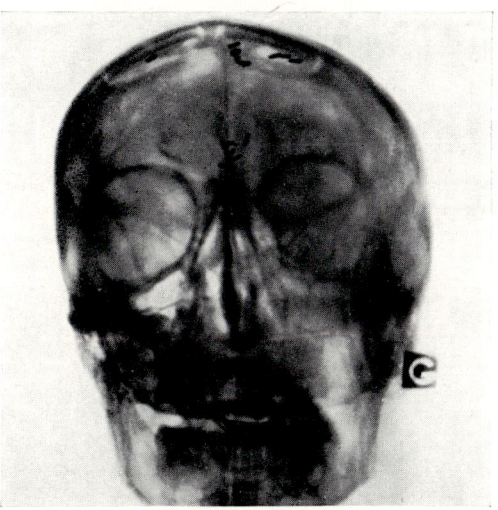

Figure 25.1 Anteroposterior roentgenogram showing the site of cingulotomy.

be differentiated from cingulectomy, which is a truly selective cortical resection of areas 24 and 25. Sections of the subcortical white matter in the cingulate area cannot be limited precisely when the operation is performed with a surgical instrument passing through some of the white matter of the parasagittal convexity. There is no doubt that the use of stereotaxis permits greater precision in cingulotomy.

It is of the utmost importance to keep in mind the location of the fronto-thalamic fibres: they run just lateral to and in front of the tip of the frontal horn, quite near the anterior thalamocingulate fibres. To deserve the name of cingulotomy the open method should enable the surgeon to see the deep face of the grey cingulate cortex quite clearly and keep the cutting instrument in close contact, down to the corpus callosum and the frontal horn. Furthermore, radiological checking is necessary, if one wants to be sure of the cingulate target (Figures 25.1,2).

In this context we cannot resist the temptation to quote the remarkable anatomic studies of Alfred Meyer at the Maudsley Hospital. In collaboration with Mrs Beck in 1954 he wrote: 'In view of the position of the thalamo-frontal projection on the lateral aspect of the anterior horn, it is possible that

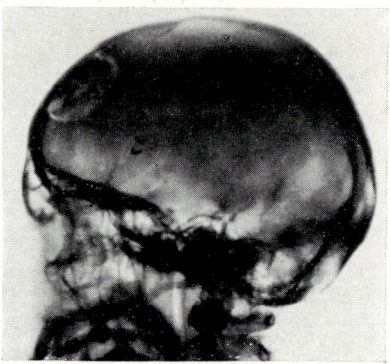

Figure 25.2 Lateral roentgenogram. The clips in the cingulate area mark the site and size of the operation.

the dramatic effect... was due rather to severance of the thalamo-frontal bundle than to other medial structures such as the fasciculus cinguli or the medial orbital convolution.'

Our series comprises 14 patients, all in satisfactory mental condition preoperatively, 7 obsessive-compulsive neurotics, 3 cases of hallucinatory psychosis, 2 cases of depression and 2 cases of hypochondriac facial pain.

Psychological tests
Our general psychological techniques have been described before (Petrie, 1952; Le Beau, 1954).

The changes in intellectual aspects of personality were investigated with the Wechsler–Bellevue test; its verbal and performance scales were used.

Changes in temperament (dimension of neuroticism) were measured on five traits for each of these traits are found in Table 25.1). A neurotic patient writes more slowly, has a high rigidity score, a high score in self-criticism, and diminished manual dexterity, and is more suggestible.

The changes in introversion–extraversion were assessed on six variables: an introverted patient exhibits a great tendency to self-blame, a high verbal score in relation to performance score on intelligence tests, and a tendency to aim at accuracy rather than speed. This last trait was measured by four subtests with the aid of the Track Tracer Machine described elsewhere (Petrie, 1952).

Table 25.1 Psychological changes after cingulotomy ($N = 14$).

Test		Mean difference between pre- and postoperative score	t-value *$p < 0.05$ **$p < 0.01$
Wechsler–Bellevue			
Verbal IQ		−2	0.71
Performance IQ		−0.8	0.43
Traits related to neuroticism (N)	N:		
Speed of writing	+	−12.6	4.23**
Disposition rigidity	−	−1.3	1.69
Self-criticism	−	−2.4	1.20
Manual dexterity			
(Highest score on track-tracer)	−	−1.2	0.53
(Time)			
Suggestibility	=	+0.05	0.05
Traits related to introversion (I)	I:		
Self-blame	−	−2.5	1.68
Total time (track-tracer)	+	+15.8	1.19
Total number of mistakes	+	−2.4	0.26
Time of penultimate trial	+	+3.9	1.43
Mistakes on penultimate trial	+	−1	0.5
Verbal IQ/Performance IQ	=	+0.02	0.25
Miscellaneous tests			
Fluency (round articles)		−1.7	2.12
First score tempo		−1.9	3.16*
Concentration		−3.4	1.5
Lowest score mistakes (track-tracer)		+0.09	0.05
Fluctuation		+0.2	0.10

Finally, five 'miscellaneous' tests are grouped together, the variation of their scores being perhaps less meaningful in psychotic or neurotic individuals.

The numerical results were analysed statistically with Student's t distribution adapted to small samples such as our series of patients. $P < 0.05$ was adopted as the limit of statistical significance.

Results

(1) *Intellect*—The very slight decrease observed for both indexes does not reach the level of significance. The same tendency is observed after other types of selective frontal psychosurgery, perhaps even less after cingulectomy, and a little more after 'convexity' operations. In later tests (6–8 weeks) the IQs are unchanged after orbital and 'convexity' operations, and slightly improved after cingulectomy.

(2) *Neuroticism*—One variable is unchanged; three show a diminution of neuroticism; one shows a significant increase, ($p < 0.01$), of neuroticism.

After cingulectomy there is practically no change in the other neuroticism variables, after 'convexity' operations two variables show a tendency to a decrease and one to an increase (speed of writing test). In later tests (6–8 weeks), all variables change in the direction of decreased neuroticism after 'convexity' operations, and four out of five after cingulectomy and after orbital resection.

(3) *Introversion*—One variable (self-blame) shows a non-significant decrease of introversion, but the other five all change in the direction of an increase in introversion, though not significantly.

Such results are similar to those published after cingulectomy, where it is perhaps interesting to note that in a group of 11 patients tested 1–4 weeks after the operation, three of the variables change in the direction of increased introversion (in one $p < 0.05$), and three in the direction of decreased introversion (in one $p < 0.05$), while there is a tendency to increased introversion in all tests performed 1–3 months postoperatively (Petrie & Le Beau, 1956).

After 'convexity' operations in a group of 14 patients submitted to postoperative tests at a relatively early date (2–4 weeks), three variables are practically unchanged, two show a tendency to an increase of introversion and one to a decrease. In 19 patients tested at a later date (6–8 weeks) a change in the direction of decreased introversion was shown by all tests. After orbital resection there is a tendency to decreased introversion or no change (Le Beau, 1954).

(4) *Miscellaneous tests*—Two were unchanged and three showed a decrease of scores (in one $p < 0.02$). It remains to be seen what are the changes in late tests. After cingulectomy early tests show a similar pattern, while in late ones (6–8 weeks) all scores are improved. After the 'convexity' operations the variables change in different directions in early as well as in later tests, without a uniform pattern.

Conclusions

First we recall that previous findings (Choppy, Le Beau & Petrie, 1955; Le Beau, 1954) allowed us to place in the same general class of psychological changes three types of frontal operations, standard lobotomy, anterior leucotomy, cortical resection or undercutting of areas 9 and 10 ('convexity'). In all three, neuroticism and introversion were decreased; intelligence was decreased after standard lobotomy, but unchanged after the other two operations.

Cingulectomy is in a different class with a slight decrease of neuroticism, no decrease in introversion, no change (or a slight increase) in intellect. The orbital operation created a pattern of changes nearer to cingulectomy than to the 'convexity' operation.

Cingulotomy, the medial operation which aims chiefly at cutting the cingulate fibres, is even nearer to cingulectomy in the pattern of psychological changes produced.

These findings bring some evidence suggesting a difference in function between the dorsal and lateral granular frontal cortices, and the agranular posterior orbital and cingulate cortices. We know that their cerebral connections are not the same, the granular cortex receiving afferents mostly from the large lateral part of the dorsomedial thalamic nucleus, the agranular and dysgranular orbital cortex from its internal part, and the agranular cingulate cortex from the anterior thalamic nuclei.

THALAMOTOMY AND PALLIDOTOMY

Of our clinical series 36 patients could be satisfactorily tested before and after stereotactic surgery. Eighteen had coagulation of the left VL thalamic area, 11 had right thalamotomy and 7 had right pallidotomy. Thirty-five were suffering from Parkinson's disease and one had congenital dyskinesia.

Methods

Burr holes are placed parasagittally, just in front of the coronal sutures. This means that cortical areas 8 or 6 and a corresponding subcortical white matter are minimally damaged by the probe. It is practically certain that such a narrow unilateral trajectory is of no psychological significance. The target is located by electrographic recording and by localized cooling (Dondey & Le Beau, 1964). Then the surgical lesion is produced by heat coagulation. Its size varies, but is always smaller in the thalamus (diameter 1 to 2 mm) than in the pallidum (3–4 mm). The thalamic target lies in the anterior part of the VL nucleus (v.o.a. and v.o.p.). The pallidal target lies in the medial part of the pallidum, close to the internal capsule. Let us emphasize once more that only the effects of a unilateral lesion are discussed in this paper.

Psychological tests

We decided to submit our patients to early postoperative testing, as soon as they seemed alert and co-operative, usually 1–4 weeks after surgery. We believe now that an average of 3 months would be more instructive. As mentioned before, early postoperative testing does not necessarily bring out the later and more permanent changes in personality.

The results of psychological examinations are summarized in Table 25.2, where $+$, $-$, or $=$ denote the change in intelligence, neuroticism or introversion. Of course, the direction of change of the variable measured can be directly or inversely related to the dimensional change in personality.

We added the results of the MMPI. It was not used on a large enough number of patients undergoing frontal surgery; therefore it was not mentioned in the first section of our paper. Levels of significance are mentioned when $p < 0.05$.

Results

(1) *Intellect*—The only significant change is in the verbal index of the patients operated on in the left thalamus. The result is not unexpected. Very likely, later tests would show a progressive return to the preoperative level, but we find here confirmation of the need for careful assessment of risks, before causing any damage, even minimal, to the deep structures of the dominant hemisphere.

(2) *Neuroticism* seems to decrease; the change was significant ($p < 0.01$) after left thalamotomy (the variable of self-criticism).

180 Surgical Approaches in Psychiatry

Table 25.2 Psychological changes after thalamotomy and pallidotomy in Parkinson's disease. The degree of significance is given in parentheses.

Test	Number of patients		
	Left Thalamus	Right Thalamus	Right Pallidum
	18	11	7
Wechsler–Bellevue			
Verbal IQ	−(0·02)	−	−
Performance	−	−	−
Traits related to neuroticism			
Speed of writing	−	+(0·01)	−
Disposition rigidity	=	=	=
Self-criticism	−(0·01)	−	−
Manual dexterity	−	=	−
Suggestibility	=	+	
Traits related to Introversion			
Self-blame	−	=	+
Total time (track tracer)	+	+	−
Total number of mistakes	−	+	+
Time of penultimate trial	+	+	−
Mistakes on penultimate trial	−	−	=
Verbal IQ/Performance IQ	−(0·05)	−	+
Miscellaneous tests			
Fluency (round articles)	−(0·05)	−	+
First score tempo	+	+	+
Concentration	+	=	+
Lowest score mistakes (track tracer)	−(0·01)	+	+
Fluctuation	=	−	
MMPI			
D (Depression)	−(0·02)	−	−(0·01)
I (Introversion)	−(0·05)	−	−
Hs, Hg, Pt	−	−	−
Mf	−	−(0·05)	=
Sc	=	+	−
Pd, Pa	+	+	−
Ma	+	+	+

(3) *Introversion* does not change. As far as reliance can be placed on early postoperative tests, it may be tentatively suggested that small lesions in the deep grey nuclei do not affect the introversion–extraversion scale, differing in this respect from the main types of limited frontal surgery.

(4) *Miscellaneous tests*—Improved test scores were seen after right pallidotomy. Changes in opposite directions for different tests were obtained after right thalamotomy. Left thalamotomy produced a significant impairment in two tests ($p < 0·01$ and $< 0·05$).

(5) *MMPI* showed an increase of depression scales in all three groups, significantly so after left thalamotomy ($p < 0·025$) and after right pallidotomy ($p < 0·01$). It should be noted that at this relatively early stage most of the patients are clinically improved and clearly aware of it.

In both thalamic groups the majority of the other scales are lowered, whereas the psychopathic, paranoid, schizophrenic and manic scales are generally raised, though not significantly. In the pallidotomy group, only the manic scale is raised; all the others are slightly lowered.

Conclusions
Generally speaking, the patterns of change after the three interventions on the basal ganglia are similar, but definitely more marked after left thalamotomy than after right thalamotomy or pallidotomy. It was to be expected that a change in personality would be more important after damage to the dominant hemisphere. Petrie (1952) found that this was so after anterior leucotomies.

The size of the lesion does not seem to be decisive, since coagulation is much smaller in the thalamus than in the pallidum.

SUMMARY

The psychological changes after cingulotomy are similar to those observed after cingulectomy. There is a tendency to an increase in introversion, some decrease in neuroticism and no significant decrease in intellect. Since Introversion is markedly decreased after 'Convexity' operations and 'Rostral' leucotomies, our findings are in favour of a functional difference between granular cortex (convexity and lateral frontal) and agranular cortex (cingular).

After stereotactic surgery of the basal ganglia (thalamotomy and pallidotomy) early psychological tests reveal changes which seem to be due to brain damage.

REFERENCES
Choppy M, Le Beau J & Petrie A (1955). Modifications de la personnalité après les opérations frontales sélectives. *Rev. neurol.*, **93**, 845
Dondey M & Le Beau J (1964). Premières observations humaines de repérage de structures cérébrales profondes par refroidissement localisé et réversible au cours des interventions stéréotaxiques. *Neurochirurgie, Stg.*, **7**, 24
Eysenck HK (1952). The Scientific Study of Personality. London, Routledge and Kegan Paul.
Le Beau J (1954). Psycho-Chirurgie et Fonctions Mentales. Paris: Masson et Cie.
Meyer A & Beck E (1954). Prefrontal Leucotomy and Related Operations. Anatomical Aspects of Success and Failure, p. 33. Edinburgh: Oliver and Boyd.
Petrie A (1952). Personality and the Frontal Lobes. London: Routledge and Kegan Paul.
Petrie A & Le Beau J (1956). Psychological changes in man after chlorpromazine and certain types of brain surgery. *J. clin. exp. Psychopath*, **17**, 170

CHAPTER 26

Combined stereotactic lesions for treatment of behaviour disorders and severe pain
Y K KIM, & W UMBACH

INTRODUCTION
The primary goal of stereotactic brain surgery is to obtain optimal therapeutic results with a minimal lesion. In our experience, a single small lesion in one target structure is not always enough to correct severe behaviour problems, whereas an extensive lesion causes undesirable side-effects such as personality changes, apathy, mental impairment and the like. Although surgery has revealed that intervention in different areas of the brain will modify the same type of behaviour disorders, the possibility of performing a selective operation for particular clinical symptoms has been little investigated.

PATIENTS AND METHODS
In this paper we report our experiences of 143 patients with epilepsy and behaviour disorders who have been operated on for the first time in a single target structure, or a second time in additional target areas. Our clinical and

Table 26.1 Stereotactic target structures selected for treatment of some behaviour disorders.

Symptoms	Primary target	Secondary target	Satisfactory improvement in %
Aggression:			
Periodic violence	Medial amygdala	Posteromedial hypothalamus	(4 patients)
Erethic oligophrenia	Posteromedial hypothalamus	Intralaminar nucleus	60
Intractable pain	Posteroventral thalamus-subthalamus	Dorsomedial thalamus	80
Anxiety states, phobias	Medial amygdala	Intralaminar nucleus	75
Obsessive–compulsive neurosis	Intralaminar nucleus	Dorsomedial thalamus	65
Obsessive pedophilia	Ventromedial hypothalamus	Intralaminar nucleus	—

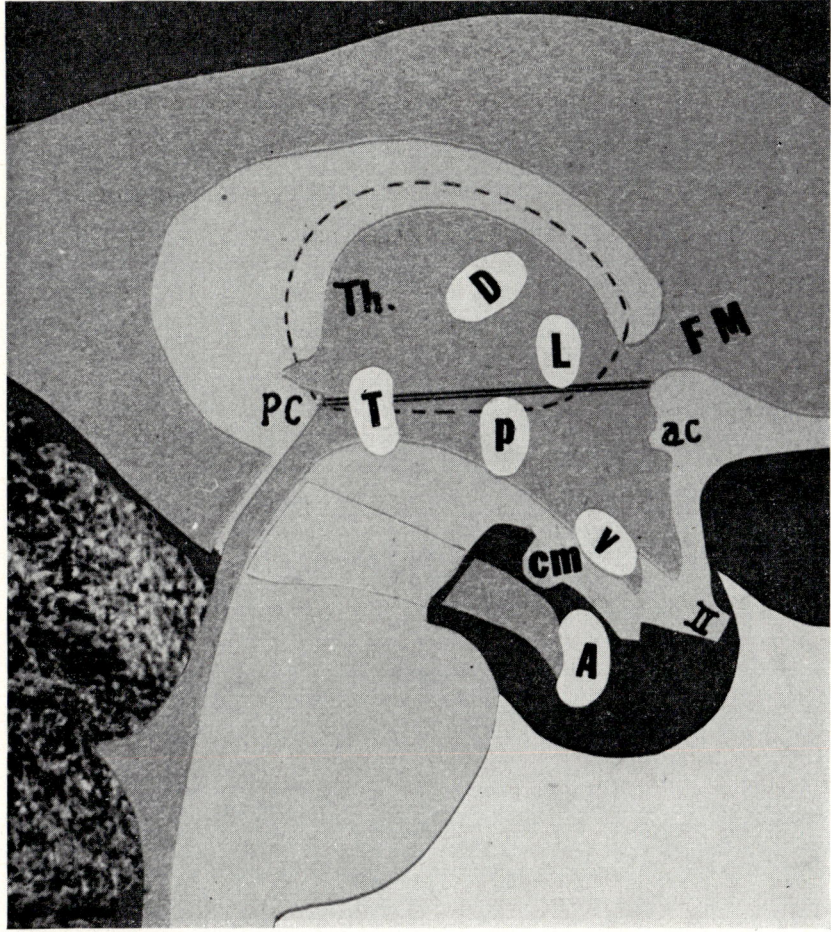

Figure 26.1 Stereotactic subcortical target structures for behaviour disorders.
A = Amygdala   V = Ventromedial hypothalamus
D = Dorsomedial thalamus   L = Intralaminar nucleus
P = Posteromedial hypothalamus   T = Tegmentothalamic area

physiological findings after surgery to different structures (Figure 26.1) are summarized and the most suitable combinations of targets are demonstrated (Table 26.1).

RESULTS
(1) *Amygdaloid complex*
Interventions in the amygdaloid complex were performed in two groups of patients: epileptic subjects, mainly with psychomotor fits, and subjects with mental disorders such as phobia and aggressiveness. Twenty-eight of our 63

patients have been investigated by special methods before, during, and after amygdalotomy. Stimulation and ablation studies in the subdivided structures of the amygdaloid complex in man show evidence of at least three functionally different areas, medial, basolateral and probably central (Kim, 1971). Electrophysiologically, the basolateral part is three times as sensitive as the medial part in spontaneous activity as well as in the propagation of stimuli applied to the adjacent temporal cortex or to both hemispheres (Table 26.2). Thus, stimulation more frequently provokes the patient's individual pattern of attacks when applied in the basolateral part than when given in the medial part, the ratio being 2 : 1. This predominance of the basolateral part can also be seen clinically, although seizure improvement occurs after both basolateral and medial amygdalotomy. Visceromotor effects are not so pronounced as those produced by stimulation of the hypothalamus or subthalamus. However, although of mild degree, they are frequent and the responses were exclusively vagotonic, as consisting of bradycardia and a fall in diastolic pressure, which is due to loss of vascular resistance and dilation of blood vessels. In some cases reactive tachycardia was seen after the end of stimulation. This occurred as a gradual shift from the primary bradycardia, and was considered to be a rebound phenomenon. These responses could be elicited from most parts of the amygdaloid complex. Apparently, the central part is the most reactive and sensitive. The plasma cortisol level increases markedly after stimulation and decreases slightly postoperatively. The most valuable features of studies in man are certainly the data obtained by plotting the subjective sensations. During stimulation the patients with psychomotor epilepsy and phobia most frequently showed sensations of anxiety and occasionally paranoid or oppressed ideas. This came up more often in the medial (50%) than in the basolateral part (14%) (Table 26.2). On the other hand, reduced vigilance, dreamy states, or vertigo, or both, are the predominant phenomena on stimulation of the lateral part (50% : 30%). These aggressive patients (two out of four) who could be operated on under local anaesthesia are also included in the test group. In these patients aggressiveness increased, whereas no aggressive reaction was observed in non-violent cases. Thus the amygdaloid complex seems not to be specific for anxiety alone or for aggression alone, and shows no specificity of the subnuclei for these emotional states. The amygdala is rather considered to be involved in all of these emotional states, probably by means of its modulating function. The autonomic responses as well as the above-mentioned subjective sensations were provoked by high-frequency stimulation of 25–50 Hz (Umbach, 1966), whereas occurrence of seizures is frequent on lower-frequency stimulation of 4–8 Hz (Kim, 1971).

Table 26.2 Effects of stimulation of the human amygdala in 28 cases (in %).

	Predominance of seizure potential	Seizure provocation	Viscero-motor responses	Anxiety aggression excitement	Reduced vigilance vertigo
Medial part	16	30	66	50	30
Lateral part	50	57	60	14	50

After coagulation of the amygdaloid complex, elated mood, increased appetite and weight gain, and elevation of sexual libido were generally observed. Seizure improvement of over 80% was found in 70% of cases after uni- or bilateral basolateral amygdalotomy in long range. Phobias and aggressive behaviour were markedly reduced. However, in cases with pronounced aggression and severe periods of violence amygdalotomies seemed less effective.

(2) *Posteromedial hypothalamus*
The sedative effect of posteromedial hypothalamotomy (Sano, 1962) is well known and was also found by ourselves. As with amygdalotomy, periodic terror or sudden outbursts of great violence cannot be influenced sufficiently at this level. Hypothalamotomy must be limited to a small area to avoid producing surgical complications and undesirable clinical side-effects such as hypokinesia or lack of bladder control in erethic oligophrenia.

(3) *Anterior and medial thalamus*
Postoperative effects within the anterior thalamus, intralaminar nuclei and dorsomedial thalamic nuclei have been reported in detail by Spiegel & Wycis (1962), Dieckmann & Hassler (1972), and ourselves (Kim, 1971; Umbach, Kim & Adler, 1972). The generalized dampening effect and liberation from obsessive ideas gave the greatest benefit in obsessive-compulsive neurosis. After a lesion of appropriate size there is no mental deficit or undesired side-effect. On the other hand, the effects are mostly non-specific and mild if a small lesion is made. This area is thus often added to other main target structures in cases with accompanying obsessive-compulsion symptoms.

(4) *Tegmentothalamic area*
In cases of visceral pain, interruption of the somatosensory system alone brings only temporary relief. Posterior ventral thalamo-subthalamotomy was performed in 24 cases of chronic unbearable pain caused by malignant tumours (Figure 26.2). This target area was chosen because coagulation in this area may interrupt the visceral afferents and efferents as well as reticulo-thalamic fibres passing nearby. At this level, the risk of any side-effects of mesencephalotomy can be avoided, while the pain-relieving effects are comparable and even better. This operation at the tegmentothalamic level, on the other hand, seems more specific for visceral pain than thalamotomy in the vcpc nucleus or centrum medianum or pure psychosurgical procedures. The most frequent effects of stimulation in this area are a sensation of warmth, a sympathotonic effect, an arousal state and disappearance of the previous pain. With stronger stimulation, patients often relate that the lights of the operating room appear brighter and hazy. The most striking immediate effect of coagulation, besides disappearance of pain, is that the patient becomes mildly euphoric. Although the patients are extremely exhausted throughout the operative procedure, they become joyful. In such cases, a mild but distinct logorrhea appears immediately after coagulation. The pain is

Surgical Approaches in Psychiatry

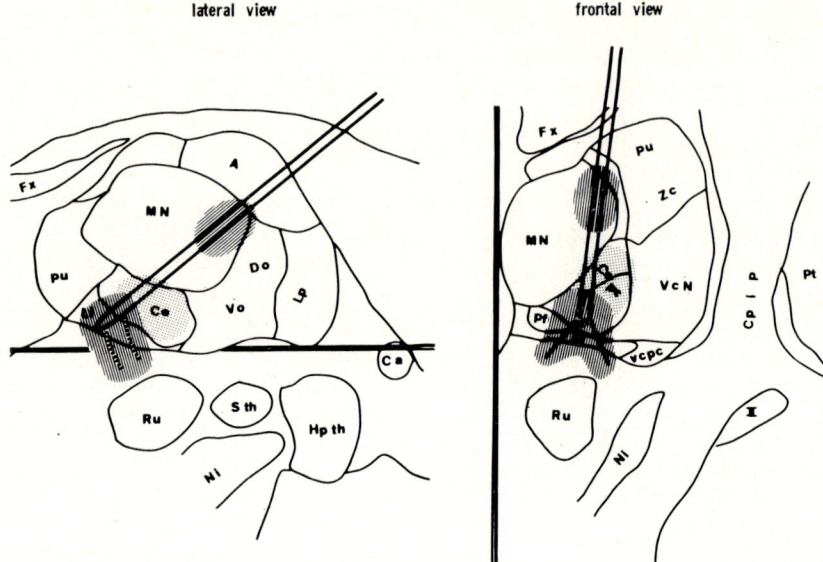

Figure 26.2 Localization of the stereotactic lesions in unbearable pain. The effect of the operation on pain is significantly better in our present targets (lined area) than in the centrum medianum (dotted area) or in the vcpc.

markedly reduced or disappears as a result of improved pain tolerance. In 70% the results were satisfactory during the 4–6 months period even after unilateral operation. Bilateral lesions are necessary in late recurrences and in cases where the first operation was unsuccessful. Especially in this operation, the size of the lesion greatly affects the outcome. A larger lesion or extension of the coagulation by means of perilesional softening, for example, causes transient postoperative confusion or hypoactivity. This is another reason why we prefer to make a small lesion in this area and additional lesion elsewhere (Figure 26.3).

Table 26.1 shows our combinations within the above-mentioned target structures, always taking into consideration the pre-existing behaviour disorders.

In cases of periodic violence, amygdalotomy (medial half) was added, since hypothalamotomy alone did not have sufficient effect. In four patients, bilateral amygdalotomy was carried out and unilateral hypothalamotomy was added. The number of cases is small and the postoperative follow-up short, but this combination seems to have been the most effective. In mentally retarded erethic children, bilateral posteromedial hypothalamotomy of Sano (1962) has had good effects. In 60% of cases the effect becomes even greater when combined with coagulation of the intralaminar nucleus. We now routinely combine the two lesions in a one-stage operation without any significant risk. Visceral pain was alleviated satisfactorily, even with unilateral lesions in the posteroventrothalamic and subthalamic areas. An additional

Part VI—Miscellaneous and Multiple Lesions 187

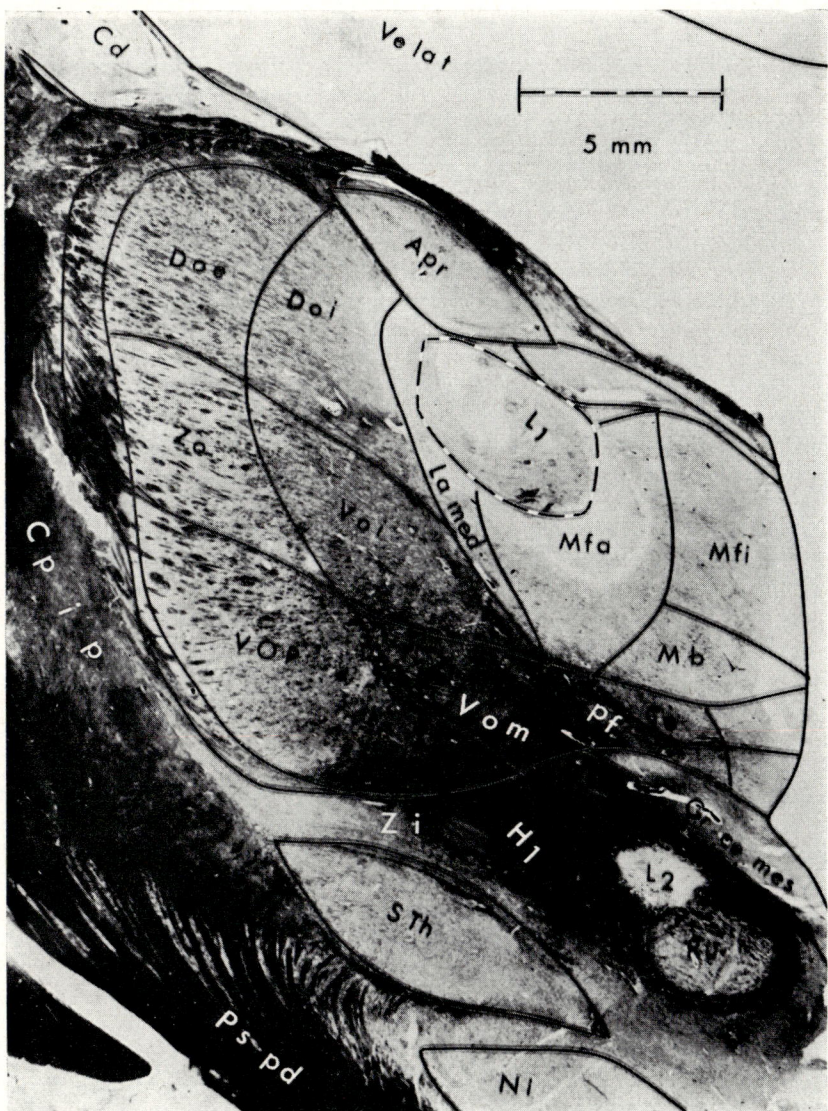

Figure 26.3 Combined stereotactic lesions in the thalamic dorsomedial nucleus (L_1) and posterior ventral thalamo-subthalamic area (L_2) of a patient with severe pain caused by terminal cancer.
L_2 is a cylindrical lesion extending from the subthalamus above the red nucleus to the ventral thalamus. The patient lived pain-free for four months postoperatively when she died of her cancer.

lesion in the dorsomedial nucleus of the thalamus was only necessary in recurrent or severe cases. Anxiety states and phobia could be influenced either by amygdalotomy or anterior thalamotomy. Because of the elation of mood after amygdalotomy, we prefer to do this first. In these cases, the medial parts of the amygdaloid complex should be the primary target, whereas for psychomotor seizure the basolateral part is indicated. Nevertheless, it depends mainly upon the primary individual reaction of the patient whether the two structures should be destroyed at one session or at separate operations. In obsessive-compulsive neurosis thalamotomy in the intralaminar nucleus extending to the anterior part of the thalamus has a lasting satisfactory effect in 65% of cases. In pedophilia with strong obsessive ideas, a combination of hypothalamotomy according to Röder & Müller (1969) and thalamotomy in the intralaminar nucleus proved to be more effective, in that the libido can be eliminated as well as the obsessive components.

CONCLUSIONS

We have summarized our clinical findings in stimulation and ablation studies with well-defined stereotactic lesions in the amygdaloid complex and in the posterior ventral thalamo-subthalamic area. Referring to these and the previously recognized effects of thalamotomy and hypothalamotomy, we have demonstrated our target combinations for specific behaviour disturbances. Psychiatric symptoms and manifestations vary greatly from patient to patient, and our expectation of postoperative results is also distinctly limited by the type of behaviour disorders we encounter. Thus, in individual cases the decision to use a combination of lesions in different subcortical areas must be made according to the behaviour manifested. In this way, we have improved our postoperative results by 20%. This method of combined lesions has definite advantages over a single extensive coagulation. It has been our aim to reduce or eliminate mental dysfunction while avoiding all deterioration of mental level or alteration of metabolic or autonomic nervous functioning. This can only be accomplished by making small well-defined lesions on carefully selected patients.

REFERENCES

Dieckmann G & Hassler R (1972). Relief from compulsion and obsession by combined intralaminary-medial thalamotomy. In: *IV European Congress of Neurosurgery*, Present limits in Neurosurgery, Avicenum, Prague.
Kim YK (1971). Effects of basolateral amygdalotomy. In: *Special Topics in Stereotaxis*, (Ed Umbach), Stuttgart: Hippokrates Verlag.
Röder F & Müller D (1969). Zur stereotaktischen Heilung der pädophilen Homosexualität. *Dtsch. Med. Wschr.* **94**, 409
Sano K (1962) Sedative neurosurgery. *Neurologia, med.-chir.*, **4**, 112
Spiegel EA & Wycis HT (1962). *Stereoencephalotomy*, Part II. New York: Grune and Stratton.
Umbach W (1966). *Elektrophysiologische und vegetative Phänomene bei stereotaktischen Hirnoperationen.* Berlin: Springer Verlag.
Umbach W, Kim YK & Adler M (1972). Follow-up study on stereotaxically treated patients with abnormal behavior. In: *Psychosurgery* (Eds Hitchcock, Laitinen & Vaernet) p. 210. Springfield, Ill.: Charles C Thomas.

CHAPTER 27

Further experience with multiple limbic targets for schizophrenia and aggression

B HUNTER BROWN

INTRODUCTION

A concept of multiple limbic targets for multiple distortions of the personality was first presented in 1970 at the 2nd International Conference on Psychosurgery (Brown, 1972). Since 1965 our major thrust has been directed to control or cure hard-core schizophrenia and sociopathic aggression. This present report records further experience with the multiple limbic approach during the past 2 years and points out worthwhile changes in target correlation and technique. Long-term statistical data will be given in the next few years.

At present patients are analysed from the standpoint of their psychodynamic distortions to ascertain the major foci of limbic imbalance. The size and placement of lesions are determined by available clinical, psychometric and electrical data and the consensus of our hospital psychosurgery committee.

BACKGROUND AND RATIONALE

In 1965 a theoretical model was conceptualized that seemed to afford reasonable prospect of success. We were convinced of the organic causation of mental and emotional illness in the electrical and neurochemical sense. The genetic, environmental, chemical, and glandular schools of aetiology were canvassed with the consensus that all were correct in part—that the syndrome of schizophrenia with its pleomorphic subtypes could result from the interaction of multiple stimuli applied to a limbic system predisposed to this type of imbalance. It appeared necessary to carefully appraise the sequence of perception–cognition–affect and avoid side-effects from those areas vital to memory, information storage, and analytical reasoning. Our final model had a striking parallel to Aaron Beck's description in 1971. One variation from his thesis in the psychopathology of certain schizophrenics relates to a seeming lack of congruity in affect-producing ideation. The incongruous chain will always require multiple targets; a consonant chain often, but not always, may be profitably treated by single targets; if there is marked primacy of one component the other links fall into place. If not, more than one target may be indicated even in the idiosyncratic chain.

Surgical Approaches in Psychiatry

TECHNICAL CONSIDERATIONS

At the 2nd Congress it was suggested that multiple targets be carried out in two stages as brain tolerance had not yet been determined. However, during the past 2 years we have found on many occasions that up to six targets in the frontal and temporal lobes may be placed at one sitting and are readily tolerated. Following pneumoencephalogram the Surgex television monitors mid-position of the head on the base plate and determines if there is adequate ventricular filling. The usual trephine locations, 4 cm anterior to the interaural line and 4 cm lateral to the sagittal plane, are used for any desired combination of targets. The development of a double probe guide that affixes to the base plate has allowed rapid simultaneous bilateral localization (Figure 27.1). Using this guide,* the average operating time for six targets including pneumoencephalography is 2 hours and 40 minutes.

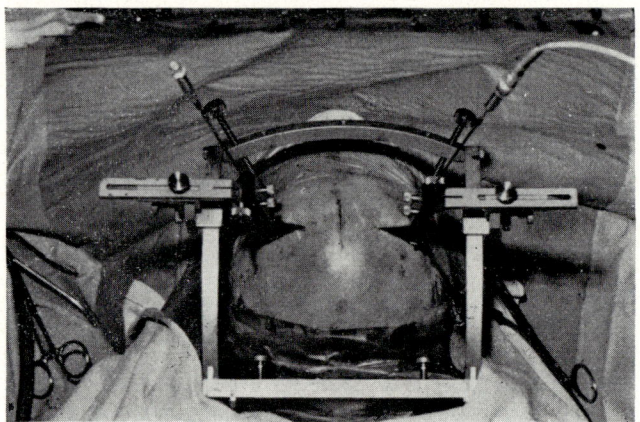

Figure 27.1 Double probe guide affixed to base plate. RFG lesion in the right amygdala.

Cingulum targets are always used, either alone or in combination with other targets in the substantia innominata and amygdaloid nucleus. Usually we place the rostral cingulotomy lesions just forward of the genu of the corpus callosum. For aggressive states or marked perceptual distortion graded tandems are made in both amygdala using 1·6 and 2·1 mm probes with 3 mm retraction (Figure 27.2). Targets in the substantia innominata likewise are always bilateral. At present we make somewhat larger targets in the dominant amygdaloid nucleus and substantia innominata.

A proportional divider is useful as a supplemental check on target localization. A chrome-plated bar notched at 1 cm intervals is placed at target depth and the divider on Surgex TV gives a rapid read-out of the enlargement ratio,

*Brown-Wells double probe guide. Available at: Mechanical Developments Co., 8120 Otis St, South Gate, California 90280, USA.

i.e. head to screen. As a function of receiver distance this enlargement may vary from 1·2 to 2·3. In addition, a size No 8 metal shot in each ear canal facilitates a true lateral projection by superimposition.

In the postoperative period Decadron is used for 1 week and Dilantin for 1 month. No mortality was experienced. There have been no problems with postoperative epilepsy and no wound infections using the plaster helmet for security (Figure 27.3).

CASE REPORTS

The following cases illustrate specific points of clinical interest in the correlation of targets with psychodynamic distortions.

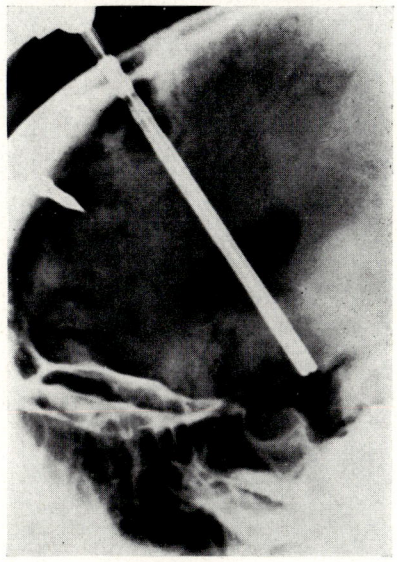

Figure 27.2 Simultaneous bilateral localization for large amygdala lesions with 2·1 mm probes.

Case 1—A 24-year-old white female with a 9-year history of intermittent depression coupled with self-mutilation, three suicidal episodes including wrist-slashing, and explosive physical violence against others without external provocation. Additionally, there were lapses into alcoholic excess and sexual promiscuity. Several years of psychotherapy with concurrent chemotherapy and two courses of ECT were not fruitful. Patient was observed in our secured unit due to marked hostility towards nurses and attendants. Psychosurgery was fractionated for research information. Following bilateral amygdalotomy on November 9th, 1970, the patient remained moderately depressed and anxious but hostility and antisocial behaviour were controlled. Subsequent cingulotomy produced good emotional balance.

192 Surgical Approaches in Psychiatry

In January 1971 she returned to work in San Francisco and has been gainfully employed without difficulty since that time.

Comment: Good control of flash rages and self-mutilation was accomplished by amygdalotomy. The patient volunteered that, 'Either this hospital has shaped up or I have. Nurses no longer bug me.' There was only a slight leavening effect on her emotional disorder, later well controlled by cingulotomy.

Case 2—A 62-year-old white female with a long history of severe mental illness dating back to 1927. During this time there were 14 admissions to private and state institutions, multiple courses of electrotherapy and a full

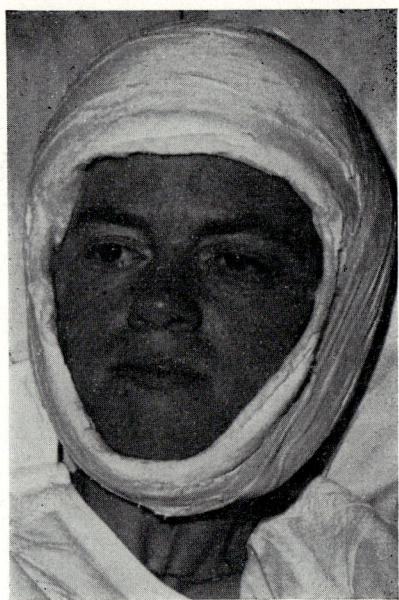

Figure 27.3 Paris plaster helmet for postoperative wound security.

complement of chemotherapy. Presenting symptoms were agitation, depression, multiple suicide attempts, and originally she was evaluated as a manic-depressive psychosis. Improvement was noted for 15 months following selective anterior cingulotomy on March 30th, 1970. Then she regressed, became withdrawn, with hallucinations in the visual sphere, delusions, and paranoia. She was hostile to her husband in a passive-aggressive sense and boasted of a continuous orgasm 24 hours a day in the absence of any physical relationship. Another course of electrotherapy gave no improvement and targets in the amygdala and substantia innominata were added bilaterally. This has entirely controlled her psychosis to date and at present she functions well in the household and enjoys her family and long-suffering husband.

Comment: A mixed schizophrenic psychosis masked as manic-depressive due to the marked primacy of presenting affective components. Circumstances in this case dictated a reverse type of personality fractionation from the sequence used in Case 1. A noteworthy feature was the increase of perceptual and cognitive distortion once the cingulum was no longer in the picture.

Case 3—TR, a 28-year-old white female, a severely disturbed young woman with an 8-year history of schizophrenia. Major presenting symptoms were marked depression, phobias, inappropriate thinking, and withdrawn, regressive behaviour. There were eight hospitalizations during this time; 2 years of analysis, all forms of chemotherapy, and two courses of ECT were of no avail. Two suicide attempts were recorded; she was one of the rare survivors after jumping from the Golden Gate bridge. Prior to hospitalization she remained locked in her home with the curtains drawn, having nightly sessions with a Ouija board for symbolic communication. The diagnosis was chronic schizophrenia of the pseudoneurotic type. Bilateral cingulo-innominotomy was carried out uneventfully on January 18th, 1972. Postoperatively the patient showed considerable but incomplete improvement. She was reasonably appropriate and outgoing, socialized and travelled to a moderate extent, but still regarded the world as a fearsome and threatening place. A few nervous twitches and mannerisms remained plus the feeling that she was unable to cope with employment. Subsequent bilateral amygdalotomy corrected these distortions and presently she appears well in all respects.

Comment: Severe schizophrenia that was considerably improved with cingulo-innominotomy but perceptual distortions persisted. Control of the latter was obtained by interruption of temporal lobe input to the amygdala.

Case 4—MH, a male aged 23 years. Admitted September 12th, 1971, with a diagnosis of chronic schizophrenia, paranoid type. He was the son of a psychoanalyst and had suffered a severe schizophrenic break in May 1969 while studying for final examinations in his second year of college. There was no initial recovery and for the next $2\frac{1}{2}$ years continuous private and public hospitalization was required. On admission he was homicidal and suicidal, attacked other patients, and at times expressed self-hate by banging his head against the wall. Thought content was paralogistic with constant ideas of reference, and he had not responded to many shock treatments or all varieties of chemotherapy. The patient received the customary six-target cingulo–innomino–amygdalotomy for established schizophrenia. On recovery from his anaesthetic he was sane, lucid and appropriate and has remained entirely well. He re-entered college in San Francisco and has maintained a straight 'A' average for three semesters.

Comment: Immediate and sustained control of a severe schizophrenic psychosis by the multiple target approach. A customary result in cases with average or better intelligence quotient in contrast to those having severe mental retardation from procrastination, overtreatment, and the unique nature of the disease process itself.

Two pilot cases of far-advanced schizophrenia with mental retardation (IQs of 51 and 58) were authorized during this past year to determine rehabilitation potential. Both cases required closed ward security and had been institutionalized for 12 and 20 years respectively prior to surgery. In one, institutionalization is still necessary and no substantial retraining has been possible; the other lives with a companion on the outside and has made some worthwhile progress in social adjustment, ability to reason, and personal happiness. The final outcome of these two pilot cases is still undetermined, but clearly the gains will be small for the effort expended. We remain convinced that it is far safer to operate than to wait in established schizophrenia after one year of competent psychiatric care.

DISCUSSION

Clinical experience with these and similar cases since 1965 lends strong support to the concept of a cerebral localization for personality. Reverberant interaction in the limbic system makes such localization somewhat less specific than for sensation, movement, vision, and the like. Presently there is a scientific consensus that the cingulum is the major monitor of man's emotional life. (Bailey, Dowling & Swanton, 1971; Brown & Lighthill, 1968). There is less awareness that other targets likewise serve their discrete purpose. A great perceptual stream enters the temporal lobes and considerable input is relayed to the lateral nucleus of the amygdala. Significant efferent tracts from the amygdala are the ansa peduncularis to the substantia innominata, the stria terminalis to the thalamus, multiple synaptic to-and-fro connections via the uncinate fasciculus and descending projections to the hypothalamus. Given a state of internal limbic imbalance, external stimuli from threatening perceptual distortions, no matter how trivial or innocuous, may trigger aggression in one form or another. This seems to hold true in the so-called explosive personality, in hysterical disassociations, paranoid schizophrenia, and sociopathic aggression, as well as the fugue states of psychomotor epilepsy. In other cases the internal discharge alone suffices with no external stimulus needed.

Similarly, the region of the substantia innominata of Reichert suggests its important role as a syllogistic monitor in the cognitive sphere. I use the term 'region' as, fortunately or unfortunately, pathological verification has not been possible in the absence of mortality. In this vein we should recall that the uncinate fasciculus courses immediately lateral to this constellation of grey matter in the medial inferior portion of the frontal lobes. Using the co-ordinates as described at the 2nd Congress meeting, our clinical observation indicates good control of pathological perceptions arising from the innominata.

SUMMARY

(1) A concept of cerebral localization for personality has been presented. This model is based on the perception–cognition–affect chain and is supported by 7 years of clinical experience with multiple limbic targets.

(2) Clinical experience indicates that the most effective procedure for established schizophrenia at the present time is a six-target bilateral cingulo–

innomino–amygdalotomy. The advantage of early surgery in these cases is again emphasized.

(3) More favourable control of aggression seems to result from bilateral cingulo-amygdalotomy than from either target alone.

REFERENCES

Bailey HR, Dowling JL & Swanton CH (1971). Studies in depression. I. Cingulotractotomy in the treatment of severe affective illness. *Med. J. Austr.*, **1**, 8

Beck AT (1971). Cognition, affect and psychopathology. *Arch. gen. Psychiat.*, **24**, 495

Brown MH (1972). Double lesions in the limbic system in schizophrenia and psychopathy. In: *Psychosurgery* (Eds Hitchcock, Laitinen and Vaernet), p. 195. Springfield Ill.: Charles C Thomas.

Brown MH & Lighthill JA (1968). Selective anterior cingulotomy: A psychosurgical evaluation. *J. Neurosurg.*, **29**, 513

CHAPTER 28

Long-term evaluation of orbito-ventromedial undercutting in 'atypical' schizophrenic patients
SADAO HIROSE

INTRODUCTION

The present concept of schizophrenia was established by Eugene Bleuler in 1911. This heading of Bleuler's included a wider range of clinical pictures than the dementia praecox of Kraepelin. The concept became increasingly confused, some psychiatrists extending it to include even neuroses and others restricting it to processes tending towards emotional deterioration. Langfeldt (1963) distinguished between typical (genuine, nuclear process, or systematic) schizophrenias and atypical ('schizophreniform') psychoses. Typical schizophrenic patients, also called 'the central group', have much in common with Kraepelin's original dementia praecox. This condition is characterized by a typical personality change, emotional blunting, lack of initiative, and so on. The central group would easily be recognized by any psychiatrist as incontestably schizophrenic patients.

On the other hand, the most important characteristics of schizophreniform psychoses are the presence of a precipitating factor, a relatively acute onset, clouded sensorium, a depressive, hysterical or paranoid colouring, and symptomatology that is often psychologically understandable. The prognosis is favourable, whereas in the typical schizophrenia it is poor.

It is clear that the atypical schizophrenic group must be recognized. From the viewpoint of clinical genetics, Mitsuda of Japan (1965) maintained that 'atypical' psychoses belong to a genetically different category from typical endogenous psychoses, including schizophrenia and manic-depressive psychoses. I think it is important for this argument that Manfred Bleuler (1963) detected inborn disharmonic personality traits in 'genuine' schizophrenia.

Since the introduction of psychotropic drugs in 1952, pharmacotherapy has contributed greatly towards improving the interpersonal relationship between psychiatrists and patients, for these drugs are effective in chronic schizophrenics as well as in patients with acute mental disorders. It also facilitated the marked development of psychotherapy and occupational therapy. However, it was found that there are limitations to the effectiveness of psychotropic drugs, and that the drugs do not cure the schizophrenia itself. Moreover, the patients often need large doses and the undesirable side-effects make them uncomfortable.

In the early years of experimentation with prefrontal lobotomy or leucotomy, these operations were performed upon an enormous number of the most hopeless and chronically disturbed schizophrenics who had not been relieved by various other somatic treatments, and expectations ran high. But the favourable results expected did not materialize, especially in chronic deteriorated schizophrenics.

A large follow-up study by Tooth & Newton (1961) surveyed a total of 10,365 lobotomized patients who had been operated on between 1942 and 1954 in England and Wales. Of these, 64% (6,634 cases) were schizophrenics and 36% (3,731 cases) fell into other diagnostic categories. After operation the discharge rate for the schizophrenic patients was lower than for those of other diagnostic categories. Of the latter, more than 60% were discharged as opposed to the schizophrenic patients, of whom only 36% had been discharged.

In Japan, I performed various kinds of psychosurgical operations between the years 1947 and 1971 on 522 patients, of whom 64.7% (338 patients) were schizophrenics. Thirty-eight per cent (96 patients) of the 255 surviving schizophrenic patients were discharged after operation. Before 1957, 70% of the patients on whom I operated had schizophrenia. Since 1957, the proportion of operations on schizophrenic patients has dropped to 40%, with a corresponding increase in a new method of orbito-ventromedial undercutting for patients suffering from affective psychoses, obsessive-compulsive neurosis, depersonalization syndrome, cenesthopathy, and epilepsy with explosive behaviour.

Recently, Freeman (1971) reported the long-range follow-up of 415 patients treated by frontal lobotomy for early schizophrenia. He showed that frontal lobotomy is much more successful in early cases of schizophrenia compared with a decline in social adjustment after illness of long duration. Freeman concludes that in a dangerous disease such as schizophrenia, operation may prove safer than expectant treatment.

It is evident to our psychiatrists that most patients with the typical schizophrenia covered by Kraepelin's concept show irreversible progress to a chronic and general personality disorganization. In my own experience, psychosurgical operation does not halt the progressive deterioration caused by the schizophrenia itself. A favourable outcome was often obtained in 'atypical' schizophrenia with preserved personality, compared with poor results in typical deteriorating schizophrenia, even in the early stages.

PATIENTS

In this report I describe the results of the long-term follow-up of my orbito-ventromedial undercutting for 15 patients with 'atypical' schizophrenia from the viewpoint of clinical psychopathology. They were a small group among the 122 patients who underwent orbito-ventromedial undercutting at the Neuropsychiatric Clinic of Nippon Medical School between 1960 and 1969,

Table 28.1 Some details of five patients with acute schizophrenic episode.

Case no.	Age	Sex	Duration of illness	Intra-familial psychoses	Precipitating cause	Premorbid personality	Symptoms	Date of operation	Follow-up after op.	Operative results
20	22	F	5 y	Yes	Yes	Oversensitive, suspicious, steady, viscosity	Periodic catatonic excitement or stupor, confusion, insomnia, hallucination, grand mal seizures	4/12/57	14½ y	Discharged (working) completely cured
47	19	F	2½ y	Yes		Oversensitive, timid, shy, suspicious, perfectionistic	Catatonic excitement, mannerism, perplexity, repeated attempts at suicide	21/9/60	12 y	Discharged (working) markedly improved
91	32	F	12 y	Yes		Cheerfulness, vivacity, steady, active, nervous	Periodic catatonic stupor, mutism, blocking of thought, repeated attempts at suicide	15/12/65	6½ y	Discharged (working) markedly improved
99	37	F	14 y		Yes	Timid, shy, suspicious, labile, emotional immaturity	Confusional state, sexual delusion, diffusion of thought, hallucination, repeated attempts at suicide	24/5/67	5 y	Discharged (working) markedly improved
100	36	M	13 y	Yes	Yes	Serious, intellectual, conscientious, hardworking, good-natured	Stupor, perplexity, delusions of reference and persecution, emotional turmoil, insomnia, excessive anxiety	28/6/67	5 y	Discharged (working) completely cured

Part VI—Miscellaneous and Multiple Lesions   199

Table 28.2 Some details of five cases of schizo-affective psychosis.

Case no.	Age	Sex	Duration of illness	Intra-familial psychoses	Precipitating cause	Premorbid personality	Symptoms	Date of operation	Follow-up after op.	Operative results
48	34	M	over 10 y	Yes	Yes	Argumentative, subject to fantasies, fanatic, suspicious, hardworking	Manic or depressive mood swing, talkative, delusion of persecution, injuring another, cenesthopathia	12/10/60	12 y	Discharged (working) completely cured
54	38	F	20 y	Yes	Yes	Timid, shy, suspicious, labile affectivity, selfish	Manic or depressive mood swing, delusion of reference, persecution, jealousy, coprolalia, insomnia	25/1/61	$11\frac{1}{2}$ y	Still in hospital moderately improved
67	43	M	$28\frac{1}{2}$ y	Yes	Yes	Sensitive, steady, bigoted, active, hardworking, good-natured	Manic or depressive mood swing, confusion, violent, restless, frequent periodic attacks	26/9/62	10 y	Discharged (working) markedly improved
68	24	F	3 y		Yes	Sensitive, obstinate, sociable, cheerful, lively or retarded, lonely	Manic elation, over-talkative, flight of ideas, eccentric idea of reference, bizarre behaviour, insomnia, irritable	7/11/62	$9\frac{1}{2}$ y	Discharged (working) completely cured
112	28	M	11 y			Timid, shy, subject of fantasies excessively cautious, eccentric, moody, lively	Manic or depressive mood swing, ecstasy, mannerism, rituals, cenesthopathy, insomnia, violent, diurnal mood variation	3/7/68	4 y	Discharged (working) moderately improved

except for case 20, treated at the Matsuzawa Mental Hospital in 1957. Patients with typical schizophrenia of Kraepelin's classification were excluded.

Details of 15 patients, 9 male and 6 female, are given in Tables 28.1,2,3,4). Their ages at operation ranged from 19–45 years (average 30 years). Age at onset ranged from 13–24 years (average 19 years), except a patient who developed paraphrenia at the age of 38. The duration of illness from the onset varied between 2 and 29 years (average 10 years). Almost all of the patients had been treated repeatedly in mental hospitals. Of course, these patients were under observation in our clinic from 2–16 weeks before operation for the purpose of psychiatric case selection. All had undergone various somatic treatments, including ECT, insulin coma treatment, continuous sleep therapy, refrigeration therapy, and pharmacotherapies (phenothiazines, butyrophenones, imipramine, amitriptyline), but with no permanent improvement and no remarkable effect on their symptoms. One patient (Case 113, cenesthiopathic state) had been treated unsuccessfully by stereotactic thalamotomy by another surgeon. The average length of follow-up after operation is over 8 years (4–14½ years).

RESULTS

As an aid to evaluating the results of the operation in each of the diagnostic subcategories of 'atypical' schizophrenia, Tables 28.1,2,3,4,5 show the present status of the patients and the degree of improvement after the operation. A favourable outcome has been obtained in the following 'atypical' schizophrenic groups with well-preserved personality:

(1) Five cases of *acute schizophrenic episode* (WHO-ICD 295.4) which compromise recurrent catatonic episodes or confusional states.
(2) Five cases of *schizo-affective type* (ICD 295.7) which show the clinical characteristics of schizophrenia, such as true paranoid delusions, bizarre behaviour, thought disorder, and incongruity of affect, but, on the other hand, exhibit an admixture of the symptoms of affective psychosis. This group is also called 'mixed psychosis'.
(3) Four cases of *chronic neurosis-like schizophrenia* (ICD 295.4) which correspond to the pseudoneurotic schizophrenia of Hoch & Polatin (1949). These patients manifest a great variety of bizarre neurotic symptoms, including pan-anxiety, obsessions, conversion symptoms, hypochondriac delusions or cenesthiopathy, idea or delusion of reference, and vegetative manifestations.
(4) A case of *paraphrenia*, which means preserved paranoid schizophrenia with progressive development of a delusional system.

Of five patients with the diagnosis of acute schizophrenic episode, all were discharged and regained social adaptability. Two of these (Case 20, a 22-year-old woman, and Case 100, a 36-year-old man), whose illnesses had lasted 5 and 13 years, respectively, before operation, recovered completely without relapse. The former, when last seen after 14½ years follow-up was keeping house, and the latter, 5 years after the operation, was employed very usefully.

Part VI—Miscellaneous and Multiple Lesions 201

Table 28.3 Some details of four patients suffering from chronic neurosis-like schizophrenia.

Case no.	Age	Sex	Duration of illness	Intra-familial psychoses	Precipitating cause	Premorbid personality	Symptoms	Date of operation	Follow-up after op.	Operative results
52	20	M	2 y		Yes	Timid, shy, steady, active, inferiority, social, hardworking	Astasia, abasia, insomnia, forced laughing, restlessness, motor and sensory conversion symptoms	30/11/60	11½ y	Discharged (working) markedly improved
56	21	M	4 y	Yes		Timid, shy, sensitive, introverted, unsociable, eccentric	Cenesthopathia, delusion of reference and observation, hypochondriac complaint, bizarre mannerism	15/3/61	11 y	Discharged (working) moderately improved
110	30	M	9 y		Yes	Oversensitive, steady, obstinate, anankastic, hardworking, reticent	Hypochondriac delusion, obsessional idea, insomnia, attempts at suicide, delusional mood, delusion of reference	22/5/68	4 y	Discharged (working) completely cured
113	19	M	6 y			Obstinate, bigoted, steady, argumentative, eccentric, perfectionistic	Cenesthiopathia, hypochondriac, delusion, mystic experience, inferiority complex, bizarre mannerism	25/9/68	4 y	Discharged (working) markedly improved

Table 28.4 Description of a patient with paraphrenia.

Case no.	Age	Sex	Duration of illness	Intra-familial psychoses	Precipitating cause	Premorbid personality	Symptoms	Date of operation	Follow-up after op.	Operative results
41	45	M	7 y		Yes	Hypersensitivity, overvalued idea, hostile, elated, mood, hardworking	Delusion of jealousy, hypochondriac delusion, insomnia, no hallucinations, irritable	23/3/60	10 y	Discharged (working) completely cured

It should be noted that the periodic catatonia disappeared completely after the operation. Another three cases showed temporary relapse, but the catatonic episodes were very mild and easily controlled by a short period of pharmacotherapy or ECT.

Of five patients of schizo-affective type, all except a 38-year-old woman (Case 54) were discharged and resumed their previous work. Concerning the degree of improvement, two patients (Case 48, a 34-year-old man, and Case 68, a 24-year-old woman), whose illnesses had lasted 10 and 3 years, respectively, recovered completely and have been followed up for 12 and $9\frac{1}{2}$ years without relapse or personality deficit. It deserves mention that a 43-year-old male patient (Case 67), whose duration of illness was $28\frac{1}{2}$ years before operation, showed marked improvement, but after psychosurgery the preoperative clinical picture of 'mixed psychosis' changed to one in which pure manic-depressive features predominated. The manic-depressive attack can be easily controlled with a combination of antidepressants and lithium carbonate. Another two patients (Case 54, a 38-year-old woman and Case 112, a 28-year-old man) were moderately improved.

Of four patients with chronic neurosis-like schizophrenia, all were discharged and could be employed adequately. A 30-year-old male patient (Case 110), whose duration of illness was 9 years, recovered completely. He was relieved from his preoperative obstinate and intractable hypochondriac delusion of bizarre type.

About the last group of paraphrenia, a 45-year-old male patient showed a favourable outcome, returning to normal life, and has worked as a taxi driver for the past 10 years.

DISCUSSION

It is very interesting to speculate on the mechanism by which psychosurgical operations cure 'atypical' schizophrenics who do not show emotional disorganization. Psychosurgery has a definite effect on periodicity and sometimes prevents a relapse (Jones & McCowan, 1949; Hirose, 1965, 1966; Sykes & Tredgold, 1964). In chronic neurosis-like schizophrenia the dominant symptom of pan-anxiety can be reduced by psychosurgery. Consequently, the various neurotic symptoms of bizarre type are relieved. Paraphrenia with well-preserved personality showed the best results. Some of these 'atypical' schizophrenic patients apparently showed a tendency to withdraw from the realities of life before the operation, but their personalities remained basically well preserved and without serious emotional blunting.

The effectiveness of the operation in 'atypical' schizophrenia was related to the preoperative mixed clinical picture, especially with combined affective traits, confusion, perplexity, obsessions, and protracted emotional tension. In a large number of these patients, some psychological, environmental, or physical precipitating factors were confirmed to have played a part prior to their nervous breakdowns. Moreover, polymorphic intrafamilial endogenous (typical or atypical) psychoses, such as schizophrenia, affective psychoses, and epilepsy, were found in the families of many patients. We found seven cases of psychosis among the 13 brothers of a patient of schizo-affective type (Case 67, a 43-year-old man), who showed marked improvement after psychosurgery.

The premorbid personality traits of those patients in whom the operation had favourable results were delicacy, oversensitivity, bigotedness, seriousness, perfectionism, fanaticism, cyclothymia, and warm-heartedness. In short, they have socially active personalities. In contrast, the premorbid personality traits of the typical schizophrenics of Kraepelin's type are in general unsociability, callousness, unfeelingness, gloominess, loneliness, and autistic tendencies, showing socially less active personalities. Usually there are no demonstrable precipitating factors. In some typical schizophrenic patients, an obvious emotional blunting was observable after psychosurgery, but such

Table 28.5 Survey of the four groups of 'atypical' schizophrenic patients subjected to orbito-ventromedial undercutting 1957–1969.

(1) Acute schizophrenic episode (ICD 295.4): 5 Patients
    Age (onset): av. 20   *Results*   Discharged (working): 5 patients
    Age (operation): av. 29   Completely cured: 2 patients
    Before op.: av. 9 y   Markedly improved: 3 patients
    Follow-up: 5–14½ y

(2) Schizo-affective type (ICD 295.7): 5 Patients
    Age (onset): av. 19   *Results*   Discharged (working): 4 patients
    Age (operation): av. 33   In hospital: 1 patient
    Before op.: av. 15 y   Completely cured: 2 patients
    Follow-up: 4–12 y   Markedly improved: 1 patient
                                              Moderately improved: 2 patients

(3) Chronic neurosis-like schizophrenia (ICD 295.5): 4 patients
    Age (onset): av. 17   *Results*   Discharged (working): 4 patients
    Age (operation): av. 22   Completely cured: 1 patient
    Before op.: av. 5 y   Markedly improved: 2 patients
    Follow-up: 4–11½ y   Moderately improved: 1 patient

(4) Paraphrenia: 1 patient
    Age (onset): 38
    Age (operation): 45   *Results*   Discharged (working)
    Before op.: 7 y   Completely cured
    Follow-up: 10 y

a personality deficit would have been masked preoperatively by the striking active symptoms. In contrast to the findings of Freeman and others, improvement in atypical schizophrenic patients was related to the preoperative mental state rather than to the duration of the illness.

Outstanding improvement has been obtained even in some 25 'atypical' schizophrenic patients treated by old-fashioned prefrontal lobotomy by myself during 1948 and 1955 at the Matsuzawa Mental Hospital. A 34-year-old high school teacher of physics developed an acute schizophrenic episode 6 years before being operated on in 1943. He underwent operation in June 1949. A month after lobotomy he returned to his job. Up to the present time, about 23 years after the operation, he has not had a single schizophrenic episode. Now, at 57 years of age, he is working as a Professor of Physics at the Institute of Technology. Recently, he published a monograph on radiological physics. He had an emotionally and intellectually well-developed premorbid personality with characteristics of delicacy, seriousness, perfectionism, and cyclothymia.

The working mechanism of psychosurgery can theoretically be summarized as follows: Psychosurgical operations do not directly cure the schizophrenic or other endogenous disease processes, or the biological conditions resulting from these. But psychosurgery changes the psychological and biological reaction patterns to the underlying pathogenetic biological conditions in accordance with the premorbid personality of each patient. The complex regulation of the autonomic functions by the activities of both limbic system and hypothalamus may change, and the pre-existing excessive psychological and biological defence mechanism, which may produce general anxiety, emotional tension, and a variety of pathological mental symptoms, may be stabilized, thus breaking the 'vicious circle'. The result is removal of or release from the pathological mental symptoms, making social rehabilitation possible.

Recently, favourable results of operations on the orbito-medial quadrants of the frontal lobe have led to recognition of the value of intervention at this site for reduction of protracted emotional tension. The orbito-ventromedial undercutting method can produce the maximum therapeutic effects without any serious side-effects. It was verified that my operative lesion had caused slight degeneration and gliosis of the uncinate fasciculus and the dorsomedial nucleus in two brains of well-improved patients. I think the very limited lesions of my operation are sufficient to interrupt both the orbito-thalamic and orbito-temporal connections at the same time. In my own experience, a patient (Case 113, a 19-year-old male, cenesthopathic state) who had been treated unsuccessfully by stereotactic thalamotomy was finally relieved from his symptoms by orbito-ventromedial undercutting.

REFERENCES

Bleuler M (1963). Conception of schizophrenia within the last fifty years and today. *Proc. Roy. Soc. Med.*, **56**, 945
Freeman W (1971). Frontal lobotomy in early schizophrenia: Long follow-up in 415 cases. *Brit. J. Psychiat.*, **119**, 621
Hirose S (1965). Orbito-ventromedial undercutting 1957–1963. Follow-up of 77 cases. *Amer. J. Psychiat.*, **121**, 1194
Hirose S (1966). Present trends in psychosurgery. *Folia psychiat. neurol. jap.*, **20**, 361
Hoch PH & Polatin P (1949). Pseudoneurotic forms of schizophrenia. *Psychiat. Quart.*, **23**, 248
Jones GN & McCowan PK (1949). Leucotomy in the periodic psychoses. *J. ment. sci.*, **95**, 101
Langfeldt G (1963). Atypical schizophrenias with special reference to the content of the term 'schizophreniform psychoses'. *Proc. III World Congr. Psychiat.*, **3**, 33
Mitsuda H (1967). *Clinical Genetics in Psychiatry*. Problems in nosological classification. Tokyo: Igaku Shoin.
Sykes MK & Tredgold RF (1964). Restricted orbital undercutting. *Brit. J. Psychiat.*, **110**, 609
Tooth GC & Newton MP (1961). Leucotomy in England and Wales 1942–1954. *Rep. Publ. Hlth. Med. Subj.*, **104**, HM Stationery Office.

CHAPTER 29

Relief of obsessive-compulsive disorders, phobias and tics by stereotactic coagulation of the rostral intralaminar and medial-thalamic nuclei

R HASSLER & G DIECKMANN

INTRODUCTION

Therapeutic surgical interventions against psychical disturbances constitute a special group in the so-called functional neurosurgery of chronic functional disorders of the central nervous system. The disordered functions have their neural correlates in definite brain structures or neuronal circuits. These neuronal correlates are in no way identical with the highly specialized neuronal structures of the teleceptive or other senses, or with the central co-ordinative apparatus for motor performances. Similarly, the neuronal circuits responsible for psychical functions are not equipotent, but specialized for definite psychical performances, such as psychomotor activity, self-assertion and self-defence, social adaptation, parental care, and affective reactivity.

Leucotomy and prefrontal lobotomy started with Moniz' theory of hyperfixed circuits for thoughts in the prefrontal areas; further development of psychosurgery should not be purely trial and error exploration, however, it should be directed by a leading idea. Since Walter Freeman's statement that many patients suffer from having too much prefrontal cortex, no other theory for psychosurgery has been put forward.

We shall try to present a new psychobiological theory for a special group of psychical disorders and shall report on the relief of these disorders by psychosurgical interventions derived from this theory.

The theory is based on the following neurophysiological and psychiatric facts: Any conscious sensual perception arises from the convergence of messages through 'specific' and 'unspecific', or truncothalamic, pathways. The cortical evoked potentials are even clearer and more elaborate during deep general anaesthesia than without anaesthesia. Narcotics suppress the messages that are elicited by the same stimulus in the reticular activating system and transferred to the basal ganglia by the unspecific projection system. Under normal conditions, they finally reach the somatosensory cortex through the so-called 'unspecific' projection system of the thalamus, which is identical with the connections of the truncothalamic nuclei in the

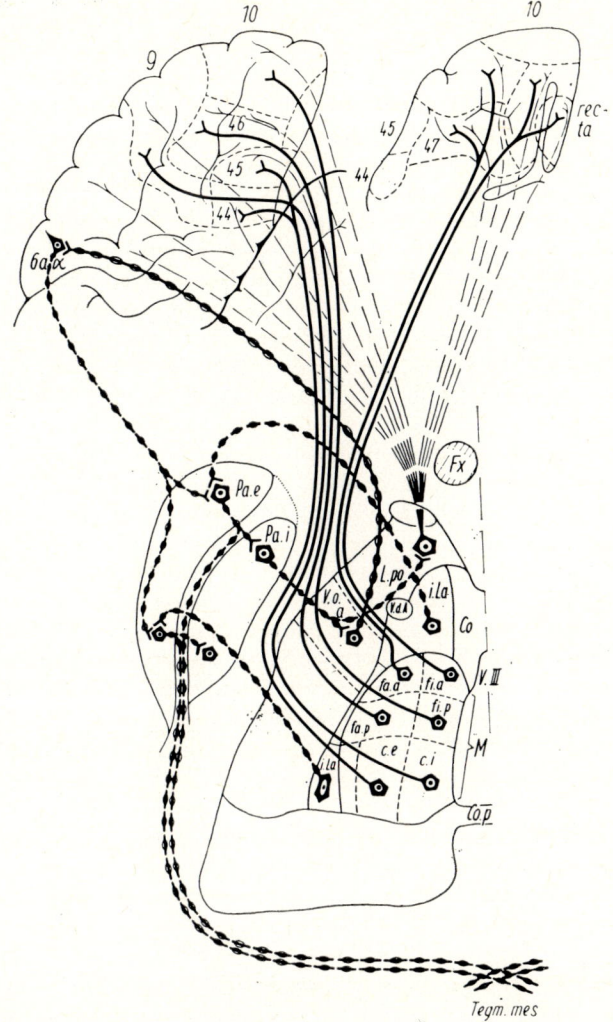

Figure 29.1 Schematic drawing of the specific and unspecific projections to the prefrontal cortex. Each of the prefrontal areas, such as area 9 or area 46 or the area recta, receives two sets of afferents, specific ones from a subnucleus of the medial territory of the thalamus, such as M.c.e (to area 8), M.fa.p (to area 46) and M.fi.a to area recta), and unspecific ones from the truncothalamic projection system, which originates from the intralaminar thalamic nuclei and passes through the pallidum to return to the frontal pole of the thalamus (L.po = VA), from where unspecific afferents run to all cortical areas, including the prefrontal one. A semispecific projection from the intralaminar nuclei goes to area 6aα, which projects to the pallidum and to the brain stem. The pallidum externum gives rise to an efferent pathway which regulates contraversive turning and muscle tone, and which has its decussation in the anterior midbrain, so that its stimulation more ventrally results in a turning to the ipsilateral side.

thalamus (Figure 29.1). Similarly, each field of the sense-independent prefrontal cortex receives not only unspecific projections from the 'truncothalamic' nuclei' (Hassler, 1949), but also the specific projection from the medial-thalamic nucleus (Hassler, 1948).

For a thought or for a multisensual emotion like hunger, sympathy or happiness, the specific complex imaginations are not in themselves sufficient to produce the actual emotion or thought. They must be joined by some activating influences, such as vigilance, directing attention, adversion, or any other kind of actualization which serves to promote objectification.

The lower neuronal level for such actualization is the reticular activating system for regulation of vigilance, the higher neuronal system is the differentiated truncothalamic system, which regulates the activity of the various cortical circuits for the senses, motility, and integrative functions. The effectory part of the truncothalamic or unspecific system is the pallidal system for adversion or direction of attention (Montanelli & Hassler, 1964) supported by the screening activity of the putamen (Dieckmann & Hassler, 1968).

Every mental activity comprises a motor or psychomotor component, which actualizes the thought or emotion, or drive. Even pathological psychical phenomena require such psychomotor components, which are contributed by the truncothalamic, activity-regulating system. In the compulsive and obsessive experiences the cogently perseverating and repetitive component may be produced by the hyperactive truncothalamic system. The same seems to be true of the compulsion to perform useless movements, expressions like tics or compulsive cries, and of compulsive fears of places or of food intake in the presence of other persons, as in phobias.

The indications for combined coagulation of the medial and intralaminar thalamic nuclei are: obsessive-compulsive neuroses, obsessive-compulsive syndromes of organic or psychopathic origin, phobias, and generalized tics with compulsive crying and echo- and coprolalia.

The theory presented has been tested by the therapeutic effects of uni- or bilateral stereotactic destruction of the intralaminar and medial nuclei of the thalamus. The truncothalamic nuclei are not compact but spread out between other thalamic nuclei, which project into the cortex. It is virtually impossible to destroy them all completely, and the objection that, if the theory held true, all conscious perceptions would be abolished after therapeutic destruction is thus invalidated. The largest extension of the intralaminar nuclei is present rostrobasal to the medial nucleus. This is the intralaminar target, rostral and medial to the mamillothalamic tract (Figure 29.2).

RESULTS

One example of a malignant obsessive-compulsive syndrome, which was almost completely relieved by intralaminar-medial thalamotomy, will be presented first. The patient has always been overaccurate, very ambitious and insistent. At the age of 18 she had severe pangs of conscience such that her father confessor felt it necessary to sooth her scruples. At 27, during her second pregnancy, an obsession to remove bloody spots, caused by a plague

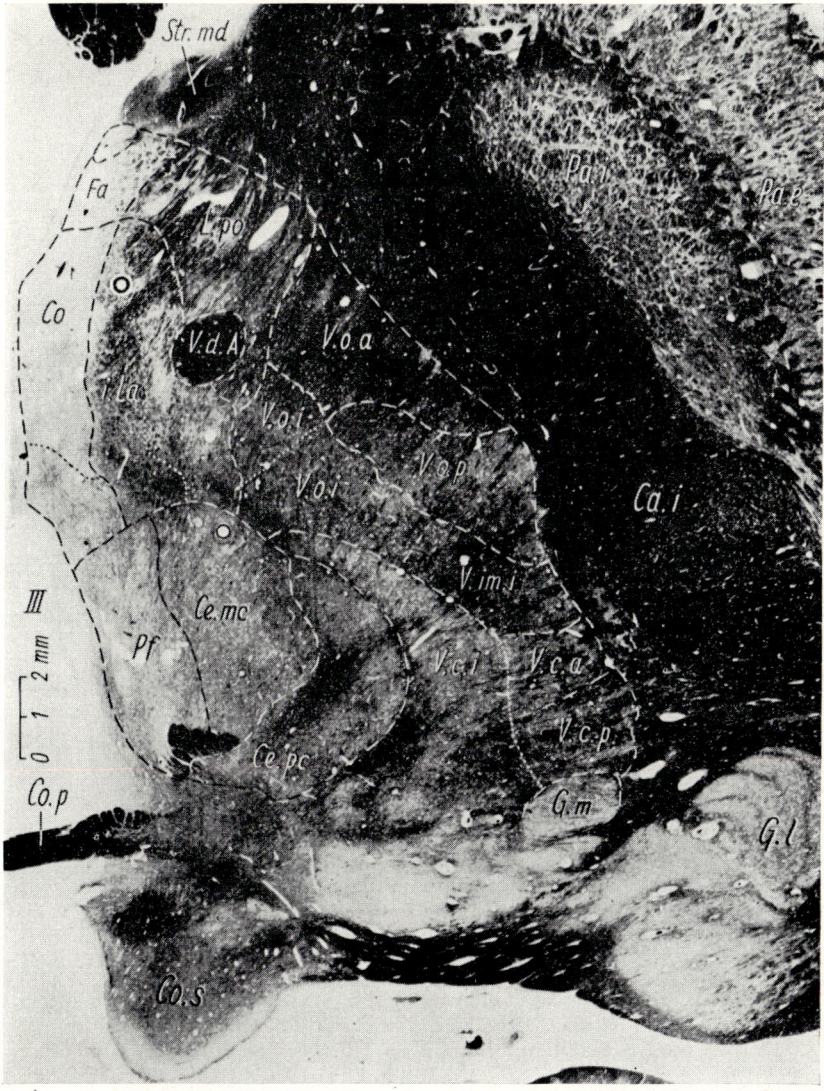

Figure 29.2 Horizontal section of the (normal) right human thalamus after fibre staining. Rostral to the centrum medianum nucleus (Ce.mc) extends the rostral, most compact part of the intralaminar nuclei (i.La), in which the intralaminar target is situated frontal and medial to the VdA (mamillothalamic tract). The downward prolongation of the target of the medial nucleus is placed in the rostral border of the centrum medianum (Ce.mc).

of gnats, from the bed-linen, became so severe that she suffered from it even though recognizing it to be nonsense. After a depressive episode, in which she was inhibited and mournful, neglecting her housework and her children on account of the obsession and other compulsions, the delusion of blood spots was replaced by a delusion of tar spots, which she felt compelled to remove even when she was aware that the spot seen was not tar. After the third delivery, fear of getting dirtied by her own excrements appeared in addition, with suppression of defecation and compulsive washing. When 22 months of psychotherapy and treatment with neuroleptics and electroconvulsions did not result in any enduring improvement, the Psychiatric University Hospital sent her for operation. During the stereotactic operation, stimulation 25–50 times per second in the left rostral intralaminar nuclei slowed down the counting backwards. After these nuclei had been coagulated by four high-frequency coagulations at 70 °C, as were also the medial-thalamic nuclei, the patient was very tired and aspontaneous, and did no longer feel the urgent need to wash each finger that had been touched.

On the 5th day after the operation, she exhibited weakness of recent memory and psychomotor akinesia. Not until the third postoperative week were the fear of getting dirty in the lavatory and the compulsive washing reduced. She wanted to return home to do her housework and to be with the three children and was able to do so, first with the help of her mother and after 6 months quite alone. Nineteen months after the operation she had completely recovered with no undesirable side-effects according to her own and her mother's judgement, so that no relapse occurred when the husband sought a divorce.

Of 40 patients with a malignant obsessive-compulsive syndrome, 27 have been treated with unilateral stereotactic coagulation of the rostral intralaminar and medial-thalamic nuclei, and 13 with bilateral operations. They were observed for more than 6 months after the interventions (Table 29.1). In 16 patients (40%) the operation has given relief (90–100%), in 14 (35%) there has been great improvement (50–80%), and in 10 (25%) the results have been poor (10–40%). Of the 16 patients with relief, the 10 who have been operated upon unilaterally have experienced no undesirable side-effects, and of the six operated upon bilaterally, three have undesirable side-effects (two, severe amnesia; one, psychomotor akinesia). Among the 14 well-improved (50–80%) patients, five have lasting, although mild, undesirable side-effects. Of the 11 unilaterally operated patients, however, only four have side-effects.

If the compulsive perseveration or iteration concerns motor behaviour only, the patients belong to the group of generalized tic disease, or Gilles de la Tourette syndrome. Of the nine patients on whom we operated for these motor compulsions, all three with a unilateral operation have almost complete relief on the contralateral side; of six with bilateral operations, three are almost completely relieved (90–100%) from the Gilles de la Tourette syndrome, and three have marked improvement (Table 29.2). One patient needed a third operation on account of a relapse during an understandable depressive reaction after the second operation. She later recovered. To abolish the cries and the verbal expressions or compulsions an additional lesion was required in the inner part of the oral ventral nuclei (V.o.i.).

With the same intralaminar-medial thalamotomy we have treated three cases of phobias. Both patients operated upon bilaterally have complete relief from the fear of food intake in the presence of others, whereas the erythrophobia of the third patient has been only partially improved by one left-sided intervention. All three are continuing to practise a demanding profession.

Thus it is demonstrated that coagulation of intralaminar and medial-thalamic nuclei always improves and often removes obsessive-compulsive neuroses, phobias, and motor compulsions like tics, cries and coprolalia (Gilles de la Tourette syndrome). The difference between these three

Table 29.1 Results of intralaminar-medial thalamotomy for obsessive-compulsive symptoms. Notice the small number of side-effects after unilateral operations.

Improvement %	Results of intralaminar-medial thalamotomy for obsessive-compulsive symptoms ( ) = with side effects		
	Bilateral operation	Unilateral operation	Total
90–100	6 (3)	10 (0)	16 (3)
50–80	3 (2)	11 (3)	14 (5)
10–40	4 (3)	6 (1)	10 (4)
Total	13 (8)	27 (4)	40 (12)

Table 29.2 Postoperative improvement of Gilles de la Tourette syndrome related to unilateral and bilateral operations and side-effects.

Improvement %	Number of patients		
	Unilateral operation	Bilateral operation	Total
90–100	1 (0)	3 (0)	4 (0)
50–80	2 (1)	3 (1)	5 (2)
Total	3 (1)	6 (1)	9 (2)

indications is that the compulsive cries and coprolalia in Gilles de la Tourette cases require an additional lesion in the thalamic nuclear area which represents articulatory movements in the inner part of the oral ventral nuclei (V.o.i.). It is remarkable that obsessive-compulsive neuroses could be completely relieved by a unilateral operation in two-fifths of the cases.

This is attained by elimination of both the disturbed regulation of the truncothalamic system and the overdominant self-representation produced by the prefrontal circuits. The disinhibition and dominance of the medio-thalamic–prefrontal circuits is the neurophysiological mechanism corresponding to the hypertrophy of conscience in obsessive-compulsive patients. The impulse component, the absurdly dominant formal perseveration and iteration experienced in all three conditions, has its neurobiological counterpart in a malintegrated actualization of different systems for impulsion and activity (Figure 29.1).

The inactivation of the rostral intralaminar nuclei of the thalamus for compulsive symptoms and of the medial nuclei for obsessive symptoms has proven to be effective.

These clear therapeutic results validate the presented psychobiological theory of compulsive symptoms.

In summary, stereotactic coagulations of intralaminar and medial-thalamic nuclei substantially improve, or even in the long run remove, obsessive-compulsive symptoms in patients with compulsive neuroses, phobias, tics and generalized tic disease, and in anankastic psychopaths. This type of stereotactic operation was developed from psychophysiological theory that compulsive symptoms are due to malintegrated regulation of the psychical activity by overdominance of the truncothalamic system, which regulates this activity.

REFERENCES

Dieckmann G & Hassler R (1968). Reizexperimente zur Funktion des Putamen der Katze. *J. Hirnforsch.*, **10**, 187

Freeman, W & Watts, JW (1950). Psychosurgery. In the treatment of mental disorders and intractable pain. 2nd. ed. Springfield, Ill.: Charles P. Thomas

Hassler, R (1948). Über die Thalamus-Stirnhirn-verbindungen beim Menschen. *Nervenarzt*, **19**, 9

Hassler, R (1949). Über die Rinden-und Stammhirn-anteile des menschlichen Thalamus. *Psychiat. Neurol, med. Psychol.* (*Lpz*). **1**, 181

Hassler, R & Dieckmann, G. (1967). Stereotaxic treatment of compulsive and obsessive symptoms. *Confin. neurol.* (*Basel*) **29,** 152

Hassler, R & Dieckmann, G (1970). Traitement stéréotaxique des tics et cris inarticulés ou coprolaliques considérés comme phénomène d'obsession motrice ou cours de la maladie de Gilles de la Tourette. *Rev. neurol.* (Paris) **123,** 89

Montanelli RP & Hassler R (1964). Motor effects elicited by stimulation of the pallido-thalamic system in the cat. In: *Lectures on the Diencephalon* (Eds Bargmann & Schade), p. 56. Amsterdam: Elsevier.

PART VII

ELECTROPHYSIOLOGICAL STUDIES IN PSYCHOSURGICAL PATIENTS

CHAPTER 30

Two-way radio communication with the brain in psychosurgical patients

J M R DELGADO, S OBRADOR &
J G MARTIN-RODRIGUEZ

The experimental study of brain functions in both animals and man requires the use of suitable methodology which should not interfere with the physiological activities to be explored. One of the significant developments in this field is the utilization of radio links for sending and receiving electrical information to and from the brain of experimental subjects while they enjoy complete behavioural freedom. In this report we discuss some recent technical innovations and describe two cases demonstrating their clinical application.

METHODS
Implantation of electrodes
This is a well-known procedure widely used in laboratories around the world in a variety of animal species ranging from rats to chimpanzees. In general, assemblies of up to 100 electrodes are implanted stereotactically within the brain and later connected with recording or stimulating instruments by means of wires, when studies are conducted in the awake animal (Delgado, 1964a).
    Similar procedures are also currently used in human patients for diagnostic or therapeutic purposes (Ramey & O'Doherty, 1960). Usually the electrodes remain implanted for a limited period of days or weeks, but in some cases the study has been prolonged up to 2 years. The main handicaps of these procedures are the presence of sockets outside the scalp and the need to employ connecting wires which restrain mobility and may interfere with the free expression of spontaneous behaviour.

Two-way radio link
An important methodological advance towards establishing two-way communication with the brain of free-moving subjects has been the use of radio links to send electrical stimulation or to record cerebral electrical activity.
    Radio stimulation of the brain in primates has been described by several workers (see bibliography in Delgado, 1964a). The method developed in our laboratory has been improved recently to increase reliability, to augment the number of channels, and to decrease the size of the instrumentation. At

present, our radio stimulator consists of a sensitive (1 μV) microminiaturized (10 mm × 10 mm × 25 mm) superheterodine receiver which controls a stimulator included in a specially designed chip of integrated circuits hermetically sealed in a ceramic capsule measuring 12 mm × 15 mm × 3 mm. Four different channels of stimulation are available with independent control of frequency (1–100 Hz), pulse duration (0·1–1 ms) and intensity (0–3 mA). Communication is established by FM radio waves in the 100 MHz band with four subcarrier oscillators working in the 100–500 kHz band. The intensity of stimulation is controlled by a constant current transistor to assure reliability of current in spite of changes in biological impedance.

EEG telemetry is accomplished by means of a miniature FM–FM amplifier–transmitter combination and a telemetry receiver working in the 216 MHz band, as described in earlier publications (Delgado, 1969).

The combination of radio stimulator and EEG telemetry constitutes the *Stimoceiver* (*stim*ulator and EEG r*eceiver*) which has been used by our group for investigation of cerebral functions in monkeys, chimpanzees, and man (Delgado, Mark, Sweet, Ervin, Weiss, Bach-y-Rita & Hagiwara, 1968).

Case report of Stimoceiver application
The Stimoceiver has been used in patient M.N., a 35-year-old white male worker with a history of epileptic attacks for more than 10 years and recent clinical evidence of a tumour in his left temporal lobe. Depth electrodes with a total of 14 contacts were stereotactically implanted in the left frontotemporal region. Duration of the study was 1 week, after which, in the light of the findings obtained, craniotomy was performed for removal of a tumour in the left temporal lobe.

During the week of studies, electrical recordings and stimulations were performed at all points, and contact 4 located in the head of the caudate nucleus was selected for repeated radio stimulation while conversation with the patient was tape-recorded. Stimulation parameters of 100 Hz, 0·5 ms of pulse duration and 0·8 mA of intensity were applied for 5 s at intervals of at least 3 min, or even longer when after-effects were evident. As shown by direct observation and by analysis of the records, within 30 s after application of caudate stimulation there was a significant change in the patient's mood. Between sessions he was reserved; his conversation was limited and he was concerned about his illness. After caudate stimulations, his spontaneous verbalization increased more than twofold and contained expressions of friendliness and euphoric behaviour which culminated in jokes and loud singing in a gay 'cante jondo' style, accompanied by tapping with his right hand, which lasted for about 2 minutes. The euphoria continued for about 10 minutes and the patient then gradually reverted to his usual, more reserved attitude. This increase in friendliness was observed after three different sessions of caudate stimulation, and did not appear when other areas were tested.

Transdermal stimulation of the brain

In the usual depth electrode implantation procedure, the leads terminate in a socket anchored to the skull and exteriorized through the scalp. The opening of the skin around the site of electrode assembly penetration and the presence of sockets on top of the head represent undesirable handicaps, especially when a programme of therapeutic chronic brain stimulation is contemplated. These problems could be solved by using totally implantable, subcutaneous stimulators activated transdermally by radio waves. With this technique, no wires pierce the skin, the risk of infection is avoided, and there is no cosmetic discomfort or possibility of breaking or dislodging the intracerebral contacts which, however, are electrically accessible at any moment.

For the last 4 years we have been developing subcutaneous stimulators, and testing them in primates, and a summary of results and the present state of the technique are presented here.

(a) *Instrumentation*—Transdermal stimulation of the brain in unrestrained subjects is performed by radio linkage of three different instrumental stages: (1) The *transmitter*, which is a console with solid-state circuitry that originates pulse trains of subcarrier frequencies which modulate the amplitude of a very-high-frequency (VHF) transmitter emitting radio signals through specially designed ground plane antenna. This console directs the remote control of the parameters of stimulation (frequency, pulse duration, intensity, and total duration in each of the four channels). (2) The intermediary *receiver-emitter*, measuring 50 mm × 20 mm × 20 mm, is battery-operated and is carried by the subject. Its role is to receive the modulated VHF signals which are demodulated, amplified, and applied to a primary coil placed on the skin above the subcutaneously implanted stimulator. (3) The final stage is the subcutaneous stimulator, measuring 30 mm in diameter by 12 mm in thickness. It is constructed with integrated circuits and is totally encapsulated in epoxy resin, covered with sylastic. This stimulator has an exposed platinum base used as indifferent electrode and terminates in four platinum leads insulated with Teflon except at the tips, to be implanted stereotactically in the preselected cerebral targets. The subcutaneous stimulator has a coil which, by transformer action, receives the electrical field of the primary coil of the receiver-emitter located outside of the skin. A voltage is thus generated at the subcarrier frequency which is used, depending on its frequency, to charge a storage capacitor in order to provide power, or to activate any of the four channels. A pulse-width modulation technique is used to transmit stimulation intensity information. In this way, gross misalignment between emitting and receiving coils is permissible without affecting the performance of the instrument. The output of the stimulator is constant current, the aim being to avoid fluctuations of intensity and to compensate for any changes in biological impedance.

(b) *Animal experiments*—Results presented here are based on studies of the following animals: (1) Chimpanzee Suzi, a 12 kg female with two subcutaneous stimulators implanted for 10 months; (2) Gibbons: Dakki a 4·6 kg female with implants for 3 months; and Coti, a 5·4 kg male with implants for

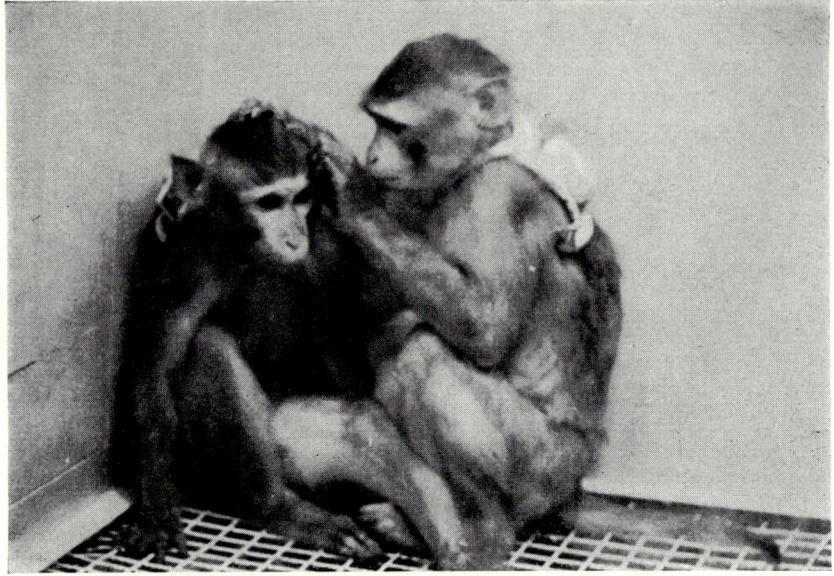

Figure 30.1 These two monkeys engaged in spontaneous grooming have brain stimulators implanted in their backs. The system is totally subcutaneous. A harness carries the electronic link which receives radio signals, sending them through the intact skin to the subcutaneous instrument. This transdermal technique permits therapeutic long-term programmed stimulation of the brain in man.

18 months; (3) Rhesus monkeys: 7 females and 4 males ranging from 3·1–5·8 kg, with total implantation times ranging from 4–25 months. Some of these animals are still alive and in good health (Figure 30.1).

(c) *Surgery for implantation*—Under diabutal anaesthesia, the animal was placed in the stereotactic instrument. Two incisions of about 40 mm were made, one on the back just below the neck and the other on top of the head. The terminal leads of the stimulator were threaded subcutaneously between the two incisions. The stimulator was then placed subcutaneously through the incision on the back and sutured to the fascia, and the wound was closed in layers. Each electrode was then implanted stereotactically according to the usual technique (Delgado, 1964b), with the difference that as there was no external plug, the wound was completely closed. Recovery was uneventful in all cases.

(d) *Tolerance*—No infections or rejections have occurred. In all cases, the implanted stimulator was enclosed in a reactive capsule of perfectly smooth connective tissue. In two cases, this capsule was surgically opened and closed again in order to replace defective instruments. Subcutaneous leads were also encapsulated with reactive connective tissue without causing any complication.

(e) *Electronic reliability*—During the initial stage of instrumental development, after a few months of successful operation, one implanted unit functioned improperly, another had a broken lead, and in a third unit the soldering point of the ground became detached. Spot-welding technique, use of ultra-flexible subcutaneous leads, and electronic improvements in circuit design solved these problems, and for the last 2 years no electronic failures have occurred. Penetration of tissue fluids inside the instrument, known to be a problem in cardiac pacemakers, has not been observed in our subcutaneous stimulators.

(*f*) *Biological reliability*—Depending on the implantation site and stimulation parameters, a variety of effects were induced in the test animals, including: (1) autonomic, such as pupillary, respiratory and cardiovascular responses; (2) somatic, such as flexion or extension of the limbs; (3) behavioural, with a wide range of emotional and social manifestations; and (4) inhibitory, including decreases in motor and behavioural reactivity.

In all cases, the patterns of response were reproducible throughout the experimentation period up to 25 months with less than 20% of variation from initial thresholds. Repetition of stimulations, which in some cases totalled several thousand, had no demonstrable effect on pattern of response or threshold, proving the reliability of both instrumental performance and biological reactivity.

(*g*) *Controls—Transdermal experiments*. As the whole stimulation system was located underneath the skin, direct testing of its electronic performance was not possible, and its proper functioning was inferred from the behavioural responses evoked. However, electronic testing in an actual biological situation was necessary, especially at the early stages of instrumental development. For this purpose, two rhesus monkeys were prepared with a transdermal stimulator implanted as usual in the back of the animal with its subcutaneous leads threaded underneath the neck skin up to the top of the head, where they terminated in a socket anchored to the skull and exteriorized on top of the head. In addition, 14 electrodes were implanted in the brain. Their terminals in two additional sockets, also anchored to the skull, were directly accessible on the head. By using jumpers between the head sockets, transdermal stimulation could be channelled to any selected intracerebral point, which also could be stimulated by direct wires connected to a standard stimulator. In this way we compared the two procedures. Voltage, milliamperage, impedance, and wave shapes were monitored in every case by means of a two-channel Taktronix oscilloscope. Spontaneous electrical activity of the brain was also recorded on different days. The total duration of these experiments was 6 months, and the following results were obtained: (1) Identical effects were recorded when the brain was stimulated with a direct wire connection and with a transdermal stimulator. (2) Frequency, pulse duration, and intensity of transdermal stimulations were reliable throughout the test period. (3) The subcutaneous stimulators functioned properly in spite of considerable variations in the position of the emitting primary coil located outside the skin, and tolerance values were as follows: Distance of the coil from the skin, up to 15 mm. Off-centre position between coil and subcutaneous stimulator, up to

17 mm. Coil inclination, up to 45 degrees. Beyond these limits, there was a quick collapse of energy and no stimulation could be applied.

Controls were also performed to test the possible accidental activation of the transdermal unit by spurious sources of energy. As transformer action was necessary, this accident was very improbable in the absence of a suitable coil at a short distance and with a proper frequency. We tested antenna effects at a distance of 1 metre, with energy up to 10 watts and frequencies from 100 kHz to 300 MHz with negative results.

(*h*) *Advantages and limitations*—The subcutaneous stimulator receives its power transdermally, and since it has no batteries and is well tolerated by the organism, it can remain implanted indefinitely, ready for use at any moment by remote control of the chosen channel and with the selected parameters of stimulation. The instrument is therefore suitable for long-term programmes of brain stimulation and can remain as standby if treatment should be resumed. Also, it offers the possibility of reaching sensory pathways or structures within the brain, circumventing damaged sensory receptors.

Transdermal stimulation shares the limitations of standard procedures for brain excitation (Delgado, 1969a), and to dispel laymen's possible fears about push-button control we must remember that electricity applied to neurons is only a monotonous, non-specific stimulus that does not carry specific messages. By electricity we can activate pre-existing functions of the brain but we cannot create them, and brain stimulation is a cruder (and far less powerful and influential) method than the normal means of reaching the brain through education and propaganda acting as physiological sensory inputs.

Another limitation is that feedback from the brain is lacking and there is no information about cerebral activity, other than the observed evoked effects. This handicap could be solved by telemetering brain waves through the intact skin with an instrument similar in size to the brain stimulator. This transdermal EEG recorder is already working satisfactorily on our laboratory bench, and it can be predicted that in the near future transdermal Stimoceivers will allow two-way communication to and from the depth of the brain through the intact skin.

CASE REPORT OF TRANSDERMAL BRAIN STIMULATION

Patient F.F. was a 30-year-old white male worker whose left brachial plexus was damaged in a car accident. The left arm was paralysed and a phantom limb appeared, causing intolerable pain that could not be alleviated with drugs or physical therapy and seriously affected the well-being of the patient. After other treatments had failed, destructive brain surgery was contemplated, and as an alternative, repeated electrical stimulation of the forebrain was proposed and accepted. After a lengthy period of thorough clinical and psychological testing, an operation was performed under local anaesthesia to implant a subcutaneous stimulator on top of the head, underneath the scalp, and its four electrodes were placed stereotactically and bilaterally, by Leksell's technique, in the septum and head of the caudate nucleus (Figure 30.2, 3). Recovery was uneventful, and these implantations did not modify the patient's

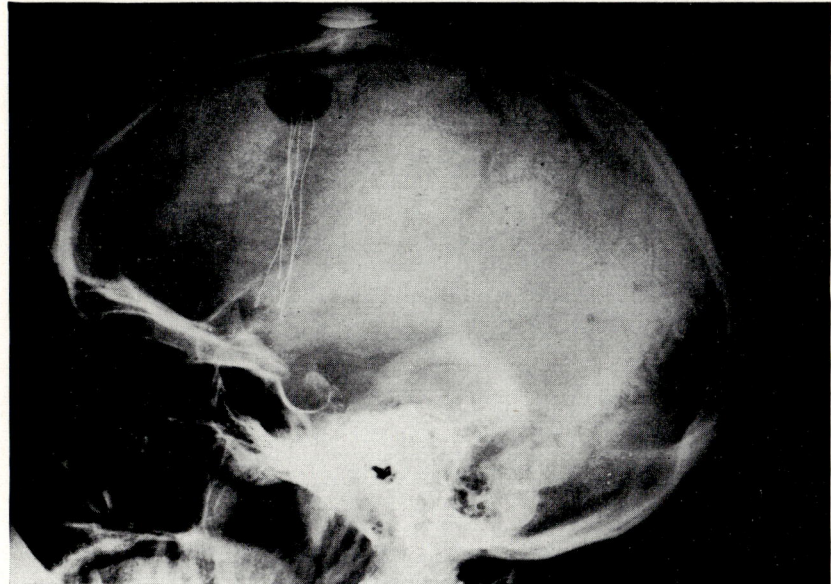

Figure 30.2 Lateral roentgenogram, showing the implanted electrodes to the multi-channel transdermal brain stimulator.

clinical situation. One week later, programmed stimulation was initiated and performed three to five times per week. During 1 hour of tape-recorded tests and interviews, about 10 stimulations were applied, including periods of 5s and two periods of 5 s 'on' 5 s 'off' stimulations, for 1 minute. These excitations were followed by a lasting improvement of the patient's state, accompanied by a notable decrease in his previous hostility.

Evaluation of clinical results and psychological changes require cautious interpretation and lengthy follow-up, but 2 months of study of this case has shown that the subcutaneous instrumentation is comfortable for the patient, being tolerated well and giving reliable performance. To our knowledge, this is the first case of clinical use of transdermal stimulation of the brain in man, and it extends the application of a technique with demonstrated usefulness in primate research.

SUMMARY

Two-way communication with the brain of free-moving subjects, for both recording and stimulation, can be established by radio link with the instrument called Stimoceiver. It has four channels with remote control of pulse duration, frequency, and intensity, plus four channels for telerecording of brain waves. In the case reported here, an epileptic patient showed lasting euphoria and increased friendliness after stimulation of the caudate nucleus.

Transdermal communication with the brain can be established by electromagnetic coupling between an instrument implanted subcutaneously and a coil placed outside of the skin and activated by a radio link. Transdermal stimulation has been tested in 1 chimpanzee, 2 gibbons, and 11 rhesus monkeys for periods of up to 25 months. Tissue tolerance, practicability of the procedure, and electronic and biological reliability were all satisfactory. As the instrument has no batteries, it can be used indefinitely.

Transdermal brain stimulation has also been used for the first time in

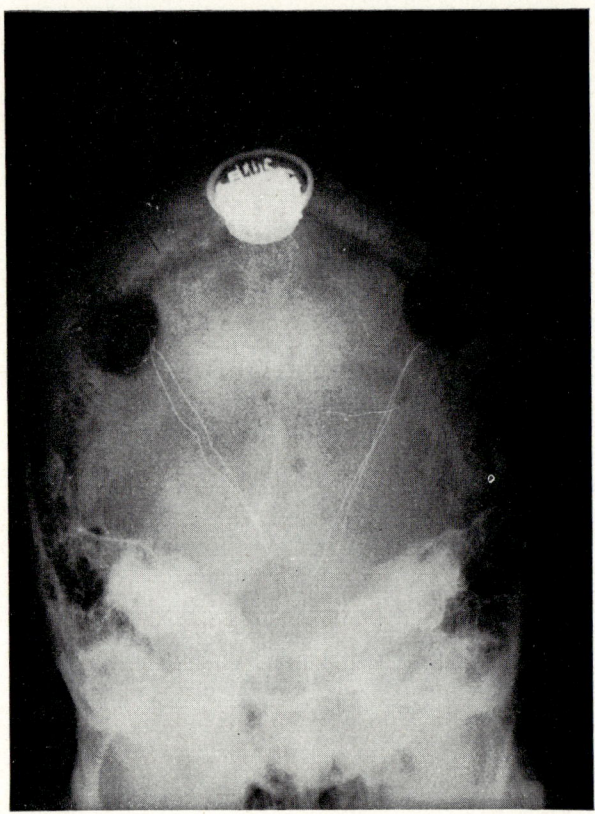

Figure 30.3 Anteroposterior view of the same case as in Figure 30.2, demonstrating the implanted electrodes and the subcutaneous brain stimulator.

a patient with a phantom limb. Programmed stimulation of the septum diminished the otherwise intractable pain and decreased the spontaneous hostility of the patient. Evaluation of therapeutic results will require a long follow-up, but the feasibility of transdermal long-term, remotely controlled, programmed stimulation of the brain is regarded as well demonstrated.

This transdermal methodology may open a new and fascinating therapeutic approach. Thus, in some patients suffering from so-called 'functional' disorders (some types of pain, psychic disturbances, etc.) transdermal long-term and programmed stimulation of different reward and pleasure areas may perhaps set up new and dominant cerebral pacemakers that could compete with the pathological activity already established in other parts of the brain.

ACKNOWLEDGEENTS

This research was supported in part by the New York Foundation, the March Foundation, and the Rodriguez Pascual Foundation. We gratefully acknowledge the collaboration of Mr Gerhard Weiss and Mr Vaino Lipponen in the development of the subcutaneous brain stimulator. We also acknowledge the collaboration of Dr J. Santo Domingo and Miss Adela Alonso in the psychological evaluation of the patients, Dr J. Carbonell in the EEG recordings and A. Parreno in the technical electronic procedures.

REFERENCES

Delgado JMR (1964a). Free behavior and brain stimulation. In: *International Review of Neurobiology* (Eds Pfeiffer & Smythies), Vol. VI, p. 349. New York: Academic Press.
Delgado JMR (1964b). Electrodes for extracellular recording and stimulation. In: *Electrophysiological Methods, Vol. V, Part A, Physical Techniques in Biological Research* (Ed Nastuk), p. 88. New York: Academic Press.
Delgado JMR (1969). Radio stimulation of the brain in primates and man. *Anesth. Analg.*, **48**, 529
Delgado JMR, Mark V, Sweet W, Ervin F, Weiss G, Bach-y-Rita G & Hagiwara R (1968). Intracerebral radio stimulation and recording in completely free patients. *J. nerv. ment. Dis.*, **147**, 329
Ramey ER & O'Doherty DS (1960). *Electrical Studies on the Unanesthetized Brain*. New York: Paul B Hoeber.

CHAPTER 31

Depth electrode investigations of the limbic system with radiostimulation, electrolytic lesions and histochemical techniques

LEOPOLD HOFSTATTER & MAKRAM GIRGIS

INTRODUCTION

Recent investigations have shown that dysfunction of the limbic system of the brain underlies many disturbances of emotion and may result in some psychotic manifestations. The interseizure symptomatology of some patients with psychomotor (limbic) epilepsy may be indistinguishable from that of paranoid schizophrenia. Medial sclerosis of the hippocampus is found in nearly all cases of limbic epilepsy. Irritative lesions in or near the limbic cortex give rise to epileptic discharges accompanied by emotional feelings of terror, fear, strangeness, unreality, sadness, wanting to be alone, and feelings of paranoid nature (MacLean, 1970). There may be also distortions of perception, again reminding one of the endogenous and toxic psychosis. MacLean thinks that of all the clinical entities there is perhaps none that has a greater potentiality for shedding light on mechanisms underlying psychic functions in man than psychomotor or limbic epilepsy.

We have undertaken an extensive study of the limbic system of the brain in the hope of better understanding its normal function and its dysfunction, both in man and in primates. It is obvious that in dealing with such questions as depersonalization, one must depend solely on subjective reports of patients, but there are some psychotic manifestations concerning which animal experimentation is helpful in elucidating the underlying neural mechanisms. Knowledge about the correlation of the site of the lesion and the symptomatology will shed a great deal of light, we hope, on the relationship of the limbic system to the psychoses.

Study of the neurophysiological correlates of emotions requires the collection of data and the introduction of experimental variables without disturbing the phenomena under consideration. Restraint of the animal, presence of human observers, and isolation from sociological and ecological surroundings represent serious artifacts in the study of emotions and have been a deterrent for research into their neuronal mechanisms. We have, accordingly, used the newly developed technique of radiostimulation for the study of the limbic system of the brain on completely unrestrained animals. By electrical stimulation of appropriate parts of the limbic system, not only can abnormal electrical activity be detected during fits of rage and induced assaultive behaviour, but it is also possible to turn off and prevent the outburst by stimulating or creating therapeutic lesions in the proper limbic structures.

The natural vulnerability of the limbic system to mechanical injury and its peculiar chemistry is a significant piece of evidence that has been observed recently. The biochemical aspect of emotional states is an area which has not been well studied. Our earlier histochemical studies have indicated a very intense acetylcholinesterase enzyme (AChE) activity in the structures of the limbic system (Girgis, 1968). Recent studies have shown that application of acetylcholinesterase inhibitors or cholinomimetics in such limbic structures as the septum, amygdala and lateral hypothalamus, caused an increased aggressiveness and hyperactivity in animals. This suggests that the changed behaviour is a result of disturbed function of neural mechanisms which are normally subject to cholinergic mediation. It can be seen from these experiments that the accumulation of acetylcholine in certain limbic structures may have significance for a clinical picture of intoxication by cholinesterase inhibitors.

METHODS
Histochemical studies
Frozen sections 50 μm thick were stained by a modification of Koelle's technique for acetylcholinesterase enzyme (for details of this technique, see Girgis, 1968). The cebus and squirrel monkeys were used for this study. Neostigmine (an inhibitor of AChE) was injected into limbic structures that showed high AChE activity in our histochemical preparations mentioned above. The rate of injection was 1 μl/min to a total volume not exceeding 10 μl. In other animals intracranial injection of a cholinomimetic drug, Mecholyl (methacholine), was initiated 1 week after surgery and made in different limbic areas.

Surgical procedures
The major part of the results reported in this study is based on investigations carried out on non-human primates. Stereotactic multilead electrodes, and in some cases chemitrodes, were placed in the monkey brain and permanently fixed to the calvarium. The precision of stereotactic localization was confirmed in other series of experiments, where small electrolytic lesions were placed in selected parts of the limbic system, such as the amygdala, thalamus, and hypothalamus, and then tracked in stained frozen sections.

Patients with temporal lobe seizures or psychomotor equivalents seen by us in the Neurology Clinic were referred to the neurosurgeon for depth electrode investigation and subsequent surgery for the relief of their conditions. Long-term medication had not been of any avail. These patients were afflicted with severe emotional disturbances, some with aggressive behaviour between or after seizures. Depth electrodes were placed in limbic structures such as the amygdala and hippocampus.

Radiostimulation of the brain
Two weeks after the surgical operation, the monkey is placed in a restraining chair, the spontaneous bioelectrical activity of its brain is recorded, and the effects of radiostimulations are tested. Then, leads connecting the terminal socket of the electrodes with a radiostimulator are strapped to the back of the monkey. This system, developed in collaboration with Dr José Delgado of Yale University, permits the independent remote control of pulse duration, frequency and intensity in four channels. This instrument has a high frequency carrier of 100 MHz. With the radiostimulator on its back and connected to a predetermined cerebral point, the monkey is released in the cage. The radiostimulation is then applied continuously for 5 s every minute to test the overall behaviour changes, and the effect of offering food, and of threatening the animal by waving leather catching gloves. Finally, the radiostimulation is applied continuously for 5–10 min or longer to determine fatiguability of brain stimulation. Behaviour was recorded throughout by time-lapse, closed-circuit video recordings and the experiment concluded with 1 h of control period. The entire procedure was repeated on at least fifteen different days, providing more than 200 stimulations of each cerebral point.

Electrolytic lesions
Very small stereotactic electrolytic lesions are placed in certain selected parts of the limbic system from which we determined the effects of stimulation. Bilateral electrolytic lesions are made by passing 3·0 mA anodal d.c. current through the uninsulated tip of a stainless steel electrode for about 20 seconds. Their behaviour is then studied. At the conclusion of the experiments, the animals are perfused with formalin, their brains removed, frozen, sectioned at 50 μm and stained with cresyl and Luxolfast-blue for reconstruction of the electrode tracts and lesions.

RESULTS
The results of all our *histochemical* studies indicate that the most intense cholinergic reaction is in the 'limbic system' of the brain (Figures 31.1,2,3). The first section (Figure 31.1) shows clearly the cingulum bundle which, arising near the orbito-frontal region from the septum, sweeps around the genu of the corpus callosum passing backwards and downwards to end in the para-hippocampal region. The magnocellular part of the basal amygdaloid nucleus shows very high activity of acetylcholinesterase enzyme. Intracerebral microinjection of Neostigmine (a cholinesterase inhibitor) in this amygdaloid nucleus (Figure 31.3) resulted in high amplitude continuous spike activity in the region of the basal nucleus (Figure 31.4). This was associated with ipsilateral smacking of the lips and contralateral jerking movements of the limbs. The bioelectrical activity mentioned above develops 2 h after the injection. In the meantime the animal becomes restless, hyperactive and will

bite hard on the gloves when presented to him. When the jerking movement starts, the animal will be less aggressive although fully awake. These activities are suppressed by atropine.

The results of *radiostimulation* of freely moving animals through implanted electrodes show that the lateral hypothalamus is a very important limbic structure for the excitation and integration of autonomic, somatomotor and endocrine effects seen in aggressive behaviour. Our experiments demonstrate clearly the paucity of evoked effects in the monkey when stimulated under restraint and the great increase in organization and complexity of the responses when the animal was free in the cage. The results of all our experiments demonstrate that restraint reduces and distorts the normal expression of

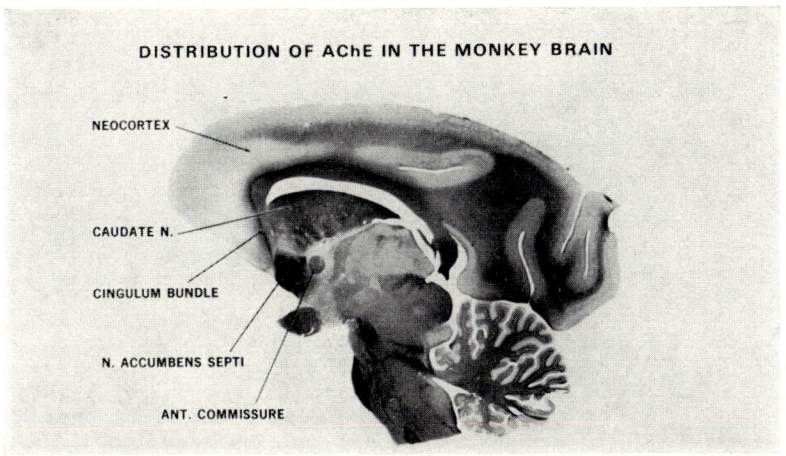

Figure 31.1 Sagittal section of the squirrel monkey brain showing cholinergic activity in the limbic structures. Note the cingulum bundle sweeping around the genu of the corpus callosum.

behavioural responses. The aggressive behaviour evoked by telestimulation of the lateral hypothalamus was well organized, skilfully performed and with properly directed attack. It was evident that brain stimulation had created a state of increased aggressiveness, but it was also clear that the animal directed its hostility intelligently and according to his previous experience, likes and dislikes, indicating an excellent processing of sensory information and demonstrating that brain stimulation had induced a 'drive' and not a stereotyped motor response. Excitation with less than 1 mA evoked offensive–defensive responses which included pupillary dilation, grimacing, threatening gesture, and attempt to escape. As after-effects, there were threatening, staring, thrusting the head forward, and opening the mouth with low tone vocalization. At this time the animal responded with restlessness and greater motor activity than usual if a glove was presented within reach attempting to grab and bite it. In these experiments seizure discharges were absent; the

228 *Surgical Approaches in Psychiatry*

observed after-effects were not related, therefore, with detectable electrical disturbances. In quite a number of these experiments it was quite clear that the animals dislike these rage-eliciting cerebral stimulations. At the height of his rage reaction, the animal would pull out the connecting wire and bite it, if he can, so as to end the stimulation experiment. Therefore, the radio receiver and the wires connected to the electrodes had to be protected by special jacket

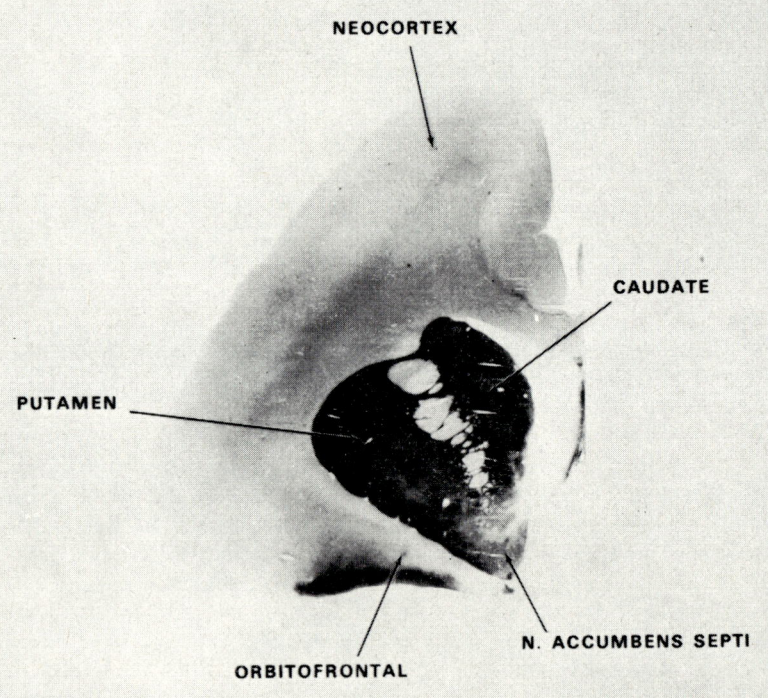

Figure 31.2 Frontal section of the monkey brain showing cholinesterase activity in the basal ganglia and nucleus accumbens septi. Note the mild activity in the posterior orbito-frontal cortex. This is the only part of the neocortex that shows clear enzymatic activity.

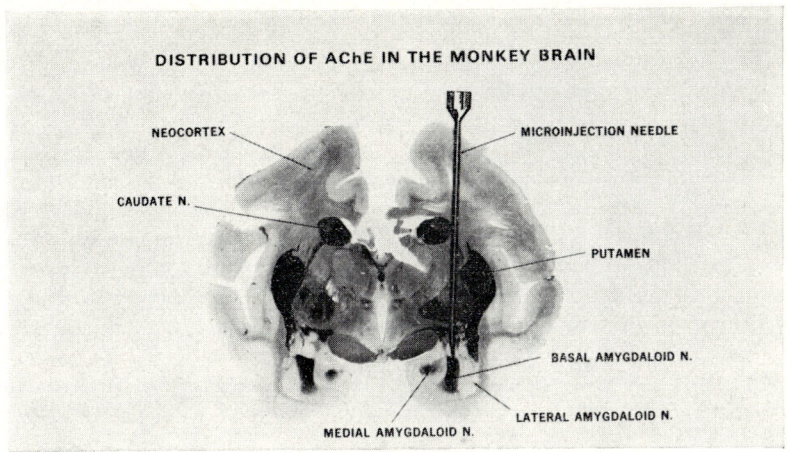

Figure 31.3 Frontal section of the monkey brain showing cholinesterase activity in the limbic structures. The arrow indicates microinjection in the basal part of amygdala.

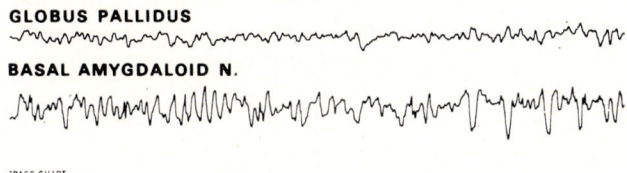

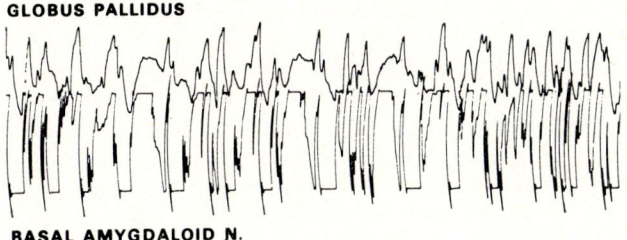

Figure 31.4 The effect of neostigmine injection in the basal part of amygdala. Note the high amplitude spike discharges appearing in the amygdala and pallidum.

and helmet. It is difficult to know how the animal feels, but we can deduce whether the animal likes or dislikes these stimulations because of its negative reinforcing properties. By adding conditioning to the experimental design, we hope to have more information, in future experiments, of how the animal feels about what we are doing to it.

The radiostimulation experiments involving the amygdaloid region were located in the most medial part of the cortical nucleus of the amygdala (the stereotaxic co-ordinates according to the atlas of the cebus monkey brain were: AP 15·5, L 6·0, H-7). Investigation of this part of the amygdala has confirmed the pacifying possibilities of electrical stimulation of the brain. During the stimulation the animal's facial expression appeared more peaceful and he performed no threatening or aggressive acts. In contrast to the aggressive animals mentioned above, radiostimulation blocked their usual aggressiveness so effectively that these animals could be caught inside the cage without danger or difficulty. From these experiments on the amygdala we have not been able so far to elicit aggressive behaviour, as was the case in the hypothalamus. However, in these experiments behavioural patterns suggesting fear have been elicited from stimulation within the amygdaloid complex.

Different areas of the brain have varying degrees of fatiguability. While the motor cortex, for example, is known to respond after a few seconds of electrical stimulation, the hypothalamic and amygdaloid structures mentioned above have been stimulated continuously for a very long time without fatigue.

Following stereotaxic *lesions* in the amygdala, the monkeys were allowed 2 weeks to recover from the lesions. With bilateral lesions the monkeys recovered very quickly and after a period of 10 days, the animals began to gain weight. The weight gain was particularly more apparent in the squirrel monkeys which looked very muscular and strong. However, these animals appeared to express a diminished aggressiveness to other animals and to humans. It was never noticed during a period of 1 y that on any occasion did a lesioned animal exhibit any aggressive posturing or behaviour directed towards other animals. In some monkeys, however, amygdaloid lesions produced restlessness, increased investigative behaviour and a tendency to run away to the highest point in the room.

On the whole, the effects of lesions aimed at the amygdaloid nucleus varied according to the site. Lesions involving the medial amygdaloid area have produced more consistent findings. After the operation, the animals were alert, active and eating well. None of the animals exhibited episodic temporal lobe seizures. Soon, however, the animals became less fearful and showed approach behaviour towards the cage. The animals did not exhibit aggressive responses, and the usual response to any social contact was avoidance by withdrawal or flight. The animals were agile and had nearly normal visuo-motor co-ordination. It is clear, however, that the animals are disinterested in engaging in social interactions and avoided other monkeys.

In the present study we have found measurable changes in monkey behaviour even after unilateral lesions, which however were much greater after bilateral lesions.

Part VII—Electrophysiological Studies

SURFACE EEG OF PATIENT WITH TEMPORAL LOBE EPILEPSY

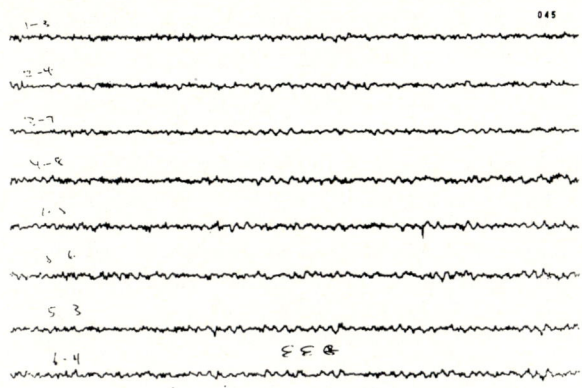

DEPTH EEG OF SAME PATIENT

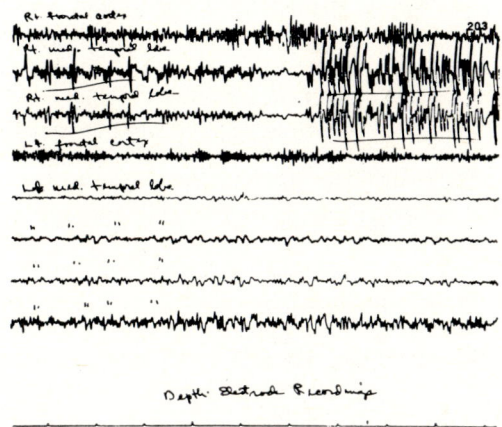

Figure 31.5 The difference between scalp EEG (upper part) and depth recording (lower part). The spike discharge in the medial temporal lobe (traces 2 and 3) is sharply limited.

The results of the surgical procedures on *the human* that are pertinent to the present investigation are as follows: Patient J.K., 27 years old, had had psychomotor seizures and behaviour problems since a very early age following a depressed fracture of the right side of the skull. Right carotid angiogram was carried out and was found to be normal. Pneumoencephalogram revealed mild ventricular dilatation on the right side. The surface EEG did not reveal any focalization. However, a recording with depth electrodes revealed almost continuous spiking in the right medial temporal lobe compatible with epileptogenic focus (Figure 31.5). Because of the clearly psychomotor character of his seizures and intractability, clear-cut spike focus with depth electrodes, and mild ventricular atrophy on the right side, it was decided to do craniotomy, electrocorticogram and anterior temporal lobectomy. The area of the amygdala was found to be tough and associated with some sclerosis.

Patient G.E., 18 years old, had an anterior temporal lobectomy because he had several grand mal seizures since childhood and later became a behavioural management problem and ended up with juvenile authorities. During the operation, the neurosurgeon encountered a large diffuse tumour extending forward towards the orbito-frontal cortex. On histopathological examination, the tumour proved to be a Grade 1 astrocytoma.

After surgery both of these patients improved considerably. Both their seizures and behaviour problems were greatly alleviated.

DISCUSSION

As indicated in the introduction, recent investigations showed that dysfunction of the limbic system underlies many disturbances of emotion and may result in some psychotic manifestations. Psychomotor seizures originating from lesions of the anterior temporal lobe or the orbito-frontal cortex may be preceded by epileptic auras characterized by strong affective or emotional feelings, most frequently of anxiety or fear, rarely of pleasure. These psychomotor seizures themselves occasionally may be accompanied by antisocial behaviour or even acts of violence. Following such seizures, combative behaviour may occur regularly in individual cases as part of a confusional state. Expanding lesions of the tip of the temporal lobe may be associated with sociopathic behavioural patterns, delinquency or psychopathology.

The clinical data presented by us suggest that both the anterior temporal and the orbito-frontal regions in the human brain may function in relation to social behaviour and its associated affective or emotional states. These may be 'models', and our forthcoming discussion on animal studies will elaborate on this. We believe that whatever goes on in the amygdala might be reflected in the orbital cortex of the frontal lobes. The uncinate fasciculus forms a two-way connection between the frontal and temporal cortices and it contains fibres orginating in the amygdala. The importance of the orbito-frontal cortex as a higher centre in the limbic system has been emphasized by us recently (see Girgis, 1971, for details). The orbital cortex as an objective in surgical treatment of mental disorders has been indicated by us quite some time ago (Hofstatter, Smolik & Busch, 1945). Also, here in the Missouri Institute of Psychiatry, a careful retrospective analysis of some of the earlier lobotomy experience has been undertaken. Most of these studies have already indicated that section limited to the autonomic effector areas of the orbital cortex was more effective in modifying psychotic and psychoneurotic disorders (Holden, Itil & Hofstatter, 1970). In a comprehensive paper, Livingston (1969) described clearly on the basis of recent evidence, how the frontal cortex occupies the apex of the major limbic circuits and suggested that a prospective 'second look' at the frontal lobes is indicated.

To investigate the cerebral mechanisms involved in aggression, the traditional approach has been to evaluate changes in behaviour following ablation of portions of nervous tissue or to observe the effects evoked by electrical stimulation of the brain. Stimulation experiments have provided valuable information about cerebral structures related to aggression. In general, however, these studies have had the handicap of the presence of trailing leads, restricted mobility, and distorted behaviour. Our studies mentioned above, using monkeys equipped with intracerebral electrodes and radiostimulators, proved to be a very useful method for studying free behaviour. Effects of brain stimulation were more complex and better organized in the free animal than in the animal under restraint.

When substances of high biological activity are found in the brain, the question of their possible function immediately comes to mind. If, furthermore, such a compound is found to be unevenly distributed, this fact suggests that the compound may take part in some specialized function attached to those regions which are particularly rich in it. A great deal of evidence has been established for tracing the cerebral cholinergic neurons histochemically by staining the brain for AChE. A good example of a system of cholinergic neurons appearing to subserve a particular function is the ascending activating system of the reticular formation (Shute & Lewis, 1967). Thus, hemisection of the midbrain in front of the activating reticular formation produces an EEG characteristic of sleep and an accumulation of acetylcholine in the inactive hemisphere. Anticholinesterases or acetylcholine given intravenously, or applied to the ventricular surfaces in moderate doses, cause arousal, which can be suppressed by atropine. Electrical stimulation of the midbrain reticular formation not only causes arousal, which also is atropine sensitive, but simultaneously increases the amount of acetylcholine released from the surface of the cortex if its destruction has been prevented by an anticholinesterase (Phillis, 1968). 'One is tempted to conclude that arousal is the result of the stimulation of cholinergic neurons in the reticular formation' (Vogt, 1971).

Other areas of the brain which show high cholinergic activity are the basal ganglia; they are very rich in acetylcholine, cholinacetylase and cholinesterase. All of our histochemical studies in mammalian brains, including the primates, point to the fact that the highest AChE enzyme activity to be found in the whole brain is in the limbic system (Girgis, 1968). The enzyme is found both in cells and in terminals. Overactivity of the cholinergic neurons of the corpus striatum appears to be causally related to some signs of Parkinson's disease. The causal relation is probably the basis for the beneficial effect of atropine-like drugs in this disease. It is thus possible to allocate specific motor dysfunctions to the over-activity of striatal cholinergic neurons. Some of the signs of Parkinson's disease are thus believed to result from uninhibited action of striatal cholinergic neurons, and dopamine is held to be the transmitter which normally keeps this activity in check. It is becoming more evident today that a combination of anticholinergic drugs and levodopa has a synergistic therapeutic effect in some patients.

Other limbic structures which show high cholinergic activity are the septal nuclei (particularly the nucleus accumbens septi), hippocampus and amygdala, areas that have been implicated in some emotional disturbances and mental disorders (see Heath, 1969). Lesions in the nucleus accumbens septi produce alterations in irritability, avoidance responses and emotionality that are consistent with schizophrenia. Psychotropic drugs appear to have some predilection of action on hippocampal function as revealed by changes in the EEG. The involvement of hippocampal regions is further supported by the high incidence of birth complications in these individuals who later became mentally ill, since the hippocampus is particularly sensitive to anoxia.

Recently the central effects of anticholinergic drugs (e.g. atropine) have been studied in detail. A comatose condition with sleep pattern (Forrer, 1956) on EEG produced by high doses (32–200 mg or more) of atropine known as 'atropine toxicity therapy' is now being used in certain clinics with some beneficial effects. Scopolamine coma therapy (1–3 mg/kg) has been found to be similarly effective with fewer side-effects. Phelps (1942) pointed out that scopolamine acts as a primary depressant of the cerebrum and causes definite psychic sedation in most cases. Atropine and scopolamine modify the EEG patterns in various pathological states. The use of these compounds in craniocerebral injuries was prompted by laboratory results that indicated a high content of acetylcholine in the cerebrospinal fluid during cerebral trauma or after electroshock therapy (Bornstein, 1946; Ward, 1950). Ward has demonstrated that atropine can be safely given to man in doses of 10 mg daily for amelioration of the symptoms of the post concussion syndrome. Ulett and Johnson (1957) reported that the high-voltage slow activity observed in the process of electroconvulsive therapy was blocked by the administration of atropine and scopolamine. Further studies by Ulett and his colleagues demonstrated that subcutaneous injection of atropine blocked the EEG changes of brain-damaged animals subjected to a series of ECS (see Fukuda, Stern & Ulett, 1959). These authors point out, however, that further studies are needed both in animals and in humans to clarify such questions as to the site and mode of action within the brain of atropine, scopolamine and ECT.

The apparent presence of cholinergic and adrenergic fibres in the limbic system suggest a certain parallel with the peripheral autonomic nervous system. In the hippocampus, for example, histochemical stains have indicated that its main afferent pathways are cholinergic type. On the other hand, radioautographic and fluorescent studies have detected a notable concentration of noradrenaline in the hippocampus and also serotinin studies have indicated a relatively high concentration in the grey matter of the hippocampus. These findings are of special interest in view of evidence that tranquillizing and psychotropic drugs known to affect the metabolism of serotonin and noradrenalin appear to have some predilection of action on hippocampal function as revealed by changes in the EEG (MacLean, 1970). MacLean also points out that the limbic system seems not only to exert powerful influences on the autonomic and neuroendocrine centres, but may also be the *reacting organ* to doubly antagonistic (and probably synergistic) innervation, which is similar in many respects to the autonomic innervation of the peripheral organs.

It is not yet quite clear why the limbic structures are so rich in cholinesterase enzyme. We believe, however, that *AChE has a proctective function, preventing the development of bizarre sensitivity in susceptible cells*. The prevalence of available AChE may ensure that the sensitivity to acetylcholine is maintained within a limited safe range. As a working hypothesis derived from the results of the work mentioned above, we would like to postulate that cerebral mechanisms underlying some emotional disturbances and psychic dysfunction may be related to cholinergic hyperactivity or hypersensitivity, of neurons of certain areas of the limbic system such as the septum, amygdala or hypothalamus. This point was elaborated in the discussion, and the analogy to the pathophysiology of Parkinson's disease was made. The mechanism of distorted neural function as manifested in mental disturbances is best described by Marrazzi: 'When resulting distortions exceed the self-correcting characteristics of the nervous system, there is a failure of cerebral homoeostasis (successful adaptation, i.e. co-ordination of output with input) whose partial or ideally complete restoration is the object of therapy' (Marrazzi, 1966).

An obvious practical conclusion that can be reached from the data reviewed above would be the development of drugs with useful degrees of stability and specificity that block excitatory or mimic inhibitory central transmitters or else agents that promote or block transmitters release, through a cholinergic mechanism or otherwise, and compounds that inhibit the metabolic destruction of inhibitory transmitters. Recent investigations have shown that facilitation of aggressive behaviour was produced by direct cholinergic stimulation of cerebral sites that normally respond to electrical stimulation by aggressive behaviour (Smith, King & Hoebel, 1970). These findings raised the practical possibility that pharmacological manipulation of the cholinergic limbic system could be used in the treatment of pathological aggressive behaviour. Every effort should certainly be made to exploit these potentialities. Koelle (1969) believes that the promising advance in the treatment of Parkinsonism, mentioned above, is a concrete example of what can be accomplished therapeutically by a basic pharmacological approach to diseases of the nervous system.

REFERENCES

Bornstein MB (1946). Presence and action of actylcholine in experimental brain trauma. *J. Neurophysiol.*, **9**, 349

Forrer GR (1956). Symposium on atropine toxicity therapy. *J. nerv. ment. Dis.*, **124**, 256

Girgis M (1968). Histochemical localization of cholinesterase in a rodent, a subprimate and a primate brain. *Histochemie*, **16**, 307

Girgis M (1971). The orbital surface of the frontal lobe of the brain and mental disorders. *Acta Psychiat. Scand.* Suppl., 222

Heath RG (1969). Schizophrenia: Evidence of a pathological immune mechanism. *Proc. amer. psychopath. Ass.*, **58**, 234

Hofstatter L, Smolik EA & Busch AK (1945). Prefrontal lobotomy in the treatment of chronic psychosis; with special reference to section of the orbital areas only. *Arch. Neurol. Psychiat.*, **53**, 125

Holden JMC, Itil TM & Hofstatter L (1970). Prefrontal lobotomy: stepping-stone or pitfall? *Amer. J. Psychiat.*, **127**, 591

Koelle GB (1969). Pharmacology of synaptic transmitters. In: *Basic Mechanisms of the Epilepsies* (Eds Jasper, Ward Jr. and Pope). Boston: Little, Brown & Co.

Livingston KE (1969). The frontal lobes revisited. *Arch. Neurol. Chicago*, **20**, 91

MacLean PD (1970). The limbic brain in relation to psychoses. In: *Physiological Correlates of Emotion*. New York: Academic Press, Inc.

Marrazzi AS (1966). Restoration of cerebral homeostasis, basis of biological treatment. In: *Biological Treatment of Mental Illness* (Ed Rinkel). New York: LC Page & Co.

Phelps ML (1942). The role of the alkaloids of the belladonna plants in clinical anesthesia. *Anesthesiology*, **3**, 71

Phillis JW (1968). Acetylcholine release from the cerebral cortex: Its role in cortical arousal. *Brain Res.*, **7**, 378

Shute CCD & Lewis PR (1967). The ascending reticular system: Neocortical, olfactory and subcortical projections. *Brain*, **90**, 497

Smith DE, King MB & Hoebel BG (1970). Lateral hypothalamic control of killing: Evidence for a cholinoceptive mechanism. *Science*, **167**, 900

Ulett GA & Johnson MW (1957). Effect of atropine and scopolamine upon electroencephalographic changes induced by electroconvulsive therapy. *Electroenceph. clin. Neurophysiol.*, **9**, 217

Vogt M (1971). Functional aspects of the localization of transmitter substances. In: *Progress in Brain Research, Histochemistry of Nervous Transmission* (Ed Eränkö). New York: Elsevier Publishing Co.

Ward A (1950). Atropine in the treatment of closed head injury. *J. Neurosurg.*, **7**, 398

CHAPTER 32

The concept of diencephalic instability
ERIC TURNER

INTRODUCTION

For 15 years sphenoid lead examination in my practice has included patterns of electrodes which show simultaneously channels at both frontal bases and both parietal convexities (Turner, 1971). As increasing numbers were examined it was realized that the records fell into defined groups. Certain records showed a striking frequency of high voltage sharp and slow wave complexes appearing synchronously at the frontal bases and parietal convexities, bilaterally, under pentothal anaesthesia. Dysrhymia is normally seen at a certain level of pentothal anaesthesia, and sharp and slow waves in themselves are no more than a reflection of the anaesthetic level. The stage of anaesthesia which shows this feature is deeper than the 'pentothal fast activity', and lighter than the stage of pentothal bursts that occur between periods of electrical flattening.

The significant feature, however, is that normally pentothal high voltage dysrhythmia appears in disorderly timing at different areas, whereas certain patients showed synchrony of both the sharp and slow wave components bilaterally at both the frontal bases and the parietal convexities. These synchronous discharges might be very numerous, moderately numerous or very rare.

When they were very numerous the patients were found to be suffering from epilepsy that from the characters of their fits and the findings in straight EEG recordings was judged to be 'centrencephalic epilepsy'.

DIENCEPHALIC INSTABILITY

Moderately numerous synchronous discharges were seen in patients with impulsive behaviour, tension and sometimes outbursts of aggression. Such a combination was termed 'diencephalic instability'. They might or might not have epilepsy. If an epileptic focus was present, say, in one temporal lobe, such patients with diencephalic instability would be more likely to have generalized attacks as well as psychomotor ones, and their temperamental disorder would probably be more severe. Frequently however, such a record would be accompanied by only personality disorder.

By contrast, normal patterns showed only very rare synchrony between the frontal bases and parietal convexities, perhaps only one or two in a whole recording, perhaps occurring only at the beginning of a pentothal burst when

238 Surgical Approaches in Psychiatry

its significance seemed to be negligible. Sometimes, when there was unilateral damage in one hemisphere, unilateral synchrony could be seen of similar high voltage sharp and slow waves at the frontal base and the parietal convexity, and it was thought that this might represent a one-sided thalamic disorder.

In order to demonstrate the synchrony, special EEG connections were made, so that the two appropriate channels were added together, halved in voltage and fed into a third channel. Electrical synchrony could then be visually demonstrated without the necessity for measurement and lining up (Figure 32.1). This arrangement proved extremely useful, and, together with the raw

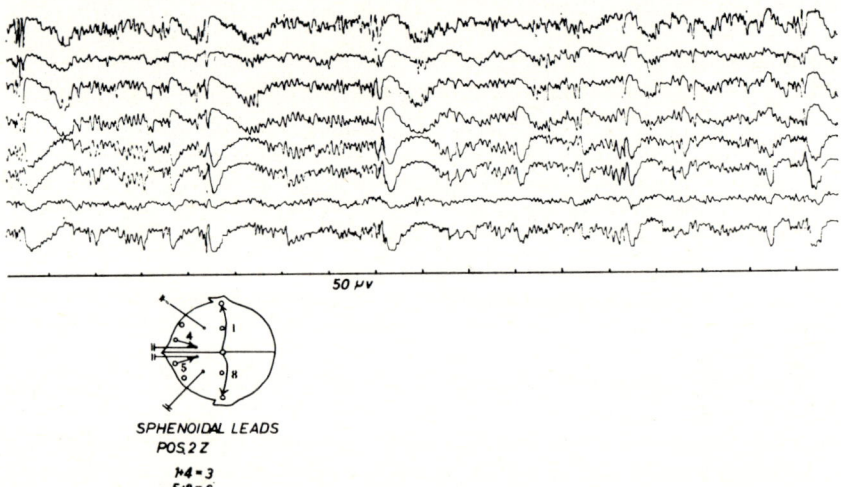

Figure 32.1 This sphenoid lead record shows high voltage sharp and slow waves appearing synchronously in channels 1, 4, 5 and 8, i.e. at the parietal convexities and the frontal bases bilaterally. This feature has been termed 'diencephalic instability'. A special electrical analysis is used in which channels 1 and 4 are added to form channel 3, and channels 5 and 8 are added to form channel 6.

patterns, formed an immediate analysis of the basic stability of the brain as a whole and also fractionally. Widespread asynchronous dysrhythmia formed a striking contrast with the synchronous type of instability.

As the concept of 'diencephalic' stability or instability emerged, analyses of the records conformed well with the clinical complaints.

The final stage was to determine whether such an analysis could be useful in the treatment and management. First, cases who showed various inadequacies of personality, but who did not show the central instability, were continued under medical and psychiatric management.

PARAMEDIAN LOBOTOMY

Secondly, cases who did show diencephalic instability, together with clinical manifestations of tension and irresistible impulsiveness, were treated by paramedian lobotomy. This operation consisted of a section of white matter

1 cm broad just in front of the genu of the corpus callosum. It extended from the subcortical layer at the vertex to the base (Figures 32.2, 3).

The operative technique was checked first by external markers on the scalp, placed 3 cm behind the lateral orbital margins and 6 cm above the zygomatic arches in a plane passing through a point 10 cm behind the nasion measured along the scalp on a sagittal line. Fifteen cubic centimetres of air

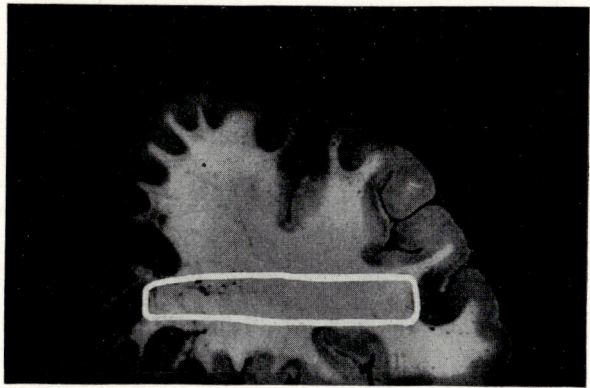

Figure 32.2 Coronal section showing the plane of paramedian lobotomy, the site and extent of which is outlined.

was insufflated by lumbar puncture with the patient in a sitting position. A lateral x-ray was then taken in the supine position, and the anterior horn of the ventricles and the sulcus of the corpus callosum identified. It was then possible to mark the correct site for a lateral burr hole (often about 1 cm behind the marker) to enable an incision, made in a para-coronal plane, to cut

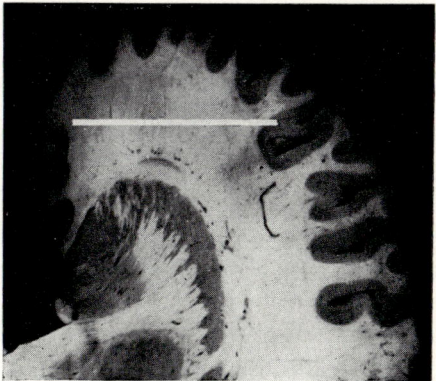

Figure 32.3 Sagittal section of the brain 15 mm from the midline indicates the site of lobotomy in this plane. Although it seems to lie well forward it is in fact just in front of the corpus callosum.

just in front of the frontal horns. Lines were drawn to get the exact angle to pass in front of the ventricle and just in front of the edge of the lesser wing of the sphenoid (Figure 32.3). When lobotomy was performed, these points were first checked directly by passage of a brain cannula in the appropriate directions.

RESULTS

As might be expected, the symptoms of tension and impulsive aggression were relieved, and this could be predicted with a high degree of confidence if the EEG showed the features of significant synchrony described above as 'diencephalic instability'.

Some patients showing these features had epileptic attacks, and an unexpected bonus was that in the early stages at least, their attacks were strikingly reduced in frequency and severity. This result is now being investigated and followed up in selected cases of uncontrollable epilepsy showing this type of EEG recording.

Altogether, 13 cases showing the EEG features of 'diencephalic instability' have been treated by paramedian lobotomy.

EEG FINDINGS

Finally, the analysis of the EEG records, and the clinical records in cases with a temporal lobe focus, psychomotor attacks, personality disorders of a temporal lobe type, namely phobic-rages, or alternatively, a paranoid type of non-temporal origin, affords valuable evidence about the prognosis, with or without surgical treatment. Such a prognosis will be valid not only regarding persistence of possible centrencephalic epilepsy but also regarding future personality disorder and specific aberrations from normal behaviour.

Patients with personality disorders are liable to have mild ventricular dilatation as shown by rounding or enlargement of the ventricular shadow. This evidence of brain atrophy shows that the borderline between functional and organic brain disorder should not be too hastily nor too arbitrarily drawn.

The analysis of sphenoidal EEG records described provides an objective test in a field that can be singularly lacking in such checks. Difficulties in psychiatric diagnosis are increased by the confusion about terms and language. What a patient understands by 'tension', 'depression' or 'being frightened' is quite variable. 'Tension' may be used as a word by a flabby self-indulgent patient, although no evidence of tension is shown to the observer. A woman may be 'frightened' to meet people, or to cross a road, in case she has a fit. This is not phobia but a rational and reasonable reaction. Under such circumstances it is of great value to have some objective support for a clinical evaluation, and a careful analysis of simultaneous patterns of sphenoid leads and isocortical channels under pentothal anaesthesia provides crucial objective information.

By and large, it is the functioning of the brain as a whole that determines behaviour. We are concerned first with large fractions of influence, secondly with their interconnections, and most important of all, with certain crucial pathways of diffuse projection. It is this kind of analysis that leads from a study of EEG records to the concept of 'diencephalic instability'.

REFERENCE
Turner E (1971). Simultaneous analysis of frontal basal and parietal areas during the use of sphenoidal leads. *Electroenceph. clin. Neurophysiol.*, **30**, 471

PART VIII

BASIC SCIENCES RELATED TO PSYCHOSURGERY

CHAPTER 33

Tentative limbic system models for certain patterns of psychiatric disorders
KENNETH E LIVINGSTON & A ESCOBAR

INTRODUCTION

Over the past three decades the rate of acquisition of new information relating to basic mechanisms of nervous system function has been revolutionary. This anatomical, physiological, biochemical and other information provides growing insight into the types of neuronal dysfunction that may be involved in some of the manifestations of major psychiatric illness. Against this background it now seems feasible to postulate tentative models for several broad patterns of psychiatric disorder.

In the Sherrington era, experimental techniques permitted the study only of nervous system events involving few neurones, particularly the afferent and efferent limbs of the reflex arc in which stimulus to response intervals were very brief (Sherrington, 1906). Only recently we have begun to acquire the tools that permit the analysis of mechanisms essential for a brain capable of feeling, learning and organizing behaviour.

In the 1930s Lorente de No's (1935) studies focused attention on the vast interneurone pool, and the mechanisms by which information might be long circuited in time and extensively modified between the entry and exit pathways. Since then the neurosciences have been increasingly engaged in exploring some of the mysteries of this central internuncial pool in which the mental process lies, and from which individualized emotional expression and behaviour must be generated.

In the 1940s the development of computer theory and technology provided a mechanical model for the complex functions of information coding, storage, and retrieval (Wiener, 1961), processes that must underlie learning, memory and behaviour. Clinical confirmation of long-term information storage and its retrieval by electrical excitation was provided in the detailed observations of temporal lobe epilepsy (Mullan & Penfield, 1959).

During the next decade major contributions to concepts of mind and behaviour followed investigations of the reticular activating system initiated by Magoun and Moruzzi (Moruzzi & Magoun, 1949; Magoun, 1950). Mechanisms of arousal and attention are clearly essential for learning, and for the 'turning on' of all emotional and behavioural activity. It seems reasonable to speculate that dysfunction within central activating circuits may contribute to patterns of 'abnormal' emotional and behavioural activity in certain psychiatric disorders.

MECHANISMS OF PSYCHIATRIC DISORDER

The most obvious disturbances might be visualized clinically in simple quantitative terms—too little activation leading to the withdrawn, apathetic, hypokinetic and mute states or conversely, too much activation leading to the restless, irritable, hyperactive and compulsive states.

It is increasingly clear, however, that the activating mechanisms are not simply quantitative 'on–off' systems operating at the brain-stem level, but that they must be selectively 'tuned' not only in reference to a continuously changing environment, but also in reference to past experience involving learning and memory. From subjective experience we know that we are aroused by sensory input that is novel, habituate to stimuli that are repetitive or neutral, and attend to and act upon information idenitfied as important through reference to past experience. If reference to past experience is an essential element in the mechanisms of attention and activation, hippocampal as well as reticular circuits must be involved. Temporary and persistent breakdown of modulatory control over such complex activating mechanisms may be the functional derangement underlying some patterns of psychiatric 'dis-ease'.

In addition the reflex responses induced by arousal stimuli—changes in blood pressure, pulse rate, vascular tone, etc., call forth counterbalancing homoeostatic responses which must also be subject to precise control if ongoing purposive behaviour such as fight or flight is not to be interrupted. For example, a cat in escaping from a dog must be able to block reflex vagal slowing that would occur under basal conditions as a response to the barrage of baroreceptor stimuli from elevation of blood pressure. It is now established that such basic homoeostatic reflex activity is subject to precise modulation by higher centres and that this modulation is dependent on the integrity of the limbic–forebrain circuits (Hockman, Talesnik & Livingston, 1969).

A similar consideration of the feedback control systems which have been shown to modulate both incoming and outgoing sensorimotor activity (Livingston, 1960), suggests that they also are dependent on reference to past experience and must involve higher limbic circuits in a similar manner. The role that derangements of feedback control may play in emotional–behavioural imbalance is suggested by observation of the wide range of psychic disturbance that can be induced in otherwise normal individuals by reduction, distortion or overload of sensory inputs.

THERAPEUTIC IMPLICATIONS

What insight do we have into the central patterning of these mechanisms that might guide our approach to therapy?

In 1937 Papez proposed an integrated 'central mechanism of emotion' based on circuits involving the hypothalamus, anterior thalamic nuclei, cingulate gyrus and hippocampus (Figure 33.1). The basic relationships of the

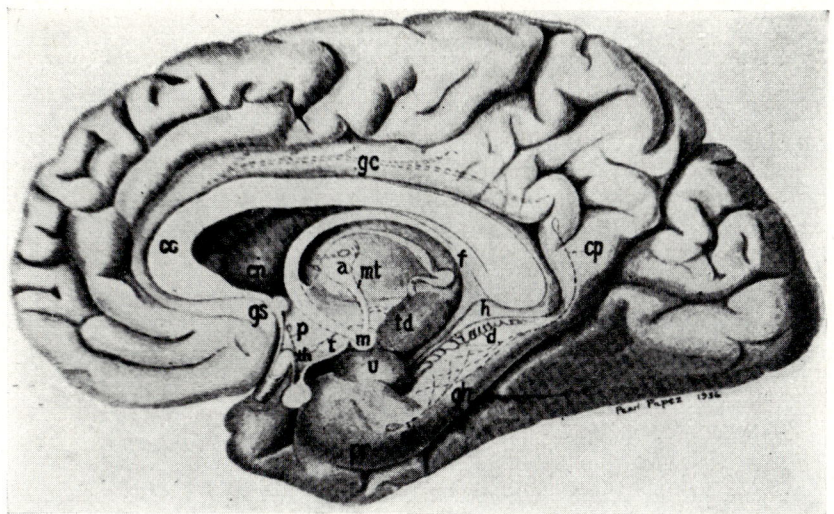

Figure 33.1 A medial view of the right cerebral hemisphere, illustrating 'the general anatomic picture I wish to propose as the probable corticothalamic mechanism of emotion'. (From Papez, 1937, *Arch. Neurol. Psychiat.* (*Chicago*), **38**, 725. Courtesy of American Medical Association, EW Beck, Exec. Managing Editor.)

'Papez' circuit have required little modification over the intervening 35 years, except for an increasing emphasis on its linkage with the brain stem reticular core (Nauta, 1958). This medial limbic circuit articulates extensively with the reticular activating apparatus throughout the brain stem from the septal region to the tegmental levels of the pons, as shown in Figure 33.2. In this circuit the great fornix pathway provides the anatomical substrate for more complex activating and feedback control mechanisms that must have access to hippocampal memory circuits. The medial-frontal cortical components of this circuit might be visualized as the highest levels of limbic modulation of these mechanisms.

In terms of clinical correlation, there is abundant evidence from both clinical and laboratory sources indicating that extensive destructive lesions of the medial limbic circuit are characterized principally as states of psychic and motor *hypo*activity. Clinical syndromes of akinesia, mutism and apathy are seen with traumatic, vascular and neoplastic lesions of these medial limbic pathways (Nielson, 1953).

Conversely, it is reasonable to postulate that irritative disorders within this circuit might produce the opposite behavioural effect—psychic and motor *hyper*activity. Psychiatric syndromes characterized by anxiety, restless irritability and obsessive-compulsive behaviour would fall in this category. In treating intractable psychiatric disturbances of this character, selective destructive lesions of the cingulate pathways and medial-frontal quadrants have been highly effective (Le Beau, 1952; Ballantine, Cassidy, Flanagan &

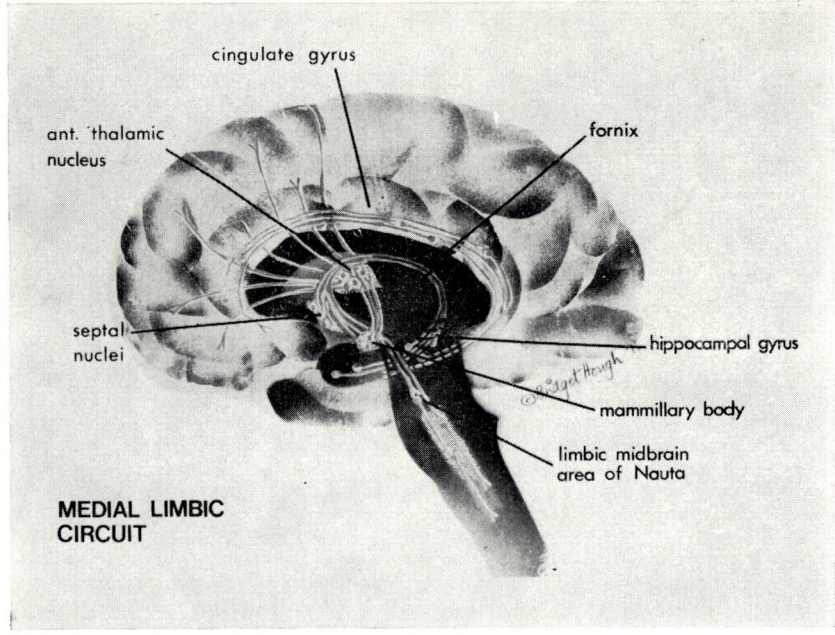

Figure 33.2 The medial limbic circuit.

Marino, 1967; Brown & Lighthill, 1968; Foltz, 1968). There is thus a good correlation between the anatomical, experimental and clinical evidence relating to functions of the medial limbic circuit.

Although the 'Papez' circuit of 1937 dominated the subsequent development of the limbic system concept, its structures constitute only the medial half of that system as it is currently recognized (Livingston & Escobar, 1971). In 1948 Yakovlev extended Papez' concept to include the cortex of the orbitofrontal, insular and anterior temporal areas, together with their connections with the amygdala and dorsomedial nucleus of the thalamus as illustrated in Figure 33.3.

The anatomical relationships of this basolateral limbic circuit with the brain stem, thalamus and neocortex, are very distinct from those of the medial circuit. In quantitative terms the major anatomical orientations of the two circuits suggest that the medial circuit is particularly concerned with activity in the reticular core of the brain stem, while the basolateral circuit through its temporal connections seems concerned particularly with the activities of the sensory-receptive and interpretative cortex (Figure 33.4). Nauta (1960) has emphasized that although there is no direct connection between the medial and basolateral circuits, both have extensive outflow converging at the septalpreoptic, hypothalamic and midbrain levels, suggesting that these two major limbic circuits must be at least in part, mutual antagonists in their influence

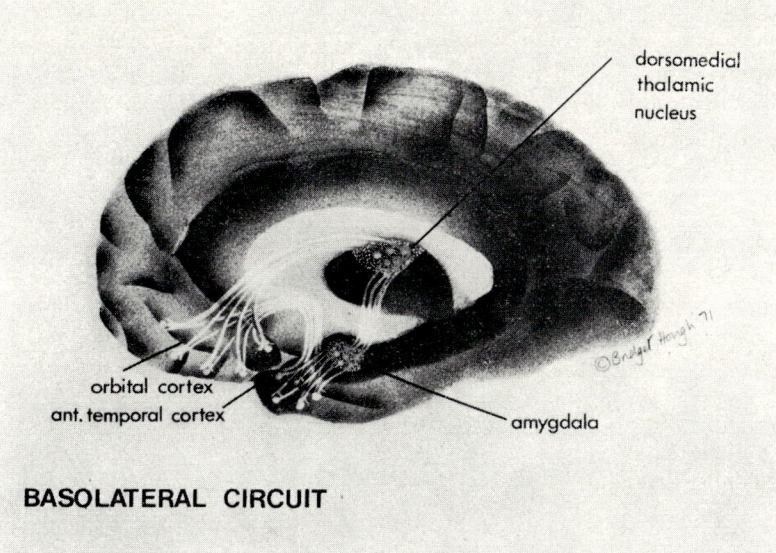

Figure 33.3 The basolateral limbic circuit.

on behavioural outflow pathways. From this evidence one might postulate that activity in these two major circuits, tends to bias behavioural outflow in different directions, and that so-called 'normal' behaviour represents a relative balance of such activity. One might predict that persisting imbalances of activity within such circuits should produce recognizable and clinically distinguishable patterns of 'abnormal' behaviour, though it is obvious that the final expression of such functional derangements will vary greatly as a reflection of the unique patterns of endowment and experience that characterize each individual.

Within the basolateral circuit structures, extensive clinical studies have demonstrated that selective lesions of the posterior orbital cortex are effective in relieving intractable depressive syndromes (Tow & Lewin, 1953; Knight, 1965) and that lesions of the amygdala and its hypothalamic connections are effective in modifying certain states of intractable aggressiveness (Narabayashi & Uno, 1966; Sano, 1962).

At present there is no direct clinical evidence as to the effects of selective 'therapeutic' lesions of the anterior temporal cortex and its pathways, but there is considerable indirect evidence that the limbic components of this interpretative cortex must be involved in the large body of psychiatric disorders in which altered sensory perception and interpretation may be considered the underlying functional disturbance, leading to complex delusional and hallucinatory experience.

250 *Surgical Approaches in Psychiatry*

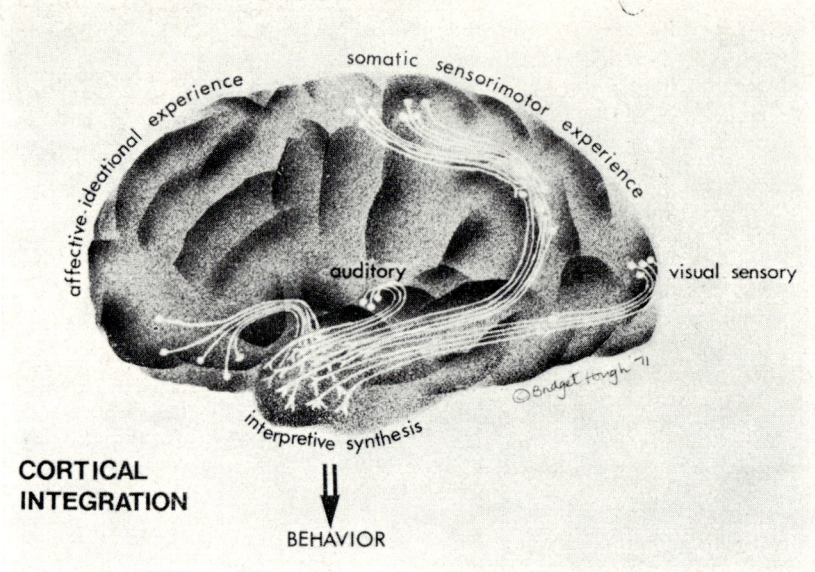

Figure 33.4 The convergence of information from the cortical sensory-receiving and association areas on to the limbic cortex of the anterior temporal region.

In this model the functions ascribed to the limbic system are broad indeed:

it monitors ongoing sensorimotor activity; it serves as the integrator of the individual's internal and external worlds, and thereby generates affect; and finally it modulates behavioural outflow.

In a sense it might be characterized as the system responsible for emotional–behavioural 'homoeostasis'.

This homoeostasis is not a static, restricted state, but rather a dynamic equilibrium within which there must be room for a broad repertoire of individualized expression and behavioural response. Transient, recurrent or persistent decompensations of these homoeostatic mechanisms are expressed as psychiatric 'dis-ease'.

The objective of therapy in terms of such a model is to assist in the process of recompensation of these homoeostatic mechanisms, by restoring balance within the limbic circuits, whether the therapeutic methods be psychological, behavioural, biochemical, pharmacological, electrophysical, surgical or several of these in combination.

As we have seen during this conference neuroanatomy and neurochemistry particularly with their newer analytical techniques, provide us with interesting clues as to the functional orientation of major circuits within the limbic system. In terms of the hierarchy of modulatory control the highest cortical components would be expected to provide the most discriminative options for modifying behavioural outflow. Thus our attention is directed to the medial-frontal, orbito-frontal and anterior temporal cortices (Livingston, 1969).

As we have seen, these are the areas in which there is the greatest correspondence of anatomical, physiological, biochemical and clinical evidence. As the analysis of dysfunction in these areas is further refined, and techniques for increasingly selective therapeutic intervention improved, we can expect to increase our effectiveness in relieving some of the crushing burden of otherwise intractable psychiatric illness.

REFERENCES

Ballantine HT, Cassidy WL, Flanagan NB & Marino R (1967). Stereotaxic anterior cingulotomy for neuropsychiatric illness and intractable pain. *J. Neurosurg.*, **26**, 488

Brown MH & Lighthill JH (1968). Selective anterior cingulotomy: a psychosurgical evaluation. *J. Neurosurg.*, **29**, 513

Foltz EL (1968). Cingular lesions: current status and use of rostral cingulotomy. *South Med. J.*, **61**, 899

Hockman CH, Talesnik J & Livingston KE (1969). Central nervous system modulation of baroreceptor reflexes. *Am. J. Physiol.*, **217**, 1681

Knight GC (1965). Stereotaxic tractotomy in the surgical treatment of mental illness. *J. Neurol. Neurosurg. Psychiat.*, **28**, 304

Le Beau J (1952). The cingular and precingular areas in psychosurgery-agitated behavior, obsessive compulsive states, epilepsy. *Acta Psychiat. Neurol. Scandin.*, **27**, 304

Livingston KE (1969). The frontal lobes revisited: the case for a second look. *Arch. Neurol. Chicago*, **20**, 90

Livingston KE & Escobar A (1971). The anatomical bias of the limbic system concepts: a proposed reorientation. *Arch. Neurol. Chicago*, **24**, 17

Livingston RB (1960). Central control of receptors and sensory transmission systems. In: *Handbook of Physiology*, Sec. I, Vol. I, p. 741. Washington D.C.: Amer. Physiol. Soc.

Lorente de No R (1935). The summation of impulses transmitted to the neurones through different synapses. *Am. J. Physiol.*, **113**, 524

Magoun HW (1950). Caudal and cephalic influences of the brain stem reticular formation. *Physiol. Rev.*, **30**, 459

Moruzzi G & Magoun HW (1949). The brain stem reticular formation and activation of the E.E.G. *Electroenceph. clin. Neurophysiol.*, **1**, 445

Mullan S & Penfield W (1959). Illusions of comparative interpretation and emotion; production by epileptic discharge and by electrical stimulation in the temporal cortex. *Arch. Neurol. Psych.*, **81**, 269

Narabayashi H & Uno M (1966). Long range results of stereotaxic amygdalotomy for behavior disorders. *Confin. neurol.*, **27**, 168

Nauta WHJ (1958). Hippocampal projections and related neural pathways to the midbrain in the cat. *Brain*, **81**, 319

Nauta WHJ (1960). Some neural pathways related to the limbic system. *Electrical Studies of the Unanaesthetized Brain* (Eds Ramey and O'Doherty). New York: Paul B Hoeber.

Nielson JM (1953). Correlation of sites of lesion with symptoms. *J. nerv. ment. Dis.*, **118**, 429

Papez JW (1937). A proposed mechanism of emotion. *Arch. Neurol. Psychiat. (Chicago)*, **38**, 725

Sano K (1962). Sedative neurosurgery. *Neurologia medico-chirurgica*, **4**, 112

Sherrington C (1906). *The Integrative Action of the Nervous System.* New York: Charles Scribner's Sons.

Tow PM & Lewin W (1953). Orbital leucotomy: isolation of the orbital cortex by open operation. *Lancet*, **2**, 644

Wiener N (1961). *Cybernetics*: Control and communication in the animal and the machine. 2nd ed. Cambridge, Mass.: MIT Press.

Yakovlev PI (1948). Motility, behavior, and the brain: stereodynamic organization and neural coordinates of behavior. *J. nerv. ment. Dis.*, **107**, 313

CHAPTER 34

Coping with stress in rats with limbic lesions
H URSIN, G C COOVER & S LEVINE

Plasma corticosterone changes during avoidance learning illustrate some of the factors that affect normal rats when coping with stress, and also the factors underlying avoidance deficits after limbic lesions. Many of the animal experiments suggesting that limbic structures are involved in the control of the emotions have employed avoidance tasks. In the typical avoidance situation, the animal learns how to avoid an electric shock or some other unpleasant or painful experience, or 'stress'. When this learning is acquired, the individual successfully avoids this stress by running away, by pressing a bar ('active avoidance'), or by not approaching food or water ('passive avoidance'). The rat has solved the problem and is successfully coping with his environment. A question of wide biological significance is whether we are still stressed when we are coping with a stressful situation.

The corticosterone in plasma rises 4–5 min after a given stressor has been applied, the delay being due to the time required to stimulate the adrenal. The peak level is reached approximately 15 min later. Thus, if blood is sampled in less than 3–4 min, it is possible to measure the corticosterone level without any interference from the sampling technique. Rats are rapidly anaesthetized with ether, and blood is obtained from the surgically exposed jugular vein. The whole procedure requires less than 2 min.

Basal samples do not change during the course of the experiment. The two-way active avoidance task was learned to an 80% criterion by the 6th day, and additional training was then given for 14 days. The post-session plasma corticosterone levels diminished slightly as the avoidance response was learned, but much more markedly when additional avoidance sessions were given. Behavioural observations showed that the animals also spent significantly less time 'freezing' during the later trials. Bolus droppings per session exhibited a continuing decline between the 6th and the 17th session. After the 20th session a forced extinction session was given. This re-established the high post-session corticosterone levels. This elevation was observed whether the forced extinction involved shock or simply blocking the crossing response.

It does not seem to be the reduction in shocks that is of primary importance for the corticosterone drop. The drop is small between the 1st and the 7th session although the number of shocks is greatly reduced. The main hormonal decrease occurs between the 6th and 17th session, although the reduction in shocks is rather small in this period.

The so-called two-factor theory of avoidance learning explains why the corticosterone level is so high on day 6, even though the animal has received so few shocks. The rats have now learned the significance of the conditioned stimulus through a classic conditioning process. This acquisition of conditioned 'fear' is the first factor in this theory. The second factor is evident from the fall in corticosterone from the 6th to the 17th session, the period in which the avoidance behaviour became stabilized. Through adequate instrumental behaviour the rat is able to control and predict the situation, and there is a corresponding reduction in acquired 'fear', indicated by the diminished pituitary-adrenal response. The corticosterones do not drop to zero, and it is impossible to conceive of avoidance behaviour occurring without any arousal. The extinction data show that when ability to predict is lost there is again an increased arousal even if no shocks are delivered.

By following the same procedure it is possible to determine the nature of the avoidance learning deficits in rats with limbic lesions. Both amygdala lesions and lesions in the cingulate cortex reduce the ability to learn active avoidance. If the reduced ability to learn avoidance is due to decreased fear (factor I), the corticosterone level should be low during the early stages. If, however, it is the second factor that is affected the levels should be high. With the two types of lesion it is possible to discriminate between these two factors.

Fifteen of our operated rats had satisfactory bilateral lesions in the basolateral amygdala nuclei, affecting both the lateral nuclei and the magnocellular basal nucleus. These rats showed a clear deficit in two-way active avoidance behaviour. The deficit was significant throughout the 20 sessions of testing. The amygdala group showed a normal basal corticosterone level, and also a normal response to ether stress. However, there was a lower steroid level than in the normals after shocks on day 1 of avoidance learning. These rats were defective in passive avoidance as well. Other deficits also suggest a general reduction in fear or arousal, less immobility in the open field and during the active avoidance intertrial intervals, and slower escape latencies during the first couple of trials on day 1. Thus, the rats with lesions of this type showed a deficit connected with the first factor, they did not acquire fear in the normal way.

Different results were obtained in the cat. Behaviour observations suggested that a cat with a lateral lesion lost only the flight reaction, but not the ability to acquire conditioned fear or passive avoidance (Ursin, 1965). The reason for this discrepancy may be differential involvement of the insula. In the rat the lesion will affect the fibres to and from the insula, but in the cat the insula is placed far too dorsally to be affected by this lesion (Figure 34.1). Insula lesions are known to produce deficits in passive avoidance.

In the 12 rats with lesions restricted to the anterior half of the cingulate cortex there was a change connected with the second factor. It was quite surprising that the animals did not show the typical deficit in two-way active avoidance. The reason may have been that the lesions were very shallow and did not interfere with the deeper layers of cingulum fibres. However, the animals with cingulate lesions exhibited no decline in plasma corticosterone level or increase in sniffing or grooming behaviour, in spite of their normal performance in the active avoidance task. The primary deficits produced by this lesion, therefore, may be failure of fear to diminish as instrumental behaviour becomes adequate. It may be that this deficit is not tied to avoidance behaviour alone, but is of importance for the acquisition of other types of instrumental behaviour as well.

In the rat, both basolateral amygdala lesions and cingulate lesions—if deep enough—produce deficits in two-way active avoidance learning, but for

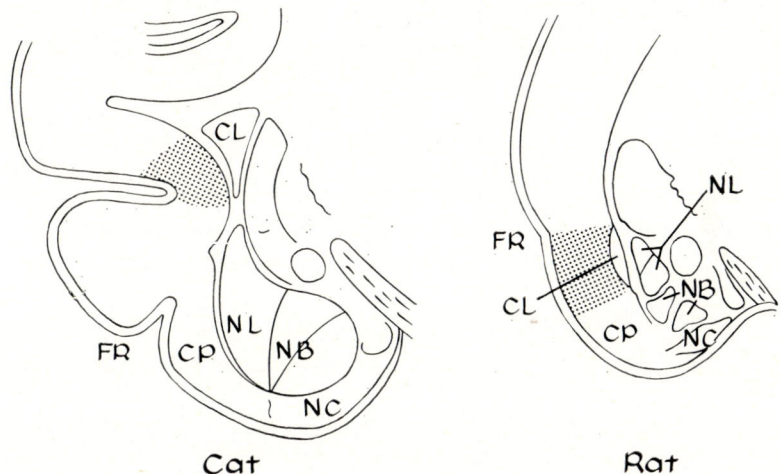

Figure 34.1 Frontal sections through the amygdala region in the cat and the rat. Basolateral amygdala lesions in the rat produce a deficit in passive as well as in active avoidance; in the cat only active avoidance is affected. This may be due to differential involvement of the insula (the cortex overlying the claustrum) in the two species. Cl, claustrum; CP, pyriform cortex; FR, rhinal fissure; NB, basal amygdala nuclei; NC, cortical amygdala nucleus; NL, lateral amygdala nucleus.

different reasons. Basolateral amygdala lesions interfere with the acquisition of the classically conditioned fear of the situation (Factor I). To obtain this effect it seems necessary to ablate two areas, one concerned with active and the other with passive avoidance. The cingulate lesion, even the shallow and ineffective one we used, interferes with the effect of adequate behaviour on the underlying, acquired drive (Factor II).

Small lesions in a small brain seem to reveal that very delicate mechanisms are involved during avoidance learning, and a relatively simple phenomenon such as two-way active avoidance deficit may derive from interference with very different psychological mechanisms. It should then be evident that terms like 'fear' include too many dimensions to be meaningful descriptions of effects on behaviour, even in a species with only 20 g of brain. Such terms may be useful, however, if large and anatomically vaguely described lesions are employed. A mass-action effect may then be the best way to predict results, since a very large number of both anatomical and psychological dimensions are being interfered with. A discrete and restricted effect on behaviour is not to be expected from such procedures.

ACKNOWLEDGEMENTS

The research reported in this paper was supported in part by Foundations' Fund for Research in Psychiatry.

REFERENCE

Ursin H (1965). Effect of amygdaloid lesions on avoidance behavior and visual discrimination in cats. *Exp. Neurol.*, **11**, 298

CHAPTER 35

Electrophysiological correlates of non-specific cortical activation by electrical stimulation of the putamen and pallidum in cats

G DIECKMANN & R HASSLER

INTRODUCTION

Usually the corpus striatum and pallidum are considered to be subcortical regulating centres of the extrapyramidal motor system. For the past 20 years neuroanatomists have also been drawing attention to their connections with the non-specific thalamic activating system (McLardy, 1948; Droogleever-Fortuyn, 1950; Hassler, 1950). As long ago as 1946 Dandy assumed that the striate might be a 'conscious centre in the brain'. While in the past some electrophysiological findings pointed to participation of the caudate nucleus in non-specific cortical activation (Shimamoto & Verzeano, 1954; Stoupel & Terzuolo, 1954; Buchwald, Wyers, Okuma & Heuser, 1961; Heuser, Buchwald & Wyers, 1961), similar experimental results concerning the putamen and pallidum have been lacking until recently.

MATERIAL

From electrophysiological and behaviour studies in a total of 122 cats reported in part elsewhere (Dieckmann, 1968; Dieckmann & Hassler, 1968; Dieckmann & Sasaki, 1970; Hassler & Dieckmann, 1967), we now present a few typical electrocortical responses following electrical stimulation of the putamen and pallidum, the appearance of which will be interpreted as a function of non-specific cortical activation.

RESULTS

In drowsy cats repetitive low-frequency stimulation of the putamen and pallidum elicits general cortical synchronization, spindle activity and recruiting responses, i.e electrophysiological correlates of behaviour inactivation. Figure 35.1 shows, at the left, such a cortical synchronization induced by low-frequency stimulation of the putamen, comparable to that produced by stimulation of the medio-thalamic nuclei.

A cortical desynchronization or an arousal reaction, i.e. an increase of frequency and reduction of amplitude, occurs during 30 Hz stimulation of the putamen and pallidum shown at the right in Figure 35.1. The electrophysiological activation does not exceed the time of stimulus application, thus indicating a phasic type of activation. As is well known, a phasic activation is induced by excitation of the non-specific thalamic activating system.

The two responses were induced by stimulation of the same points within the putamen and pallidum, but at different stimulation frequencies, as shown

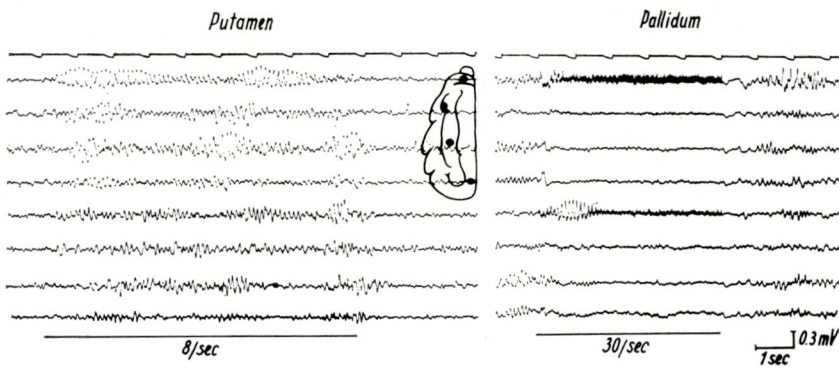

Figure 35.1 Cortical synchronization (left) and desynchronization (right) due to repetitive stimulation of the putamen and pallidum depending on stimulation frequency. Monapolar recording.

in Figure 35.2. This is a schematic drawing of the cat diencephalon in sagittal section, where dark half-circles indicate production of synchronization and white half-circles mean production of desynchronization. These stimulation points with reversed function have been found mostly within the putamen, pallidum and entopeduncular nucleus, the latter corresponding in cats to the internal part of the pallidum of primates. The dark spots indicate sites at which stimulation did not give these responses.

Low-frequency repetitive stimulation of the putamen and pallidum produces characteristic laminar field potentials in the cerebral cortex, indicating the pure recruiting nature of the responses. Examples of such field potentials generated by the putamen (A), pallidum (B) and centrum medianum (C) are given in Figure 35.3, according to the depth of the cortex from which they were recorded. In the uppermost row electrocorticograms (S.R.), and in the lowest row intracellular potential changes (I.R.) of the same cortical region are presented.

The traces in column C (Figure 35.3) recorded during centrum medianum stimulation correspond in all respects to the standard cortical potentials of thalamic-induced recruiting responses in surface cortical, intracellular and laminar field potentials. In the electrocorticogram, thalamic stimulation sets up the well-known slow negative waves. In laminar field potentials, superficial slow negative and deep positive waves reveal the typical recruiting nature of the response first reported by Li, Cullen & Jasper (1956) and

Spencer & Brookhart (1961). Intracellular recordings show EPSPs with spike potentials followed by IPSPs.

Stimulation of the putamen (A) and pallidum (B) give much the same responses as those produced by centrum medianum stimulation.

However, the cortical distribution of recruiting responses generated by putamen and pallidum stimulation differs from that produced by medio-

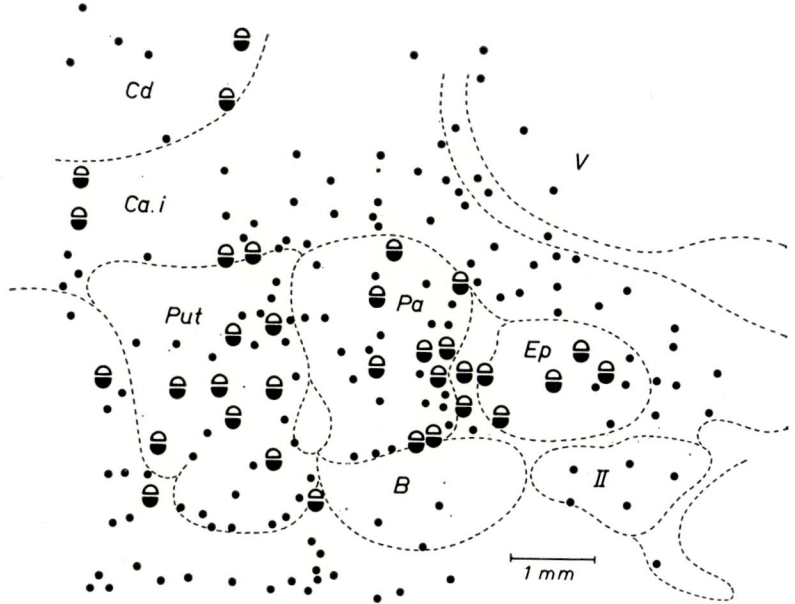

Figure 35.2 Localization of stimulation points producing cortical synchronization (dark half circles) and desynchronization (white half circles) respectively. They are mainly situated within the putamen and pallidum. Dark points indicate stimulation sites from which such reversed cortical responses could not be obtained. B, basal nucleus; Ca.i, internal capsule; Cd, caudate nucleus; Ep, entopeduncular nucleus; Pa, pallidum; Put, putamen; V, ventral thalamus; II, optic nerve.

thalamic stimulation. While the usual EEG recruiting responses appear bilaterally in the sigmoid and suprasylvian gyruses, the field potential analysis in Figure 35.4 reveals that putamen and pallidum stimulation set up typical recruiting responses only in the medial part of the ipsilateral sigmoid gyrus (area 6a). Now responses appear in the lateral sigmoid gyrus (area 4γ). In the suprasylvian gyrus (area 7), in contrast to centrum medianum stimulation, which gives good recruiting responses in the premotor (area 6a) and association (area 7) cortex, putamen and pallidum stimulation only occasionally induce some dubious responses. Stimulation of the cerebral peduncle (P.c.), which sets up antidromic spike potentials in the pyramidal tract neurones in areas 6a and 4γ, will not be discussed here.

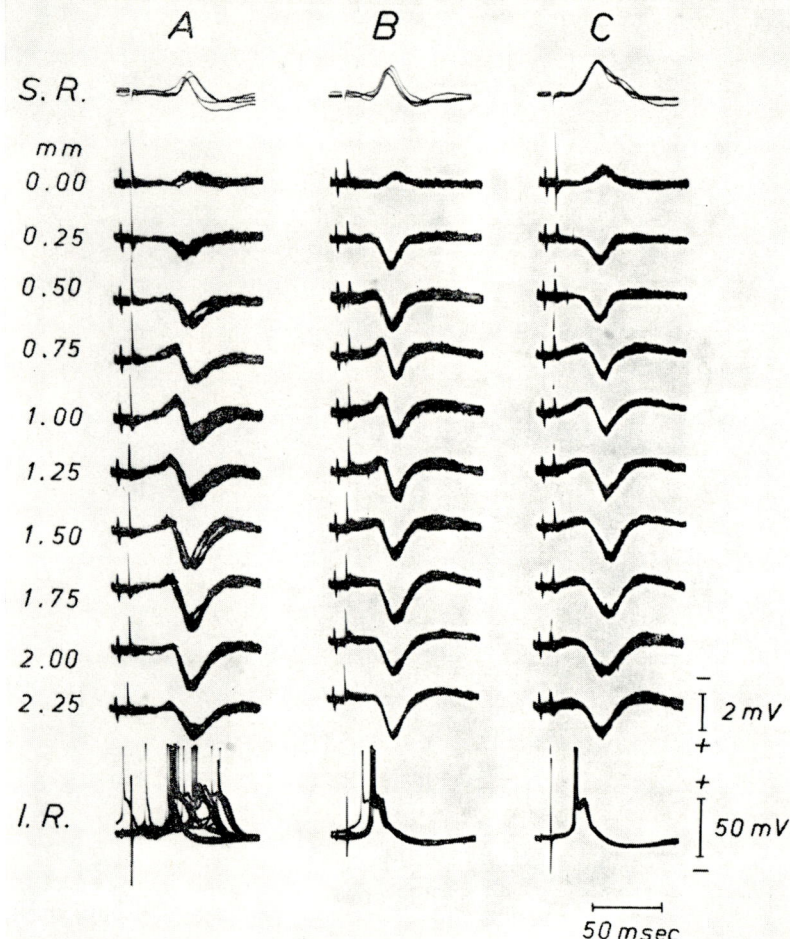

Figure 35.3 Laminar field potentials, surface cortical potentials (S.R.) and intracellular potential changes (I.R.) elicited by repetitive (7/sec) stimulation of putamen (A), pallidum (B) and centrum medianum (C). Recordings from cortical area 6aβ. Numbers on the left indicate depths of the microelectrode in the cortical layers. (From Dieckmann & Sasaki, 1970, by courtesy of Springer-Verlag, Berlin.)

It is a striking feature that putamen- and pallidum-induced non-specific activation does not excite more cortical fields but obviously only a motor field. One may assume that this non-specific activation is only responsible for a motor neuronal system, and recedes in other systems.

Since the putamen and pallidum are surrounded by the internal capsule, spread of stimulating current to this adjacent structure had to be ruled out by special investigation. Stimulation of the internal capsule, even very close to

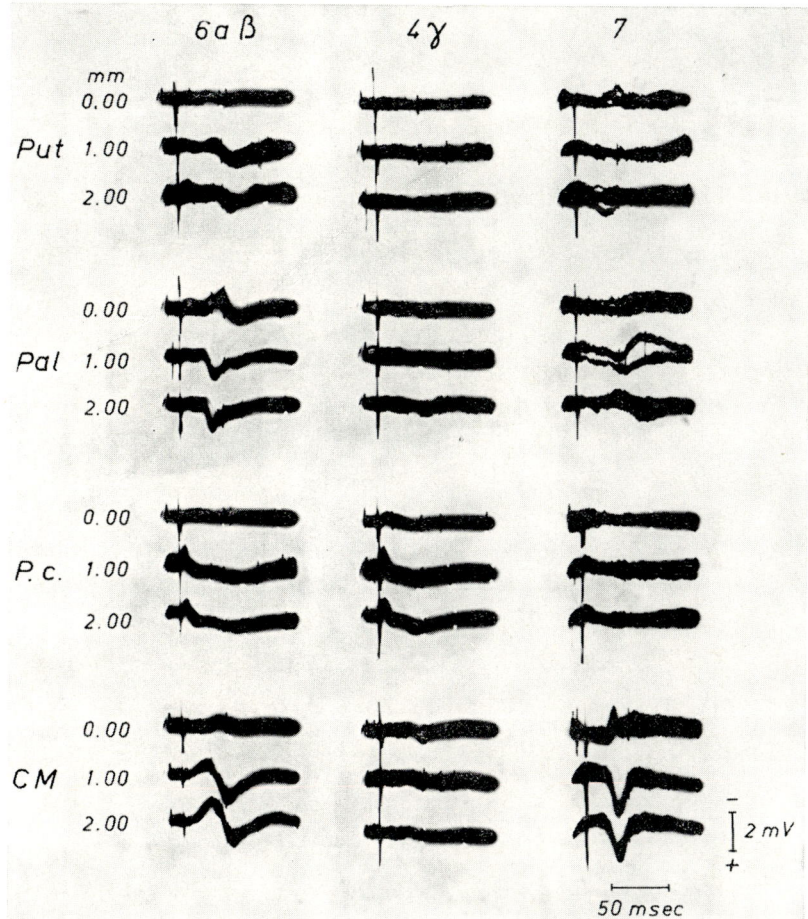

Figure 35.4 Field potentials recorded from different cortical fields (areas 6aβ, 4γ and 7) and elicited by 7/sec stimulation of putamen (Put), pallidum (Pal), cerebral peduncle (P.c.) and centrum medianum (Cm), respectively. (From Dieckmann & Sasaki, 1970, by courtesy of Springer-Verlag, Berlin).

the putamen and pallidum, elicited laminar field potentials of an entirely different type (Dieckmann & Sasaki, 1970).

The putamen- and pallidum-induced recruiting and spindle responses were suppressed by a coagulation lesion in the rostral thalamic reticulate nucleus which represents the rostral end of the thalamic non-specific activating system. As an example, the upper trace (Ia) in Figure 35.5 shows a recruiting response evoked by pallidum stimulation. After a lesion in the thalamic reticulate nucleus, demonstrated in the histological picture above, repeated pallidum stimulation was no longer followed by a recruiting of the cortical

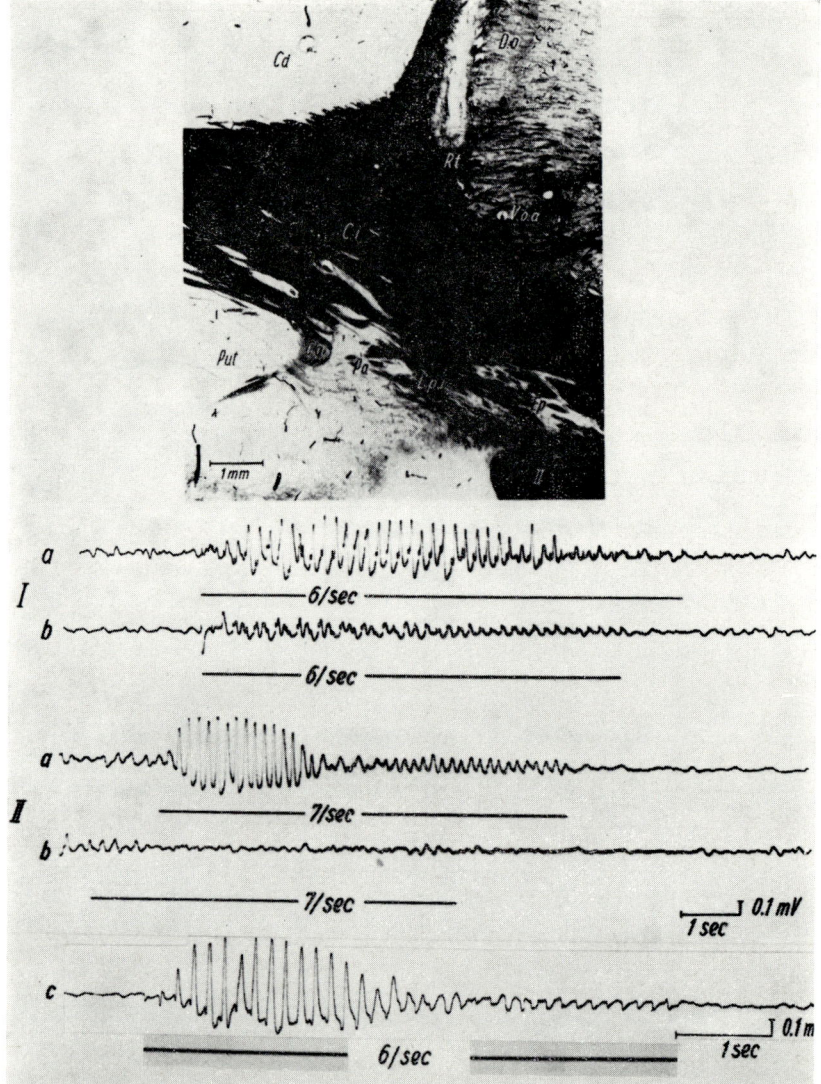

Figure 35.5 Abolition of a pallidum-produced recruiting and spindle response by high-frequency lesion in the rostral thalamus. In Ia, cortical activity (recruiting) before, in Ib after lesion of the thalamic reticulate nucleus as shown in the histological picture above. In IIa, cortical activity (spindling) before, in IIb after thalamic lesion. In IIc, the spindle response obtained by low frequency stimulation of the internal capsule rostrally of the thalamic lesion. Ca, anterior commissure; Cd, caudate nucleus; C.i., internal capsule; D.o., dorsal oral nucleus; Ep, entopeduncular nucleus; L.p.i., lamella pallidi interna; Pa, pallidum; Put, putamen; Rt, thalamic reticular nucleus, rostral part; V.o.a., thalamic oroventral nucleus; II, optic nerve. (Staining after Heidenhain-Woelcke. Magnification 19:1.)

activity (Ib). The same happened with the spindle response (IIa and b). However, stimulation of the internal capsule rostral to the thalamus after the thalamic lesion again produced a spindle response with a positive predeflection (IIc). Obviously, the non-specific pallidum impulses to the cortex have been interrupted by the reticulate nucleus lesions, as is to be expected from the known anatomic connections.

THE ROLE OF THE PUTAMEN AND PALLIDUM IN MAN

The experimental evidence of participation of the putamen and pallidum in non-specific activation is also relevant in human beings. The important role of the pallidum in maintaining psychic activation is known from the results of bilateral pallidal lesions due to poisoning or produced in the early period of stereoencephalotomy (Hassler, 1964). In contrast, prolonged therapeutic stimulation of the pallido-thalamic activating system by means of chronically implanted electrodes in patients with a post-traumatic apallic syndrome induced a clinical and electrophysiological arousal reaction (Hassler, Dalle Ore, Dieckmann, Bricolo & Dolce, 1969).

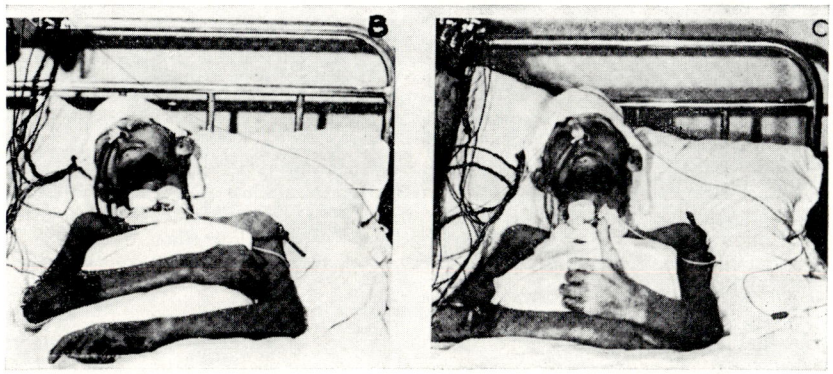

Figure 35.6 Patient with a post-traumatic apallic syndrome with chronically implanted electrodes placed in the right pallidum and left VA nucleus. B: before; C: during stimulation. Bilateral stimulation induces a clinical arousal reaction. (From Hassler, Dalle Ore, Dieckmann, Bricolo & Dolce, 1969 by courtesy of Elsevier Publishing Co.)

Figure 35.6 shows such a patient with stimulating electrodes *in situ*. To the left, the patient is seen before stimulation. To the right, one sees clinical arousal during stimulation of the right pallidum and the left basal VA nucleus, which is the end of the pallido-thalamic pathway. Stimulation induces opening of the eyes, mydriasis, moving of the head and pseudo-intentional movements of the left arm and hand. The patient also shows affective reactions and some vocalization to his relatives during stimulation. After cessation of each stimulation the comatous state recurs.

Figure 35.7 shows the corresponding EEGs. Above, one sees the EEG monitoring before (A) and 2 days after intermittent stimulation (B). At this

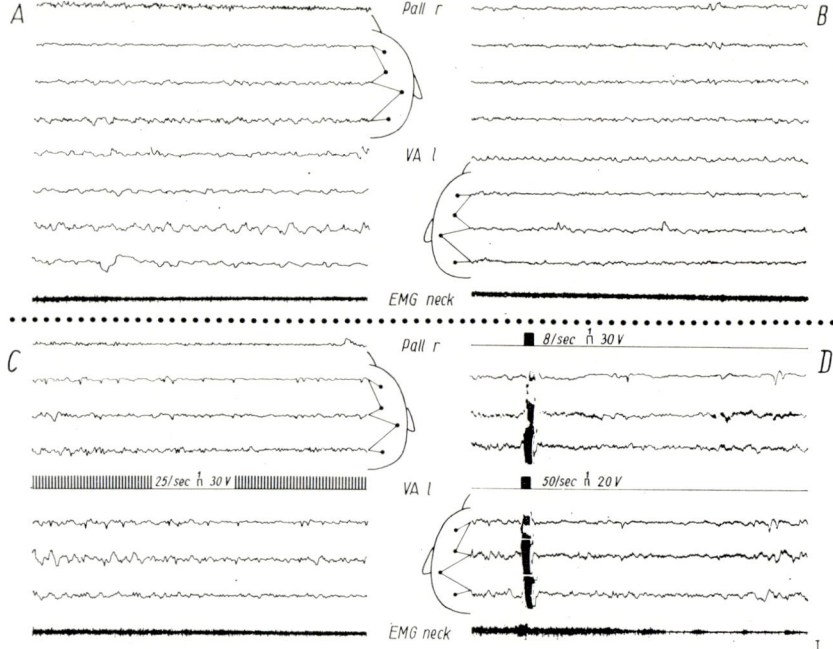

Figure 35.7 Electrocorticogram and subcorticogram of patient shown in Figure 35.6. A: before stimulation; B: 2 days after intermittent stimulation. Background activity modified to desynchronized pattern. C: during VA stimulation; D: during bilateral stimulation (right pallidum and left VA nucleus). Note the immediate desynchronization in D. (From Hassler, Dalle Ore, Dieckmann, Bricolo & Dolce, 1969 by courtesy of Elsevier Publishing Co.)

time background activity is already modified to a desynchronized pattern. The pictures below show the change of activity during stimulation. In C, stimulation of the left VA alone produced predominantly ipsilateral acceleration of spontaneous activity. In D, bilateral stimulation of the right pallidum and left VA evoked immediate desynchronization in all traces.

SUMMARY

To summarize, with an electrophysiological investigation technique in cats, the functional role of the putamen and pallidum in controlling the activity level of the cerebral cortex can be verified. This control seems to be more restricted, particularly to motor neuronal systems, than that of thalamic origin.

REFERENCES

Buchwald NA, Wyers EJ, Okuma T & Heuser G (1961). The 'caudate-spindle'.
   1. Electrophysiological properties. *Electroenceph. clin. Neurophysiol.*, **13**, 509

Dandy WE (1946). The location of the conscious center in the brain—the corpus striatum. *Bull. Johns Hopk. Hosp.*, **79**, 34

Dieckmann G (1968). Cortical synchronized and desynchronized responses evoked by stimulation of putamen and pallidum in cats. *J. neurol. Sci.*, **7**, 385

Dieckmann G & Hassler R (1968). Reizexperimente über die Funktion des Putamen der Katze. *J. Hirnforsch.*, **10**, 187

Dieckmann G & Sasaki K (1970). Recruiting responses in the cerebral cortex produced by putamen and pallidum stimulation. *Exp. Brain Res.*, **10**, 236

Droogleever-Fortuyn J (1950). On the configuration and the connections of the medioventral area and the midline cells in the thalamus of the rabbit. *Folia psychiat. neerl.*, **53**, 213

Hassler R (1950). Contribution morphologique à la physiologie des lobes frontaux. *Compt. Rend., I. Congr. mond. Psychiat.*, Vol. III, p. 118. Paris.

Hassler R (1964). Limbische und diencephale Systeme der Affektivität und Psychomotorik. In: *Muskel und Psyche* (Ed Hoff), p. 3. Basle and New York: Karger.

Hassler R, Dalle Ore G, Dieckmann G, Bricolo A & Dolce G (1969). Behavioural and EEG arousal induced by stimulation of unspecific projection systems in a patient with post-traumatic apallic syndrome. *Electroenceph. clin. Neurophysiol.*, **27**, 306

Hassler R & Dieckmann G (1967). Arrest reaction, delayed inhibition and unusual gaze behaviour resulting from stimulation of the putamen in awake, unrestrained cats. *Brain Res.*, **5**, 504

Heuser G, Buchwald NA & Wyers EJ (1961). The 'caudate-spindle'. 11. Facilitatory and inhibitory caudate-cortical pathways. *Electroenceph. clin. Neurophysiol.*, **13**, 519

Li CL, Cullen C & Jasper HH (1956). Laminar microelectrode analysis of cortical unspecific recruiting responses in the cerebral cortex. *J. Neurophysiol.*, **19**, 131

McLardy T (1948). Projections of the centromedian nucleus of the human thalamus. *Brain*, **71**, 290

Shimamoto T & Verzeano M (1954). Relations between caudate and diffusely projecting thalamic nuclei. *J. Neurophysiol.*, **17**, 278

Spencer WA & Brookhart JM (1961). Electrical patterns of augmenting and recruiting waves in depths of sensomotor cortex of cats. *J. Neurophysiol.*, **24**, 26

Stoupel N & Terzuolo C (1954). Etude des connexions et de la physiologie du noyau caudé. *Acta neurol. belg.*, 54, 239

CHAPTER 36

Sensory convergence in the cerebral cortex
T P S POWELL

Although my title is concerned with sensory convergence within the cerebral cortex, I should like to consider some of our recent experimental work on the cerebral cortex in the broader context of corticohypothalamic connections. This will mean that it will overlap to some extent with Dr Nauta's talk but I am sure he will agree that there is room for more than one discussion of this difficult problem. It will receive a slightly different emphasis from each of us.

There is a good deal of evidence that changes in emotional and psychological states can affect secretions of the anterior pituitary gland, and the suggestion has been made that the hypothalamus integrates 'not only patterns of endocrine activity but also patterns of emotional behaviour' (Harris, 1959). The marked changes in higher mental functions and personality brought about by leucotomy stimulated considerable interest in the possibility of direct connections from the neocortex to the hypothalamus in the late 1940s, and indeed Le Gros Clark & Meyer (1950) described such connections using the Glees technique. Those results were never written up in detail however, and a few years later when Cowan and I were asked to re-examine the material we were forced to question the validity of the findings and even the validity of the technique itself because in the experimental material a similar distribution of degeneration was always found in the hypothalamus despite marked differences in the size and the site of the lesion in the neocortex, and also because an exactly similar appearance and distribution of 'degeneration' were observed in sections of normal brains (Cowan & Powell, 1956). That interpretation received certain criticism but it simply means that the Glees technique cannot be used in the hypothalamus. At present the only direct projections from the neocortex to the hypothalamus which have been established are those from the orbital surface of the frontal lobe and from a restricted part of the lateral surface, probably from the region of area 46 (Nauta, 1962, 1971). During the next decade, in the 1950s, most neuroanatomical work on the connections of the hypothalamus was concentrated upon elucidating the details of the projection to this region from the hippocampus and the amygdala, and was done mainly by Nauta and his associates in the United States, by Cragg, Hamlyn and Guillery at University College London, and by Le Gros Clark and his colleagues in Oxford. As a result of those investigations there is probably general agreement now about the details of these pathways, and also that the fibres coming from the hippocampus and amygdala form the most massive set of afferents to the hypothalamus. Despite this anatomical knowledge there was little known about the functional significance of these big fibre tracts, and this ignorance was largely due to the fact that we did not know the functional significance of the afferent fibres which in turn were going to the hippocampus and amygdala. This recalls the fundamental truth of the statement of Elliot Smith many years ago that the key to the understanding of the neocortex lies in an intensive study of the thalamus; in other words, before we can understand the significance of a particular part of the brain we usually have to know the details of the afferent pathways going into it. On the other hand, there is extensive functional evidence for important influences of the sensory systems upon the hypo-

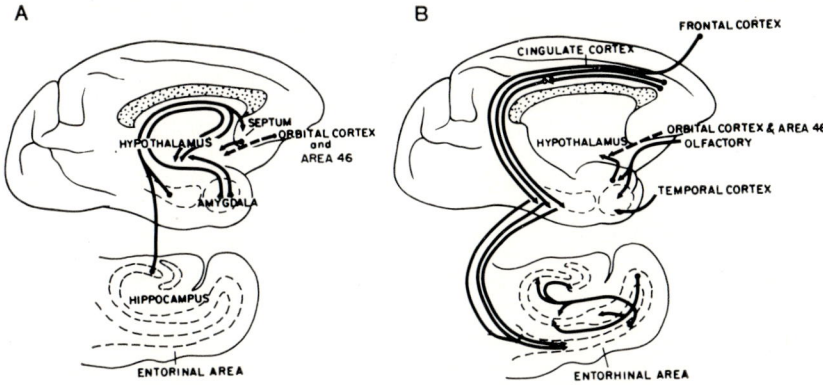

Figure 36.1 Diagrammatic representation of the major fibre pathways from the hippocampus and amygdala to the hypothalamus (A), and of the main afferent connections of the hippocampus and amygdala (B). The broken lines indicate the direct connections to the hypothalamus from the orbital cortex and area 46 of the neocortex.

thalamus but with the exception of the olfactory pathway (Powell, Cowan & Raisman, 1965) little is known about the fibre connections by which these sensory systems exert their effects, as few, if any fibres are known to pass directly to the hypothalamus from the sensory pathways. The most massive connections to the hypothalamus are from the limbic forebrain, and Figure 36.1 outlines the pathways to and from the hippocampus and amygdala. The fornix-fimbrial system projects to the septum and hypothalamus, and from the amygdala there are two pathways to the hypothalamus, the stria terminalis and the ventral projection system. The afferent pathways to the entorhinal area, which is in turn the major source of afferent fibres to the hippocampus, come from the cortex of the frontal, cingulate and temporal regions. Into the amygdala are passing fibres from the neocortex of the temporal lobe and from the olfactory pathway.

In 1957 Scoville & Milner showed that the bilateral removal of the medial parts of the temporal lobes resulted in persistent loss of recent memory. To the experimental neurologist here was an important puzzle or paradox: one would have predicted that a structure importantly concerned in memory would have strong connections from the sensory systems, but at that time, and until relatively recently, there was not only no evidence for such connections but as far as I know this problem has not been emphasized, although Cragg (1965) commented that 'it is surprising that the neocortical connections of the allocortex are not more prominent'. With this in mind in 1963 I examined an extensive collection of rabbit brain material which had been used for mapping out the projections of the neocortex to the striatum (Carman, Cowan & Powell, 1963), hoping to find a connection from the neocortex to the vicinity of the entorhinal area. In this material I did find some degeneration in the vicinity of the entorhinal area but as I could discern no organization in it nor define the origin of the degenerating axons I did not pursue it further. Then in 1965 came the important paper of Cragg; using the cat he described projections from a localized region of the suprasylvian gyrus or parietal cortex going into the cingulate cortex, and he also confirmed projections from the prefrontal cortex and from the equivalent of the temporal cortex to the entorhinal area. At that time we were working on the association connections of the sensory cortical areas in the cat; after lesions in the somatic sensory area we always found a projection back into area 5 of the parietal cortex (Jones & Powell, 1968) and after similar lesions of the auditory cortex degeneration was found in the suprasylvian gyrus (Diamond, Jones & Powell, 1968). Together with Cragg's finding these observations gave us a clue: it was possible that the sensory pathways were coming together in this parietal cortex and from the site of final convergence there were projections into the limbic system. For this reason Jones and I turned to the larger brain of the monkey and placed lesions systematically in discrete functional and architectonic areas and traced the degenerating fibres with the Nauta technique (Jones & Powell, 1970).

At this point I would like to pay a tribute to Dr Nauta as he is here with us. His technique is probably the most sensitive and reliable method in use for tracing connections of the central nervous system today. During the last twenty years it has contributed enormously, and I am sure that in the history of experimental neurology his name will rank with others of the past such as Nissl, Golgi, and Marchi.

After lesions in the somatic sensory area of the post-central gyrus of the monkey (Figure 36.2), degenerating fibres pass back into area 5, and forward into area 4 and the supplementary motor area; so that from the somatic sensory area there is one projection back into the parietal lobe and another forward into the frontal lobe. If the lesion is in area 5, degeneration is found in area 7 of the parietal cortex and in area 6 of the frontal lobe. A lesion in area 7, in turn, as a third step, produces degeneration in the walls of the superior temporal sulcus and again in the frontal lobe, in the vicinity of the upper bank of the principal sulcus, area 46, and on two aspects of the medial surface—in the cingulate cortex, and in the immediate vicinity of the entorhinal area,

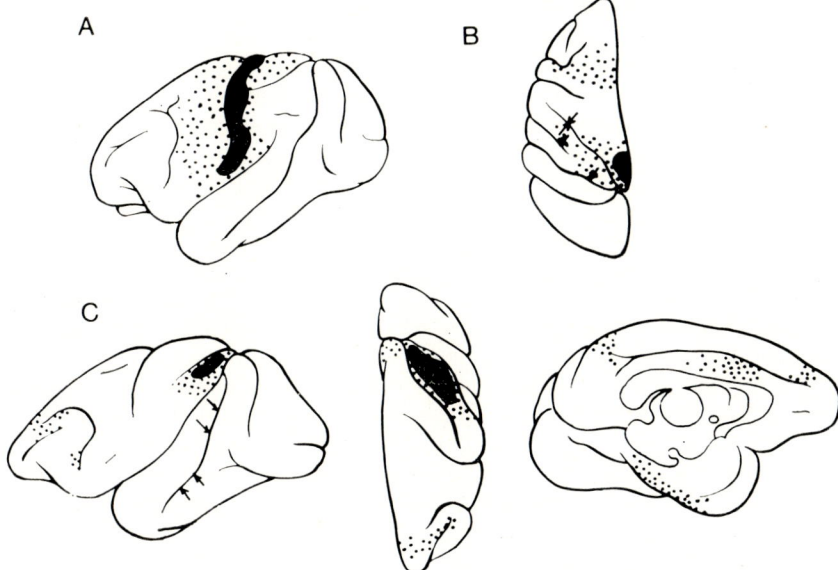

Figure 36.2 The distribution of axonal and terminal degeneration in the ipsilateral cortex of the monkey brain following lesions of the somatic sensory cortex of the post-central gyrus (A), in area 5 (B) and in area 7 (C). In this and subsequent figures the lesion is indicated in black, terminal degeneration by stippling and degenerating fibres by short lines. The arrows point to degeneration in the walls of sulci.

the perirhinal region on the medial part of the temporal lobe. So parietal cortex is projecting into limbic areas—cingulate and perirhinal, and this is the equivalent, in the primate, of Cragg's experiment in the cat. The sequence in the frontal lobe is shown in Figure 36.3. The somatic sensory cortex projects forward into area 4, and a lesion in area 4 shows that as well as projecting back into the somatic sensory cortex it also sends fibres forward into area 6; a lesion in area 6 in turn indicates that it projects back to area 4 and also forward into the region (area 46) which is connected with area 7. Damage in the vicinity of area 46 shows that it is in turn connected with area 7 of the parietal region. The two lesions here close to the frontal pole result in degeneration in the cingulate gyrus and the small area of degeneration in the superior temporal gyrus is related to involvement of area 10 of the frontal pole. The important points from the experiments which have been described so far are that the somatic sensory areas project into *both* parietal and frontal cortical regions, there is a step-by-step sequence in each lobe and each new step in the parietal cortex is interlocked with the corresponding one in the frontal region.

There is a similar progression from the visual cortex (Figure 36.4). From area 17 fibres go out to the peristriate cortex (areas 18 and 19) and to a separate region in the posterior wall of the superior temporal sulcus. Only when the peristriate region of 18 and 19 is involved is an appreciable projection found to frontal cortex, area 8, and down into area 20 of the temporal lobe. A lesion in the latter area results in degenerating fibres passing forward into area 21 of the temporal lobe and into a new region of the frontal lobe, the agranular precentral cortex; there is also a projection into the basolateral group of the amygdala indicating that there is an earlier connection from the visual areas to the amygdala than from other pathways. From area 20 there is also a pathway to the perirhinal region. Damage of the cortex of area 21, the next step in the sequence of visual connections in the temporal lobe, results in degeneration in several sites in the parieto-temporal lobe: at the tip of the superior temporal gyrus, in the walls of the superior temporal sulcus where it is co-extensive with the area affected after a lesion of area 7 on the somatic sensory progression but distinct from that involved after a lesion of area 17, in the basolateral nuclei of the amygdala and in the perirhinal region. There is also degeneration in the cortex of the frontal lobe, in the part of area 46 below the principal sulcus and in area 25 on the medial surface.

The auditory progression in the cortex is difficult to trace in the monkey. We do not have lesions restricted to the primary auditory cortex, but Figure

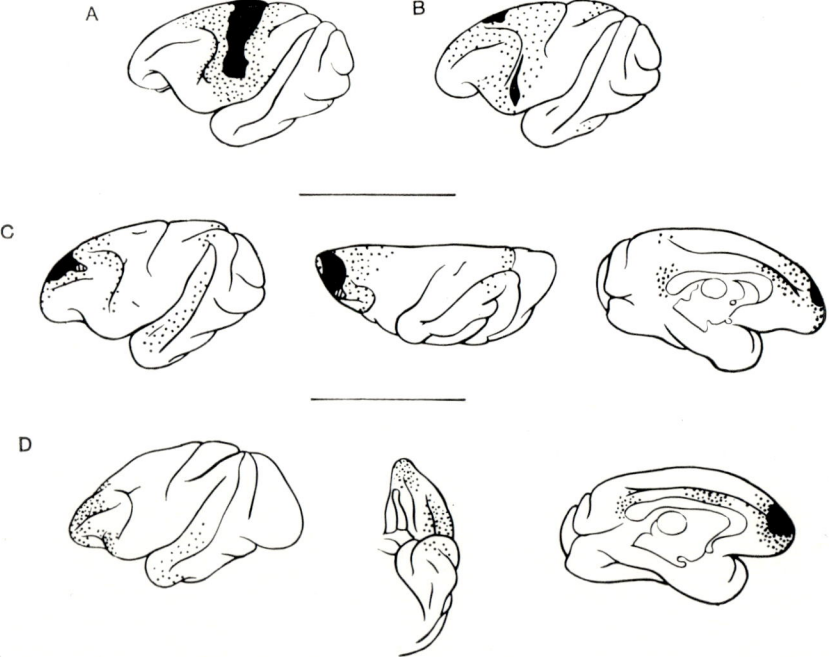

Figure 36.3 The distribution of degeneration due to damage of area 4 of the motor cortex (A), of area 6 and the supplementary motor area (B) and of area 9 (C and D), but with undercutting of the upper part of area 46 in C and with involvement of area 10 of the frontal pole in D.

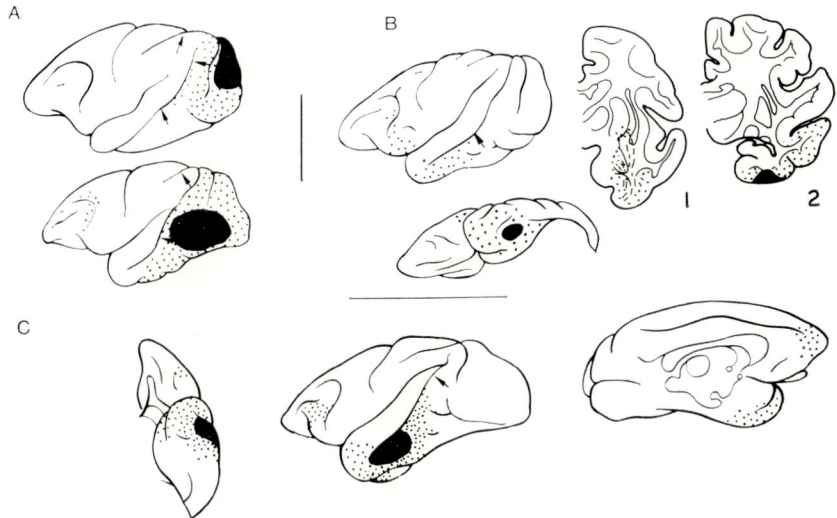

Figure 36.4 The lesion and degeneration in experiments done to determine the sequence of connections from the visual cortex. In A the first brain has a lesion confined to area 17, and in the second areas 17, 18 and 19 are damaged. In B area 20 of the temporal lobe has been damaged and in section 1 degeneration can be seen in the baso-lateral group of the amygdaloid nuclei. In C the lesion is in area 21.

36.5 shows an experiment with a lesion involving the supratemporal plane and area 22 which has resulted in degeneration throughout area 22 in the superior temporal gyrus and in three parts of the frontal lobe: at the frontal pole and adjoining medial surface (areas 10 and 25), at the junction of the lateral and orbital surfaces (area 12), and on the lateral surface from the upper end of the arcuate sulcus forwards around the principal sulcus. When area 22 in turn is selectively damaged (Figure 36.5) there is axonal degeneration throughout this area, and it extends forward to the temporal pole and medially into the perirhinal region. Convergence of the three sensory pathways is indicated by the presence of degeneration in the depths of the superior temporal sulcus, in the same area affected by a lesion of area 7 (somatic) and area 21 (visual). In the frontal lobe degeneration is present in the same sites as in the previous brain *except* close to the principal sulcus.

Finally, lesions of the frontal and temporal poles (Figure 36.6) show that both these regions are interlocked with each other, and that both send heavy projections into the cortex on the orbital surface of the frontal lobe, to the anterior part of the cingulate cortex on the medial surface and to area 45 and the orbito-frontal cortex close to the ventral part of the lateral aspect of the same lobe. From the frontal pole fibres also pass back to the cortex in the depths of the superior temporal sulcus.

If the sequential progressions of the sensory pathways in the parietal lobe are considered diagrammatically, they are seen to run in parallel: somatic sensory

272 *Surgical Approaches in Psychiatry*

cortex to area 5, area 5 to area 7 and area 7 to the superior temporal sulcus and to the cingulate and perirhinal cortex on the medial surface (Figure 36.7). There is a comparable progression in the visual and auditory pathways. It is in the walls of the superior temporal sulcus that somatic, visual and auditory come to overlap. They all ultimately send fibres into the cingulate cortex and to the perirhinal region immediately adjoining the entorhinal cortex; this region is closely related to that which Scoville removed in human patients in 1957. There is a comparable sequence of connections in the frontal lobe from the somatic sensory cortex to area 4 and the supplementary motor cortex; area 4 to the whole precentral motor cortex (area 6, the supplementary motor area and the precentral agranular field) and area 6 to the upper part of area 46 (Figure 36.8). It is similar in the visual progression. It is interesting to note that when connections cease going into areas 4 and 6 of the motor cortex they begin to go into the cingulate region, and one interpretation of this observation could be that these are the two major outflows of the neocortex: through areas 4 and 6 the somatic motor influence, and from levels 'beyond' this into the cingulate and hippocampal pathways to the hypothalamus for emotional and visceral regulation. In summary it can be said that there is a step by step sequential spread from each of the main sensory cortical areas in *both* the

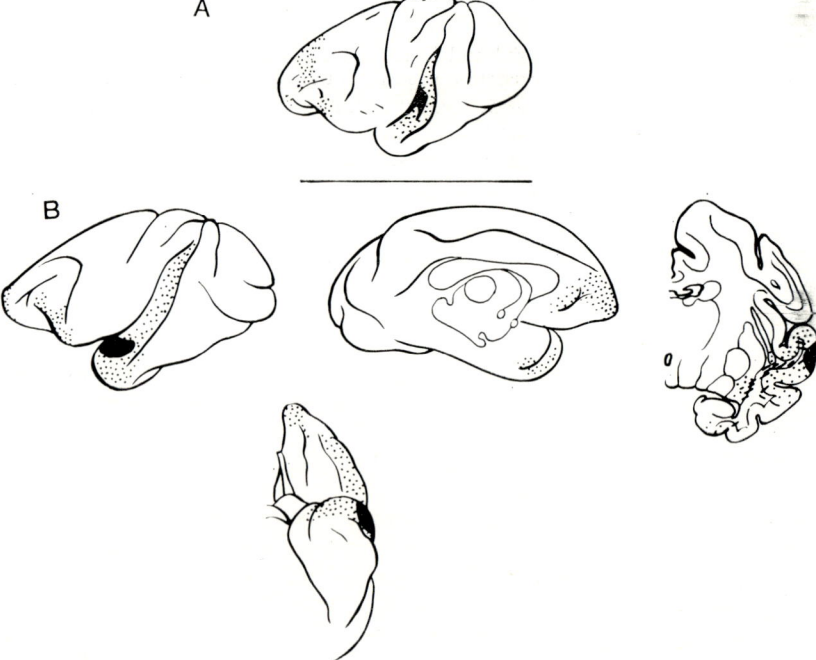

Figure 36.5 The distribution of degeneration following damage of the supratemporal plane and area 22 of the auditory areas (A), and after a lesion confined to area 22 (B).

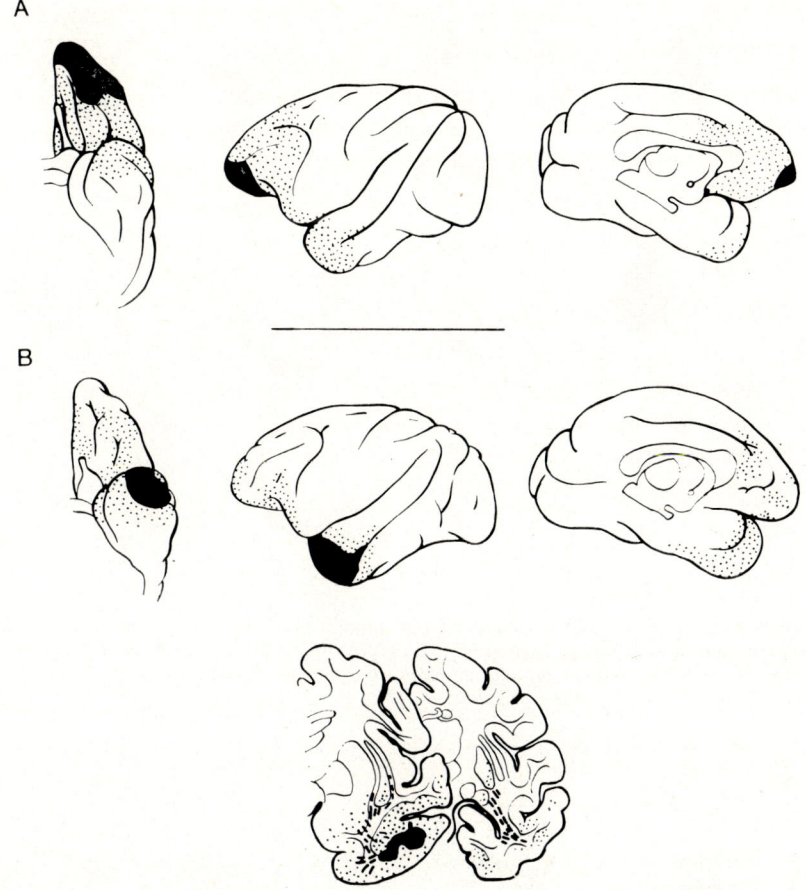

Figure 36.6 The lesions and degeneration in experiments in which the frontal pole (A) and the temporal pole (B) have been involved.

parieto-temporal and frontal lobes, and these steps in the two lobes are interlocked with each other. When connections cease going into areas 4 and 6 from both frontal and parieto-temporal lobes they begin to go into limbic regions. The regions of final convergence, in the frontal pole and the orbito-frontal cortex of the frontal operculum project heavily into the orbital cortex of the frontal lobe, and are interlocked with the temporal pole and superior temporal sulcus.

Figure 36.9 is taken from the paper of Penfield (1966) in which he summarizes his findings on stimulation of the temporal lobe; this shows the sites at which electrical stimulation elicited what Penfield calls 'experiential' or psychic responses in the dominant and non-dominant hemispheres in the conscious patient. The auditory responses are predominantly in the superior

274 *Surgical Approaches in Psychiatry*

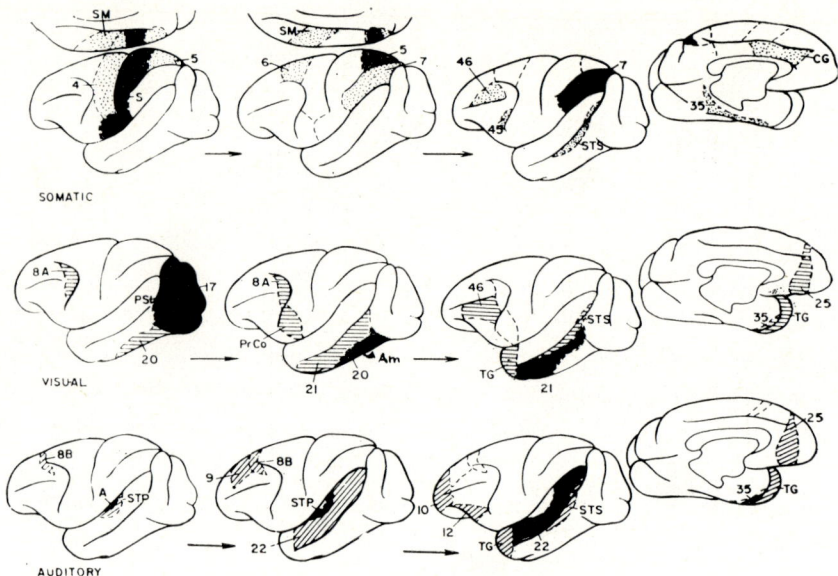

Figure 36.7 A schematic summary of the sequence of connections from the somatic, visual and auditory areas. Each new local step is shown in black and the further connections by stippling or hatching. Note that all sensory pathways converge in the depths of the superior temporal sulcus.

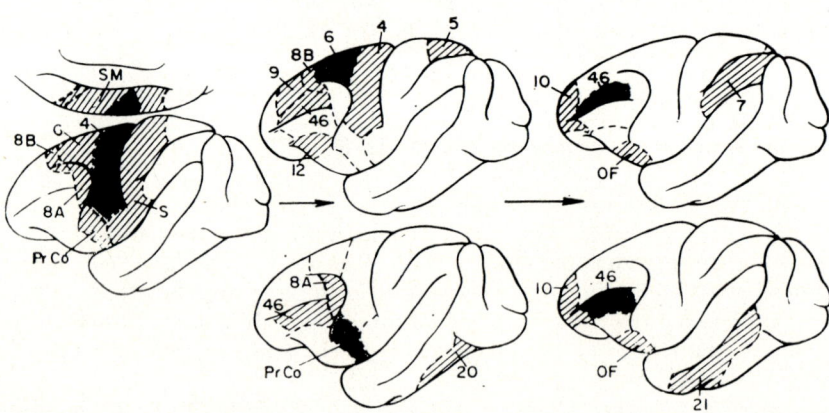

Figure 36.8 The stepwise progression of connections of the somatic (above) and visual (below) pathways in the frontal lobe, and the reciprocal connections with equivalent steps in the parietal and temporal lobes. Note the regions of convergence in area 10 and the orbito-frontal cortex (OF).

Part VIII—Basic Sciences 275

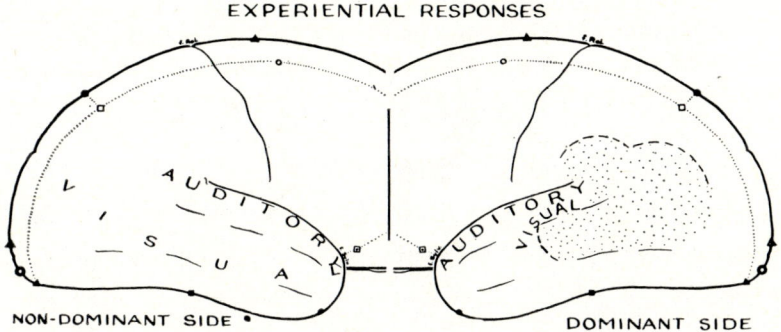

Figure 36.9 Summary of experiential responses. The dotted zone indicates ideational speech area. (From Penfield & Perot, 1963).

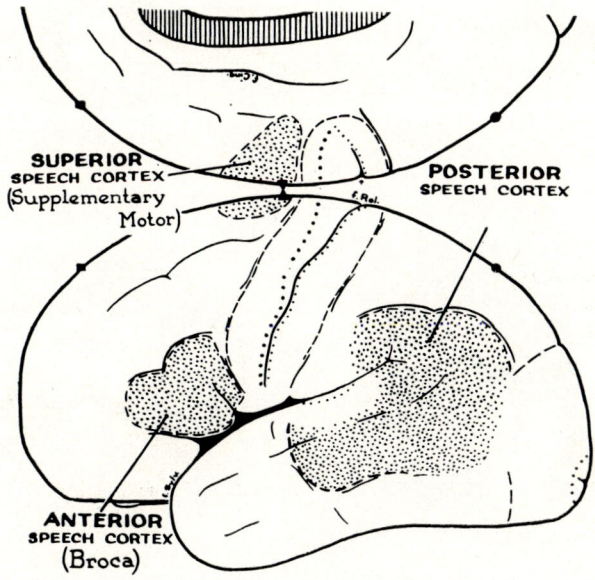

Figure 36.10 Cortical speech areas of dominant hemisphere as determined by the method of aphasic arrest or electrical interference. (From Penfield & Roberts, 1959).

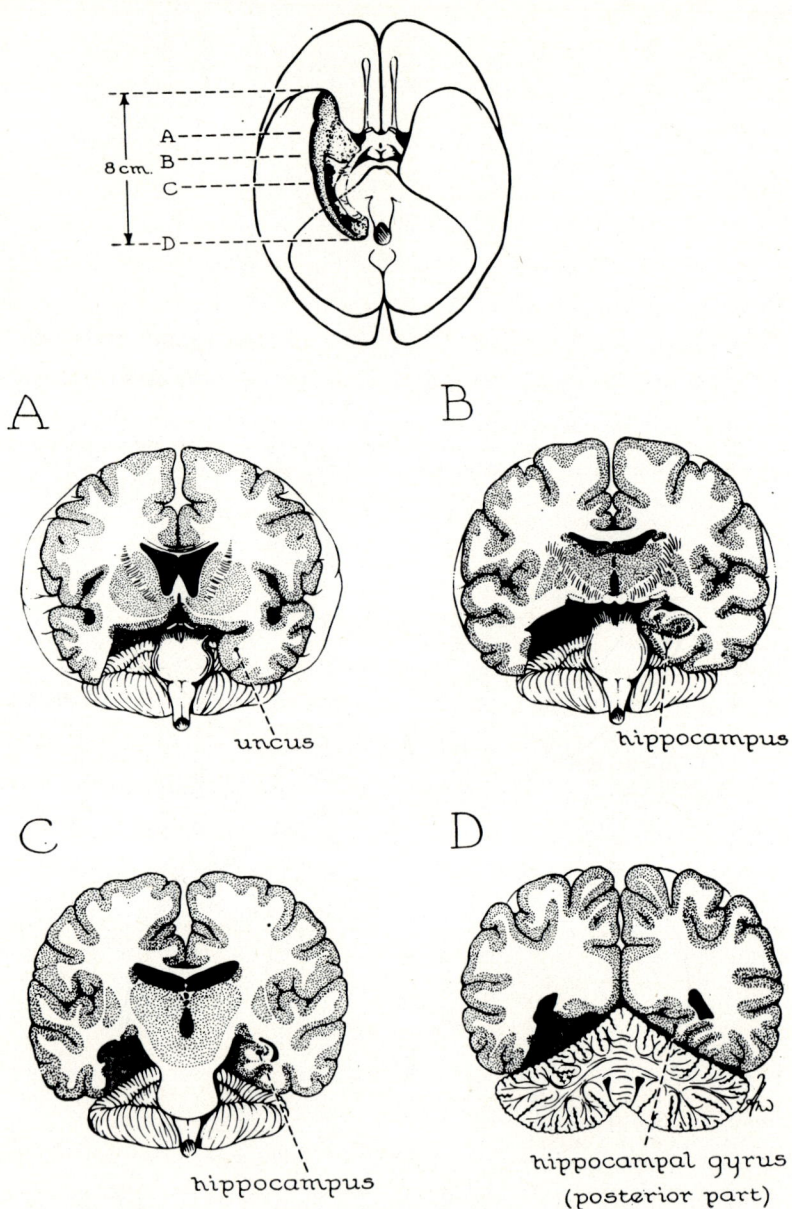

Figure 36.11 Diagrammatic cross-sections of human brain illustrating extent of attempted bilateral medial temporal lobe resection in the radical operation. (For diagrammatic purposes the resection has been shown on one side only). (From Scoville & Milner, 1957).

temporal gyrus, and the visual responses, which are more frequent on the non-dominant side than on the dominant, are mainly in the middle temporal gyrus. They are in those regions where the visual and auditory pathways have been shown to make connections in the monkey brain. It is significant that Penfield also got a few similar responses on the inferior surface of the temporal lobe in the immediate vicinity of the entorhinal cortex. Figure 36.10 is also taken from the same paper by Penfield and shows the anterior and posterior speech areas; it may be tentatively suggested that the regions of convergence of the sensory pathways in the monkey, in the walls of the superior temporal sulcus and in the ventro-lateral region of the frontal lobe below the arcuate sulcus, are the bases for the two speech areas which have so markedly expanded in the human brain. Figure 36.11 is taken from the paper of Scoville & Milner (1957) and shows the extent of the removal of the medial temporal lobe, in a transverse section, and this includes the perirhinal cortex adjoining the entorhinal area.

So far I have dealt with the somatic, visual and auditory pathways within the neocortex but some recent work on the olfactory system suggests that its relationship may be somewhat similar (Price & Powell, 1971). Figure 36.12 shows outlines of sagittal sections of the brain of the rat after a lesion of the olfactory bulb. While for some years it has been agreed that the degeneration resulting from such a lesion of the bulb spreads up on to the posterior surface of the hemisphere, there has been debate as to whether this represents a direct projection from the bulb to the entorhinal cortex. If one maps out precisely the site of these degenerating fibres on the posterior surface and compares it with a Nissl section or with the original figure of Cajal, (Figure 36.13) in which it may be seen that the true entorhinal cortex is characterized by a well-marked deep plexiform or IVth layer, it can be seen that the

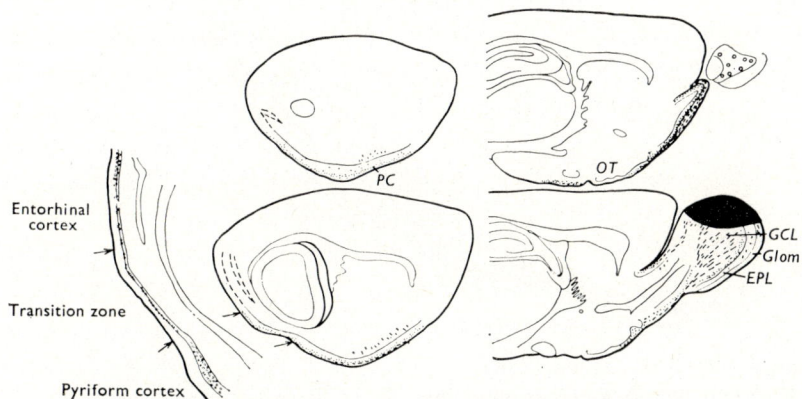

Figure 36.12 The lesion of the olfactory bulb and the resulting degeneration in sagittal sections of the rat brain together with a tracing of an alternate, thionin-stained section of the transition region between the entorhinal cortex proper of Cajal and the pyriform cortex.

278 *Surgical Approaches in Psychiatry*

degeneration never spreads into the region occupied by the deep plexiform layer. The degenerating fibres extend only into a transition zone on the posterior surface, between the true olfactory, pyriform cortex and the entorhinal area, and it has therefore been suggested that the olfactory pathway is similar to the other main sensory pathways in sending fibres to a region immediately around the entorhinal cortex proper, but not into the entorhinal area itself.

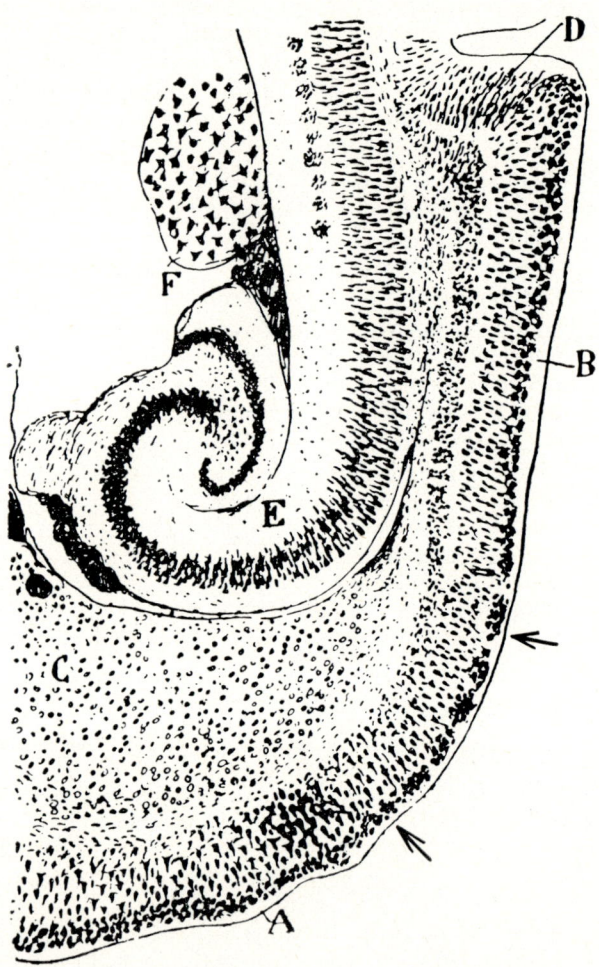

Figure 36.13 Reproduction of Figure 451 of Cajal (Volume 11, 1911) to show his interpretation of the structure and limits of the 'true olfactory sphenoidal cortex' (A) and of the 'spheno-occipital ganglion' (entorhinal cortex) (B) in a 'central sagittal section of the pyriform lobe of the cat'. D is the superior limit of the spheno-occipital ganglion, E is the hippocampus and C the lenticular nucleus. The arrows have been inserted to indicate our interpretation of the presence and site of the transition zone, although it was not identified as such by Cajal.

Figures 36.14 and 36.15 summarize these findings. The main sensory areas of the neocortex send fibres into the parietal cortex *and* into the frontal cortex in a step by step progression until they finally overlap and converge in the superior temporal sulcus, in the region of the frontal pole and in the orbito-frontal cortex of the frontal operculum. These parietal and frontal regions are interconnected with each other, and they project into the cingulate cortex medially and into the perirhinal region below. The frontal and temporal poles are also interconnected and from these regions there are strong projections to the orbital surface of the frontal lobe, from which there are direct connections to the hypothalamus. The amygdala receives fibres from quite an early step on the visual progression in the temporal lobe. The olfactory pathway contributes fibres to the amygdala, directly to the hypothalamus and to a transition zone around the entorhinal cortex. The olfactory

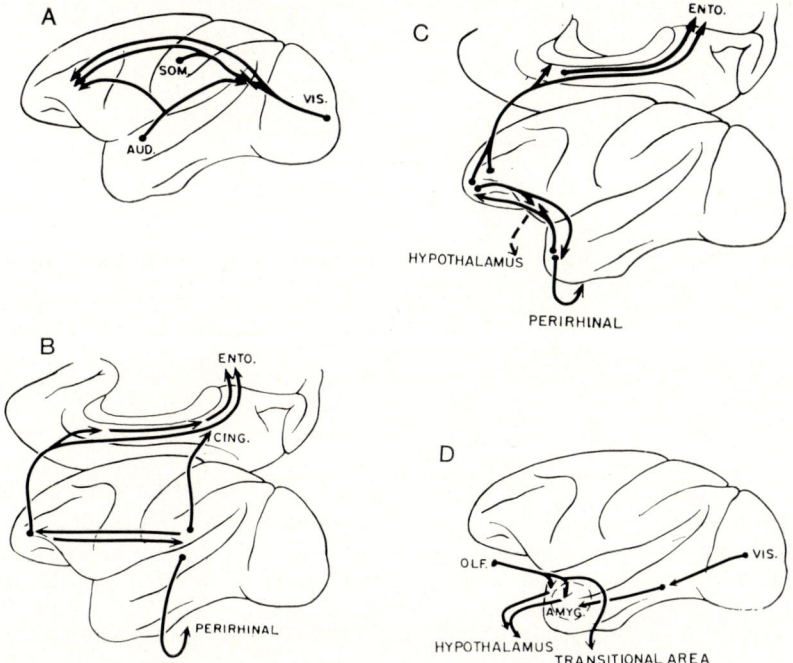

Figure 36.14 Schematic summary of the experimental findings on convergence of the sensory pathways within the neocortex. The three pathways from the somatic, visual and auditory areas project into and converge in *both* the parietal and frontal lobes (A). The frontal and parietal areas are interconnected and project into the cingulate and perirhinal regions (B). The frontal and temporal poles are interconnected, and both send fibres to the orbito-frontal cortex in the frontal operculum and into the cortex of the orbital surface (from which fibres pass directly to the hypothalamus) (C). The olfactory pathway is connected with the pyriform cortex (from which fibres go directly to the hypothalamus), with the transition zone and with the amygdala; the amygdala also receives connections from an early step in the cortical progression from the visual cortex (D).

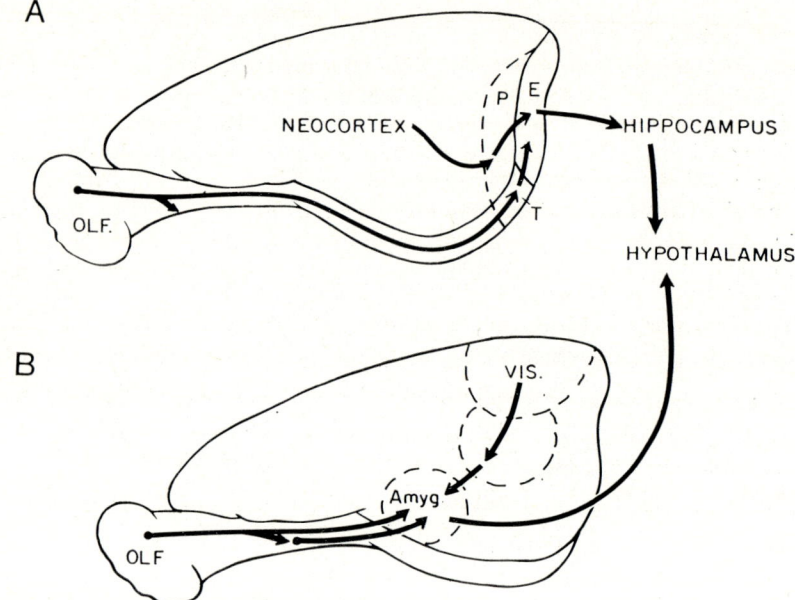

Figure 36.15 A. Diagram of a typical mammalian brain to summarize the suggested relations of the projection from the neocortex to the perirhinal area (P) and of the olfactory pathway to the transition zone (T), and of the further connections, through the entorhinal area (E) and hippocampus, with the hypothalamus. B. The afferent connections of the amygdala from the olfactory and visual pathways, and the direct projection of the amygdala upon the hypothalamus.

input to the amygdala is related to the cortico-medial group of nuclei and the visual to the basolateral group; the latter connection is probably the basis for the expansion of the basolateral group in the primate in which there is a corresponding enlargement of the temporal cortex. It appears that immediately around the entorhinal area there is a region of cortex which receives projections from the olfactory and other main systems, and it is possible that the final integration of sensory information occurs here: this region was included in the medial part of the temporal lobe removed by Scoville. The neocortex may influence the hypothalamus by direct connections from the orbital surface and area 46 of the frontal lobe, and indirectly by connections to the cingulate and perirhinal areas (and thence through the hippocampus) and to the amygdala.

REFERENCES

Carman JB, Cowan WM & Powell TPS (1963). The organization of the cortico-striate connexions in the rabbit. *Brain*, **86**, 525

Cowan WM & Powell TPS (1956). A note on terminal degeneration in the hypothalamus. *J. Anat. (Lond.)*, **90**, 188

Cragg BG (1965). Afferent connexions of the allocortex. *J. Anat. (Lond.)*, **99**, 339

Diamond IT, Jones EG & Powell TPS (1968). The association connections of the auditory cortex of the cat. *Brain Res.*, **11**, 560

Harris GW (1959). Central control of pituitary secretion. In *Handbook of Physiology—Neurophysiology II* (Eds J Field, HW Magoun & VE Hall) Washington, D.C.: American Physiological Society.

Jones EG & Powell TPS (1968). The ipsilateral cortical connexions of the somatic sensory areas in the cat. *Brain Res.*, **9**, 71

Jones EG & Powell TPS (1970). An anatomical study of converging sensory pathways within the cerebral cortex of the monkey. *Brain*, **93**, 793

Le Gros Clark WE & Meyer M (1950). Anatomical relationships between the cerebral cortex and the hypothalamus. *Brit. Med. Bull.*, **6**, 341

Nauta WJH (1962). Neural associations of the amygdaloid complex in the monkey. *Brain*, **85**, 505

Nauta WJH (1971). The problem of the frontal lobe. A reinterpretation. *J. Psychiat. Res.*, **8**, 167

Penfield W (1966). Speech, perception and the cortex. In *Brain and Conscious Experience* (Ed JC Eccles) Berlin: Springer-Verlag.

Powell TPS, Cowan WM & Raisman G (1965). The central olfactory connections. *J. Anat. (Lond.)*, **99**, 791

Price JL & Powell TPS (1971). Certain observations on the olfactory pathway. *J. Anat. (Lond.)*, **110**, 105

Scoville WB & Milner B (1957). Loss of recent memory after bilateral hippocampal lesions. *J. Neurol. Neurosurg. Psychiat.*, **20**, 11

CHAPTER 37

Cholinergic pathways of the brain
C C D SHUTE

A number of methods are possible for investigating cholinergic mechanisms in the central nervous system: none of these can be regarded as complete in itself, and in each case the findings should be evaluated in relation to those obtained with other types of approach. One such approach is through acetylcholine (ACh) assay: changes in ACh concentration may be estimated in different brain regions, or ACh release can be measured from, for instance, the cerebral cortex in response to reticular stimulation. Drugs that affect cholinergic transmission can be administered either systemically or locally, e.g. by iontophoresis. Drugs that promote cholinergic activity include cholinomimetics such as carbachol which produce effects similar to ACh, cholinogogues such as tremorine which promote ACh release, and anticholinesterases such as eserine which prevent destruction of ACh. Anticholinergic drugs such as atropine or scopolamine depress cholinergic activity by blocking receptor sites. Although responses to the administration of such drugs may throw much light on cholinergic function in the brain, it must be remembered first, that the effects produced may be dose-dependent according to the extent to which the amount of ACh made available at the site of action approaches the physiological optimum, and secondly, that the drug may have actions of its own unrelated to cholinergic function.

In order to study how neurones utilizing a particular transmitter are organized into actual pathways, it is necessary to use a histochemical method which can be considered to be specific for that transmitter. In the case of monoaminergic systems this is now straightforward at light microscopy level, since with the formaldehyde–fluorescence method the transmitters themselves can be visualized. In the case of cholinergic neurones this is not possible, so a technique must be adopted which will reveal enzymes associated with ACh rather than ACh itself. Histochemical methods designed to locate the synthetic enzyme choline acetyltransferase (ChA) are only moderately successful, since this enzyme is probably not membrane-bound. The lytic enzyme acetylcholinesterase (AChE), on the other hand, is strongly bound to membranes and very stable. Its specificity, however, with respect to cholinergic neurones requires careful consideration.

The thiocholine method for AChE was devised by Koelle & Friedenwald (1949) and applied to sections of normal rat brain by Koelle (1954). Other workers have modified the method in attempts to increase its specificity, and a version suitable for electron microscopy was used by Lewis & Shute (1966). The Karnovsky ferricyanide method has been adopted by a number of workers, but in our opinion is inferior, owing to the poor penetration of the reagents. We applied the thiocholine method, in a version designed to show large amounts of AChE only, to lesioned rat brains, and on the basis of our results were able to publish a map of the main AChE-containing pathways (Shute & Lewis, 1963). Subsequently a close correlation was found between AChE and ChA levels in the afferent innervation of the hippocampus (Lewis et al., 1967); these findings provided a justification for the hypothesis that the AChE-containing pathways revealed by our methods were indeed cholinergic.

The histochemical criteria for cholinergic and cholinoceptive neurones can be summarized as follows. In cholinergic neurones large amounts of AChE are present in the rough endoplasmic reticulum (ER) of the cell cytoplasm, in the nuclear envelope and sometimes on the plasma membrane. In sectioned peripheral motor neurones the enzyme disappears temporarily from the cell body during chromatolysis. AChE is also present on the axolemma of cholinergic neurones along the whole length of the axon as far as its terminals, and is particularly obvious in preterminal neuropil. The enzyme disappears permanently from sectioned axons distal to the cut, and piles up on the proximal side in the region of the axon immediately adjacent to its cut end. Electron microscopical studies of the fornix after lesions intercepting its fibres have shown that AChE pile-up occurs mainly in unmyelinated preterminal axons. Recently we have been trying to quantify some of these changes, using the method of x-ray emission microanalysis.

In some sensory nerves including optic nerves (Lewis & Shute, 1965) a small proportion of fibres (up to 5%) contain AChE. Such fibres in the dorsal roots respond to sectioning by producing AChE pile-up (Gwyn & Flumerfelt, 1972): whether they represent a cholinergic element of the sensory pathway is unknown. There is evidence that cuneate cells respond, albeit weakly, in an inhibitory fashion to ACh (Galindo et al., 1967), and dorsal horn cells have the histochemical appearance of being cholinoceptive. It is possible that the AChE-containing fibres have the function of modulating transmission by release of ACh at sensory relays, rather than that of setting up a postsynaptic action potential.

In non-cholinergic cholinoceptive neurones AChE is present on the plasma membrane of dendritic spines. Cholinergic endings on such neurones are predominantly axodendritic (Shute & Lewis, 1966). Cholinoceptive neurones also typically possess small to moderate amounts of AChE on the rough ER of the cell cytoplasm, but the enzyme is absent from the axonal membrane and from the terminals. Occasionally AChE is present in large amounts in the cell cytoplasm, as in the inhibitory Golgi type II interneurones of the hippocampus and cerebellum, and in the cells of the hypothalamic paraventricular nucleus and the locus coeruleus, all of which are probably non-cholinergic and cholinoceptive.

Cholinergic pathways within the brain that can be detected and traced by histochemical means include the roots of peripheral motor nerves, the fornix afferents to the hippocampus, and components of the ascending reticular activating system (ARAS). A peripheral motor nerve whose status has been disputed, partly on account of its unusual response to strychnine, is the olivo-cochlear bundles, but evidence has accumulated that this too is cholinergic (Comis, 1970). AChE is present in the cells of origin in the superior olivary region of the brain stem, along the axons and on the endings which terminate presynaptically on (predominantly) the outer hair cells of Corti's organ. Although the nerve is inhibitory, that is to say it produces a diminution in the responses of the auditory nerve to click stimuli, it probably functions to sharpen auditory perception. Where a narrow band high intensity signal is partly masked by a wide band of low intensity noise, the widespread inhibition produced by the olivo-cochlear bundle on the low threshold outer hair cells will tend to suppress the noise preferentially and so increase signal-to-noise ratio (Dewson, 1967).

The cholinergic hippocampal afferents arise in the nuclei of the medial septum and diagonal band, travel via the fimbria and dorsal fornix and terminate in all hippocampal regions axodendritically, especially on the basal dendrites of hippocampal pyramids, which have the histochemical characteristics of cholinoceptive cells (Shute & Lewis, 1966; Lewis & Shute, 1967). This input is apparently excitatory, since hippocampal firing is accelerated by ACh and anticholinesterase (Green et al., 1960; Salmoiraghi & Stefanis, 1966), and is probably antagonized by an inhibitory monoaminergic input.

The cholinergic portion of the ARAS arises mainly from the midbrain reticular formation (scattered neurones) and projects to all forebrain areas, although the density of innervation differs greatly in different regions. There is a particularly heavy projection to the non-specific thalamic nuclei and to the striatum (areas which may have inhibitory functions). The ARAS can be divided into a dorsal tegmental pathway supplying metathalamus (including visual areas) and medial thalamus, and a ventral tegmental pathway supplying subthalamus, hypothalamus and basal telencephalon (Shute & Lewis, 1963, 1967). The main final cholinergic relays to cortical areas other than hippocampus are in the lateral preoptic area, which appears to be equivalent to the primate substantia innominata and supplies olfactory and cingulate cortex, and the globus pallidus and interpeduncular nucleus, which supplies neocortex via the external capsule, and also the striatum. The cholinergic input to the striatum is mainly facilitatory (Bloom et al., 1965) and is opposed by the nigro-strial dopaminergic pathway. Imbalance of the two apparently forms the basis of Parkinsonism. The cholinergic input to cortical pyramidal cells is also mainly excitatory (Krnjević & Phillis, 1963a,b). Recent experimental work (Shute & Lewis, 1972) has shown that a recurrent pathway from the globus pallidus travels via the reticular thalamic nucleus to supply the lateral thalamus and hypothalamus. These fibres may correspond to the descending cholinergic hypnogenic pathway described by Hernández-Peón et al., (1963) although the cholinergic system is probably concerned physiologically with alerting and attentive mechanisms, and with paradoxical sleep, rather than with the induction of slow-wave sleep.

Some other workers, e.g. Karczmar (1971) have tended to lay special emphasis on the inhibitory effects which result from cholinergic activity. It would seem truer to say that the role of cholinergic innervation in the brain is rather to produce a combination of facilitation and inhibition that will subserve the process of selective attention. Selective reticular stimulation by the sensory input may be such as to set up a 'facilitatory centre' promoting dominant responses, with an 'inhibitory surround' where competing responses will be eliminated. Some degree of inhibition superimposed on facilitation may help to improve signal-to-noise ratio. Unselective reticular stimulation, on the other hand, is likely to result in hyperexcitability, as in the morphine abstinence syndrome believed by Crossland (1971) to be due to ACh release. The excitatory and inhibitory effects of the cholinergic system can often be matched by contrary effects exerted by amines of the monoaminergic systems. Monoaminergic transmitters through inhibition of inhibitory centres can also give rise to general excitation.

Some of the effects of cholinergic input on sensory transmission are most clearly seen in the special sense systems. For instance, in the visual system, there is evidence that in the lateral geniculate body geniculo-striate neurones are excited by ACh while interneurones (presumably inhibitory) are inhibited (Salinsky, 1967). These responses provide a double means by which transmission at the geniculate relay may be facilitated. There is also an atropine-sensitive excitatory reticular input to visual cortex (Spehlmann, 1963, 1971), and in the superior colliculus evoked responses to visual stimuli are facilitated by a high degree of arousal (Pickering & Freeman, 1967). In the auditory system, there is a facilitatory cholinergic input to the cochlear nuclei (Comis & Whitfield, 1968; Comis & Davies, 1969) which is opposed by a non-cholinergic inhibitory input (Comis, 1970). In the medial geniculate body, supplied by AChE-containing fibres of the dorsal tegmental pathway, there is pharmacological evidence of cholinergic facilitation of geniculo-cortical neurones and depression of other neurones (Tebĕcis, 1972). Thus a double excitatory mechanism operates here as in the lateral geniculate body, through direct facilitation and through inhibition of inhibition.

The hypothalamus is a region where the histochemical method is particularly useful for studying cholinergic pathways because of the comparative paucity of AChE-containing fibres. In the more medial regions, i.e. those concerned with control of the anterior pituitary gland, monoaminergic mechanisms would appear to be dominant, and are probably concerned with inhibiting the production and discharge of releasing factors. In the arcuate nucleus, the tubero-infundibular dopaminergic neurones described by Ungerstedt (1971), which may be responsible for inhibiting the secretion of gonadotrophin (Gallo et al., 1971), have the histochemical appearance of cholinoceptive cells (Shute, 1970). The lateral and dorsal regions of the hypothalamus contain some neurones of cholinergic type which may be concerned with thirst mechanisms and emotional responses. The supraoptic and paraventricular nuclei are both histochemically and pharmacologicallly cholinoceptive. Atropine-sensitive (muscarinic) cholinoceptors cause release of anti-diuretic hormone (ADH), while inhibition of ADH is produced by β adreno-receptors (Bharyaja *et al.*, 1972). The reason for the exceptionally high concentration of AChE in the neurones of the paraventricular nucleus is obscure, unless it is related to the low spontaneous firing rate in those cells (Sundsten *et al.*, 1970).

The hypothalamus receives an afferent innervation not only from the cholinergic and monoaminergic systems, but also from the hippocampus. There is considerable evidence for a functional interaction between the cholinergic reticular system and the hippocampus, and this may be of a mutually sustaining facilitatory nature, rather than inhibitory as has often been suggested. It has already been stated that the cholinergic input to the hippocampus, which travels entirely by the fornix route, is facilitatory. The initial hippocampal fornix output is also, so far as is known, facilitatory. That is to say, hippocampal neurones are excitatory to the lateral septal nucleus; inhibitory effects are polysynaptic, being produced by inhibitory interneurones (De France *et al.*, 1971, 1972). Excitatory effects in the hypothalamus are reported by Poletti *et al.* (1969, 1970). Evidence that the hippocampus may have an activating and sustaining effect on the cholinergic reticular formation is as follows: (1) The electrocortical desynchronization which normally results from stimulation of the midbrain reticular formation is difficult to produce after hippocampectomy, and does not continue after the stimulus ceases (Green, 1960). (2) Cholinergic and anticholinergic drugs produce similar effects whether they are injected into the septum or ventral hippocampus, or into the region of the ventral tegmental pathway of the ARAS, which would argue against the reticular and hippocampal systems acting in opposition (Warburton, 1972). Nevertheless, inhibitory responses are produced in the hypothalamus and elsewhere by hippocampal stimulation as various workers have observed (e.g. Dafrey & Feldman, 1969). Possibly such concomitant inhibitory effects, which may be produced by interneurones or by inhibitory nuclei, serve to depress less intense, irrelevant stimuli (noise, that is), and so form part of the attentive mechanism. Functional suppression resulting from hippocampal activity may extend to locomotion and hormonal secretion. Thus, locomotor activity has been found to increase in rats following the administration of intrahippocampal atropine (Leaton & Rech, 1972). Hippocampal stimulation can depress release of luteinizing hormone (LH) by the anterior pituitary due to activation of inhibitory neurones in the arcuate nucleus (Gallo *et al.*, 1971), and the diminished LH release produced by the administration of progesterone is abolished by fornix section (Velasco & Taleisnik, 1971).

We are now in a position to consider various behavioural correlates of cholinergic innervation. First, alertness and selective attention. It has been shown that ACh is released from the cerebral cortex during the desynchronization that results from high-frequency stimulation of the midbrain reticular formation (Kanai & Szerb, 1965). We may presume that the effects of the cholinergic system in alertness and attention are exerted by an appropriate combination of facilitation and inhibition on motor and sensory systems.

In the latter, signal-to-noise ratio may be increased, and competing inputs manipulated in an advantageous manner. A cholinergic input may also operate on reward systems to help to determine behaviour. Thus it has been shown (Margules, 1971) that the suppressant effect of punishment is abolished by atropine applied to the entopeduncular nucleus, which as we have seen is a source of cholinergic projections to neocortex and subcortex.

The cholinergic system appears to be highly active during paradoxical sleep (rapid eye movement sleep, dreaming sleep). During rapid eye movement (REM) sleep midbrain reticular neurones have been shown to have a high firing rate, whereas during slow-wave sleep their firing rate is low (Manchar et al., 1972). Hippocampal neurones fire steadily both in REM sleep and in arousal (Noda et al., 1969). There is evidence that the auditory input is reduced in REM sleep (Mori et al., 1972), possibly as a result of activity of the olivo-cochlear bundle. REM sleep is potentiated by eserine and abolished by atropine (Jouvet, 1962). Eserine has been shown by Magherini et al. (1972) to produce postural atonia together with bursts of rapid eye movements in the decerebrate cat. The preparation differs from the normal sleeping animal in that the REM bursts occur at regular intervals. The authors suggest that two pathways are involved; an excitatory one causing increased neuronal discharge, and an inhibitory one causing rhythmical interruption of discharge. Possibly in the normal animal this rhythmicity is abolished by cortical influences. Eserine will also produce paradoxical sleep in animals which have been depleted of amines by the administration of reserpine (Karczmar et al., 1970).

According to the theories of Jouvet (1967, 1969) the essential brain-stem structures involved in sleep are the tryptaminergic (5-HT releasing) raphe nuclei which produce slow-wave sleep, and the noradrenergic (NA-releasing) locus coeruleus which produces REM sleep. The locus coeruleus is histochemically cholinoceptive; all its cells contain large amounts of AChE, which does not, however, extend into the axons. ACh when applied to the region of the locus coeruleus has been shown to induce REM sleep (George et al., 1972). It is possible, therefore, to fit cholinergic influences into the system as follows: 5-HT from the raphe nuclei inhibits REM sleep and promotes slow-wave sleep. Reserpine depletes 5-HT, thereby enabling eserine to produce REM sleep. NA from the locus coeruleus inhibits an inhibitory centre which depresses the ARAS. ACh activates the locus coeruleus and so produces excitation of the ARAS. The locus coeruleus with its wide projections throughout the brain (Ungerstedt, 1971) may be an important link in reticular excitation by cholinergic agents.

There is evidence that cholinergic processes are crucially involved in learning and memory. Deutsch (1971) has investigated the effects of an anticholinergic drug (scopolamine) and of a fluorophosphate anticholinesterase (DFP) on the performance of a learned task in rats. The anticholinergic drug during its period of action always produced an impairment of performance consistent with memory block. DFP facilitated a poorly remembered habit, but blocked a well-remembered habit. Deutsch suggests that an increase in sensitivity to released ACh occurs during training, so that at the peak of sensitivity anticholinesterase will produce an excess of ACh causing memory block. Eventually sensitivity declines, and this is the basis of forgetting. Extinction, that is to say suppression of a habit when the reward is withdrawn, can be regarded as equivalent to learning a new habit and, therefore, also involves cholinergic mechanisms.

Experiments supporting the view that the ARAS is involved in learning include the following. Reticular stimulation during the consolidation period has been found to enhance memory storage in rats (Bloch et al., 1970). Lesions of the ventral tegmental pathway, on the other hand, impair learning (Thompson & Hawkins, 1961; Olds & Hogberg, 1964; Santacana & Delacour, 1968). Electrocortical arousal patterns may be necessary for consolidation of the memory trace, as evidenced by the association reported between desynchronization and the active phase of learning (Thompson & Obrist, 1964), and by investigations into the memory storage of sentences presented during sleep (Koukkou & Lehmann, 1968). Total bilateral lesions of the globus pallidus, which could destroy the corticopetal cholinergic radiations, have been shown to produce loss of conditioned reflexes in cats, which are then re-established, if at all, only with the greatest difficulty (Gambarian et al., 1971). Similar results occur after hippocampal damage (Gambarian et al., 1972). Effects similar to those produced by hippocampal lesions are also seen following the administration of anticholinergic drugs. High doses lead to actual memory impairment and low doses to behavioural perseveration (Bignani & Rosić, 1971).

In addition to those already mentioned, other centrally acting drugs may produce some at least of their effects through influencing cholinergic pathways. Many central depressants, e.g. morphine (Crossland, 1971), barbiturates, chloral, etc. (Matthews & Quilliam, 1964) have been shown to inhibit the release of ACh. Mathews & Quilliam suggest that such drugs block the access of choline to the site of acetylation. Conversely, a mild central stimulant such as caffeine may act by increasing ACh release (caffeine is said to augment the release of ACh by potassium ions in perfused ganglia—Birks, quoted by Matthews & Quilliam, 1964). The more intense central stimulant, amphetamine probably acts through monaminergic systems. Its effects are enhanced by anticholinergic drugs and antagonized by cholinergic drugs (Arntred & Randrup, 1968). This may be regarded as providing further evidence of a balance of cholinergic and monoaminergic modulating influences in the brain.

The precise setting of the cholinergic-monoaminergic balance could be the basis of the Pavlovian concept of a 'strong' and 'weak' nervous system (see Gray, 1964). A 'weak' nervous system is a highly reactive one: the weaker the system, the more intense is the excitatory process set up by a given physical stimulus. Important factors in determining the reactivity of the system could be the amount of ACh released by cholinergic neurones and the sensitivity to ACh of cholinoceptive relays. In 'weak' nervous systems either ACh release or ACh sensitivity might be increased. If such were to occur on the human brain, in certain personality types perhaps, it is conceivable that overstrong or overprolonged stimulation such as may be set up in stressful situations could lead to the sort of disruption of psychic function which is termed neurosis.

Finally it is pertinent to consider whether the concept of opposed cholinergic and monoaminergic modulatory systems can explain the development of psychoses and provide a rationale for pharmacological or surgical measures designed to relieve them. It may be that of the two systems, the monoaminergic is the one that is most vulnerable and most liable to malfunction, and that Parkinsonism is only one of several conditions characterized by localized cholinergic dominance. There is suggestive evidence that in schizophrenic states, for instance, some disorder of monoaminergic function may be implicated, which may be either a primary biochemical lesion, or a secondary factor intensifying the original condition. In either case, it would be reasonable to suppose that, as in Parkinsonism, the resultant imbalance might be improved by drugs or lesions having the effect of diminishing cholinergic activity. It is notable that the main target areas of psychiatric surgery are the site of cell bodies (e.g. those in the globus pallidus and substantia innominata), axons (e.g. in the cingulate white matter and deep to the orbital cortex) or terminals (e.g. in the medial thalamus and amygdala) of neurones believed to be cholinergic. The beneficial effects of amygdalotomy on aggressive states may be due to the suppression of the input to cholinergic centres in the posterior hypothalamus. Anterior cingulate lesions and orbital undercutting will both disrupt part of the cholinergic input to frontal cortex, as well as its output back on to the cholinergic centres of the basal forebrain. If the hypothesis is correct that the therapeutic effects of surgery derive, at least in part, from a diminution of cholinergic activity, this might go some way towards explaining the similar results achieved from differently sited lesions. At the same time, a knowledge of the cholinergic pathways involved should help in the task of determining what sites could be expected to provide maximum benefit with a minimal disturbance of psychic function.

REFERENCES

Arntred T & Randrup A (1968). Cholinergic mechanism in brain inhibiting amphetamine-induced stereotyped behaviour. *Acta pharmacol. et toxicol.*, **26**, 384

Bharyaja KP, Kulshrestha VK & Srivastava YP (1972). Central cholinergic and adrenergic mechanisms in the release of antidiuretic hormone. *Brit. J. Pharmac.*, **44**, 617

Bignani G & Rosić N (1971). The nature of disinhibiting phenomena caused by central cholinergic muscarinic blockade. In: *Advances in Neuropsychopharmacology* (Eds Vinar O., Votava Z & Bradley PB), pp. 481–96. Amsterdam: North Holland.

Bloch V, Deweer B & Hennevin E (1970). Suppression de l'amnésie rétrograde et consolidation d'un apprentissage à essai unique par stimulation réticulaire. *Physiol. and Behav.*, **5**, 1215

Bloom FE, Costa E & Salmoiraghi GC (1965). Anesthesia and the responsiveness of individual neurons of the caudate nucleus of the cat to acetylcholine, norepinephrine and dopamine administered by microelectrophoresis. *J. Pharmac. exp. Ther.*, **150**, 244

Comis SD (1970). Centrifugal inhibitory processes affecting neurones in the cat cochlear nucleus. *J. Physiol. Lond.*, **210**, 751

Comis SD & Davies WE (1969). Acetylcholine as a transmitter in the cat auditory system. *J. Neurochem.*, **16**, 423

Comis SD & Whitfield IC (1968). Influence of centrifugal pathways and unit activity in the cochlear nucleus. *J. Neurophysiol.*, **31**, 62

Crossland J (1971). Neurohumeral substances and drug abstinence syndrome. In: *Advances in Neuropsychopharmacology* (Eds Vinar O, Votava Z & Bradley PB), pp. 497–507. Amsterdam: North Holland.

Dafney N & Feldman S (1969). Effects of stimulating reticular formation hippocampus and septum on single cells in the posterior hypothalamus. *Electroenceph. clin. Neurophysiol.*, **26**, 578

DeFrance JF, Shimono, T & Kitay ST (1971). Anatomical distribution of the hippocampal fibers afferent to the lateral septal nucleus. *Brain Res.*, **34**, 176

DeFrance JF, Shimono T & Kitay ST (1972). Hippocampal inputs to the lateral septal nucleus: patterns of facilitation and inhibition. *Brain Res.*, **37**, 333

Deutsch JA (1971). The cholinergic synapse and the site of memory. *Science*, **174**, 788

Dewson JH (1967). Efferent olivocochlear bundle: some relationships to noise masking and to stimulus attenuation. *J. Neurophysiol.*, **30**, 817

Galindo A, Krnjevic K & Schwartz S (1967). Micro-iontophoretic studies on neurones in the cuneate nucleus. *J. Physiol. Lond.*, **192**, 359

Gallo RV, Johnson JH, Goldman BD, Whitmoyer DI & Sawyer CH (1971). Effects of electrochemical stimulation of the ventral hippocampus on hypothalamic electrical activity and pituitary gonadotropin secretion in female rats. *Endocrinology*, **89**, 704

Gambarian LS, Garibian AA, Sarkisian JS & Ganodian VO (1971). Conditional motor reflexes in cats with damage to the globus pallidus. *Exp. Brain Res.*, **12**, 92

Gambarian LS, Koval IN, Garibian AA & Sarkisian JS (1972). Conditional motor reflexes in cats with damage to the hippocampus. *Exp. Brain Res.*, **15**, 15

George R, Haslett WL & Jenden DJ (1964). A cholinergic mechanism in the brain stem reticular formation: induction of paradoxical sleep. *Intern. J. Neuropharmacol.*, **3**, 541

Gray JA (1964). *Pavlov's Typology*. Oxford: Pergamon.

Green JD (1960). The hippocampus. In: *Handbook of Physiology*, Section I Neurophysiology, **2**, pp. 1373-89. Washington: American Physiological Society.

Green JD, Maxwell DS, Schindler WJ & Stumpf C (1960). Rabbit EEG 'theta' rhythm: its anatomical source and relation to activity in single neurones. *J. Neurophysiol.*, **23**, 403

Gwyn DG & Flumerfelt BA (1971). Acetylcholinesterase in non-cholinergic neurones: a histochemical study of dorsal root ganglion cells in the rat. *Brain Res.*, **34**, 193

Hernández-Peon R, Chevez-Ibarra G, Morgane PJ & Timo-Taria, C (1963). Limbic cholinergic pathways involved in sleep and emotional behaviour. *Exp. Neurol.*, **8**, 93

Jouvet M (1967). Recherches sur les structures nerveuses responsable de differentes phases du sommeil physiologique. *Arch. ital. Biol.*, **100**, 125

Jouvet M (1967). Neurophysiology of the states of sleep. *Physiol. Rev.*, **47**, 117

Jouvet M (1969). Biogenic amines and the states of sleep. *Science*, **163**, 32

Kanai T & Szerb JC (1965). Mesencephalic reticular activating system and cortical acetylcholine output. *Nature Lond*, **205**, 80

Karczmar AG (1971). Neurophysiological, behavioural and neurochemical correlates of the central cholinergic synapses. In: *Advances in Neuropsychopharmacology* (Eds Vinar O, Votava Z & Bradley PB) pp. 455–80. Amsterdam: North Holland.

Karczmar AG, Longo VG & Scotti de Carolis A (1970). A pharmacological model of paradoxical sleep: the role of cholinergic and monamine systems. *Physiol. and Behav.*, **5**, 175

Koelle GB (1954). The histochemical localisation of cholinesterases in the central nervous system of the rat. *J. comp. Neurol.*, **100**, 211

Koelle GB & Friedenwald JS (1949). A histochemical method for localizing cholinesterase activity. *Proc. Soc. exp. Biol. Med.* **70**, 617

Koukkou M. & Lehmann D. (1968). EEG and memory storage in sleep experiments with humans. *Electroenceph. clin. Neurophysiol.*, **25**, 455

Krnjević K & Phillis JW (1963a). Acetylcholine-sensitive cells in the cerebral cortex. *J. Physiol. Lond.*, **166**, 296

Krnjevic K & Phillis JW (1963b). Pharmacological properties of acetylcholine-sensitive cells in the cerebral cortex. *J. Physiol. Lond.*, **166**, 328

Leaton RN & Rech RH (1972). Locomotor activity increases produced by intra-hippocampal and intraseptal atropine in rats. *Physiol et Behav.*, **8**, 539

Lewis PR & Shute CCD (1965). Fine localisation of acetylcholinesterase in the optic nerve and retina of the rat. *J. Physiol. Lond.*, **180**, 8p

Lewis PR & Shute CDD (1966). The distribution of cholinesterase in cholinergic neurones demonstrated with the electron microscope. *J. Cell Sci.*, **1**, 381

Lewis PR, Shute CDD & Silver, A (1967). Confirmation from choline acetylase analyses of a massive cholinergic innervation to the rat hippocampus. *J. Physiol. Lond.*, **191**, 215

Magherini PC, Pompeiano O & Thoden U (1971). The neurochemical basis of REM sleep: a cholinergic mechanism responsible for rhythmic activation of the vestibulo-oculomotor system. *Brain Res.*, **35**, 565

Manchar S, Noda H & Adey WR (1972). Behaviour of mesencephalic reticular neurones in sleep and wakefulness. *Exp. Neurol.*, **34**, 140

Margules DL (1971). Localisation of anti-punishment actions of norepinephrine and atropine in amygdala and entopeduncular nucleus of rats. *Brain Res.*, **35**, 177

Matthews EK & Quilliam JP (1964). Effects of central depressant drugs on acetylcholine release. *Brit. J. Pharmacol.*, **22**, 415

Mori K, Mitani H, Fujita M & Winters WD (1972). Multiple unit activity of dorsal cochlear nucleus and midbrain reticular formation during paradoxical phase of sleep. *Electroenceph. clin. Neurophysiol.*, **33**, 104

Noda H, Manochar S & Adey WR (1969). Spontaneous activity of cat hippocampal neurons in sleep and wakefulness. *Exp. Neurol.*, **24**, 217

Olds ME & Hogberg D (1964). Subcortical lesions and maze retention in the rat. *Exp. Neurol.*, **10**, 296

Pickering SG & Freeman WJ (1967). Variations of the superior colliculus evoked response in cats. *Exp. Neurol.*, **19**, 127

Poletti CE, Kinnard MA & MacLean PD (1969). Effect of hippocampal stimulation on unit activity of hypothalamic, preoptic and basal forebrain areas. *Electroenceph. clin. Neurophysiol.*, **27**, 686

Poletti CE, Kinnard MA & MacLean PD (1970). Analysis of hippocampal influence on units of mammillary region in awake, sitting squirrel-monkeys. *Electroenceph. clin. Neurophysiol.*, **29**, 322

Salinsky D (1967). Pharmacological responsiveness of lateral geniculate nucleus neurones. *Int. J. Neuropharmacol.*, **6**, 387

Salmoiraghi GC & Stefanis CN (1965). Patterns of central neurons responses to suspected transmitters. *Arch. ital. Biol.*, **103**, 705

Santacana MP & Delacour J (1968). Effets, chez le rat, des lesions de la zona incerta et des corps mamillaires, sur un conditionnement defensif. *Neuropsychologia*, **6**, 115

Shute CCD (1970). Distribution of cholinesterase and cholinergic pathways. In: *The Hypothalamus* (Eds Martini L, Motta M & Fraschini F) pp. 167–79. New York: Academic Press.

Shute CCD & Lewis PR (1963). Cholinesterase-containing systems of the brain of the rat. *Nature. Lond.*, **199**, 1160.

Shute CCD & Lewis PR (1966). Electron microscopy of cholinergic terminals and acetylcholinesterase-containing neurones in the hippocampal formation of the rat. *Z. Zellforsch.*, **69**, 334

Shute CCD & Lewis PR (1967). The ascending cholinergic reticular system: neocortical, olfactory and subcortical projections. *Brain*, **90**, 497

Shute CCD & Lewis PR (1972). Cholinergic pathways. In: *International Encyclopedia of Pharmacology and Therapeutics* (Ed Hornykiewicz O), Section 25: Pharmacology of the Extrapyramidal System. Chap. 6. Oxford: Pergamon.

Spehlmann R (1971). Acetylcholine and the synaptic transmission of non-specific impulses to the visual cortex. *Brain*, **94**, 139

Spehlmann R (1963). Acetylcholine and prostigmine electrophoresis at visual cortex neurones. *J. Neurophysiol.*, **26**, 127

Sundsten JW, Novin D & Cross BA (1970). Identification and distribution of paraventricular units excited by stimulation of the neural lobe of the hypophysis. *Exp. Neurol.*, **26**, 316

Tebecis AK (1972). Cholinergic and non-cholinergic transmission in the medial geniculate nucleus of the cat. *J. Physiol. Lond.*, **226**, 153

Thompson LW & Obrist WD (1964). EEG correlates of verbal learning and overlearning. *Electroenceph. clin. Neurophysiol.* **16**, 332

Thompson R & Hawkins WF (1961). Memory unaffected by mamillary body lesions in the rat. *Exp. Neurol.*, **3**, 189

Ungerstedt U (1971). Stereotaxic mapping of the monoamine pathways in the rat brain. *Acta physiol. scand.* Suppl., **367**, 1

Valasco ME & Taleisnik S (1971). Effects of the interruption of amygdaloid and hippocampal afferents to the medial hypothalamus on gonadotrophin release. *J. Endocrinol.*, **51**, 41

Warburton DM (1972). The cholinergic control of internal inhibition. In: *Inhibition and Learning* (Ed Boakes RA & Halliday MS), Chap. 17. London: Academic Press.

CHAPTER 38

The subcortical monoaminergic systems
O HORNYKIEWICZ

INTRODUCTION

The topic of my presentation 'The Monoaminergic Systems in the Brain' brings us back to basic sciences again.

My approach to this discussion will be an eclectic one, that is to say I will be confining myself to subcortical monoaminergic systems only and even within the area I will be discussing only a few of the most important monoamines which are involved in such subcortical systems.

A. DOPAMINERGIC SYSTEMS

There is no question but that the major recent discovery in the field of monoaminergic systems in the brain is the existence of large dopamine-containing neuronal systems located in the midbrain and the subcortical telencephalic nuclei and also to some extent in the diencephalon (for references, cf. Hornykiewicz, 1966, 1971).

Dopamine is a catecholamine chemically very closely related to noradrenaline, being the immediate precursor substance in the biosynthesis of the latter. Therefore, small amounts of dopamine can be expected to occur in all noradrenaline-rich tissues. In the brain, however, dopamine has a completely different localization from noradrenaline and this fact by itself suggests that dopamine's functional significance in the brain may be different from that of noradrenaline.

Table 38.1 shows the brain areas which contain detectable amounts of dopamine and/or its metabolite homovanillic acid. Dopamine is not a very stable substance in post mortem material; therefore the estimation of homovanillic acid is quite useful as an indicator of the *in vivo* occurrence of dopamine in the brain. It can be seen that the highest amounts of dopamine occur in the so-called extrapyramidal subcortical centres, namely the caudate nucleus, the putamen, the substantia nigra and the globus pallidus. The distribution of homovanillic acid is on the whole similar to that of dopamine, although some of the dopamine-containing areas contain higher concentrations of the metabolite than of dopamine itself.

Besides the above extrapyramidal areas, dopamine has been detected in other important brain areas (cf. Table 38.1). Thus, in the rat, dopamine has been found in fairly large concentrations in areas which can be classified as limbic structures—namely the olfactory tubercle, the nucleus accumbens,

Table 38.1 Distribution of dopamine and homovanillic acid in discrete brain regions.

Brain region	Species	DA	HVA
		(μg/g)	
Caudate nucleus	Rhesus monkey	9·6	10·1
Putamen	Rhesus monkey	11·4	28·9
Subst. nigra	Rhesus monkey	1·2	4·9
Gl. pallidus	Rhesus monkey	1·1	8·9
Thalamus			
'whole'	dog	0·03	1·6
'massa intermedia'	sheep	0·34	?
Olfactory tubercle +			
Nucl. accumbens +	rat	1·3	?
Septum + Nucl. interstit. striae termin.			
Hypothalamus	dog	0·3	?
Medial eminence	cat	1·3	?
Retina	rabbit	5·3	?

the septum, nucleus interstitialis striae terminalis, and the nucleus amygdalae centralis. In man we have found recently in the amygdala detectable amounts of homovanillic acid. In addition, the thalamus contains detectable concentrations of dopamine; although the present literature does not suggest which of the thalamic nuclei contains the dopamine, the ventral portions of the thalamus seem to contain higher concentrations of homovanillic acid than the other parts of this nuclear mass.

Other brain parts containing dopamine are the hypothalamus (here probably mainly as precursor of noradrenaline), the medial eminence and the associated nuclei (where dopamine seems to play an important role in endocrine control) and the retina.

In the last decade the development, by Falck and Hillarp (Falck, Hillarp, Thieme & Torp, 1962), of the elegant histofluorescence technique for the visualization of monoamines in fresh tissue slices has made it possible to trace the course of many monoaminergic pathways in the animal brain. By means of this method, four major dopamine-containing pathways have been detected in the animal brain (cf. Fuxe, Hökfelt & Ungerstedt, 1970): (1) The nigro-striatal dopamine pathway, originating in the compact layer of the substantia nigra and projecting to the caudate nucleus and putamen; (2) The 'meso-limbic' dopamine system which originates in cell bodies found in the region of the nucleus interpeduncularis and projects to the nucleus accumbens, tuberculum olfactorium and nucleus amygdalae centralis; (3) The tuberoin-fundibular dopamine system consisting of short neurones which originate in the anterior part of the nucleus arcuatus, and terminate in the external layer of the medial eminence and (4) the retinal dopamine system which is localized within the inner plexiform layers of this tissue.

It is quite obvious that it would be of considerable importance to know something more definitive about the functional role of the meso-limbic and

Part VIII—Basic Sciences 295

thalamic dopamine systems. This would be of special relevance to the theme of this conference. Unfortunately our knowledge as to the functional role of these extra-striatal dopaminergic systems is very scanty.

In the human brain (post mortem material), to which the histofluorescence method is not easily applicable, the distribution of dopamine is very similar to that in the animal brain. As shown in Figure 38.1, highest concentrations of dopamine are contained in the caudate nucleus and putamen, followed by

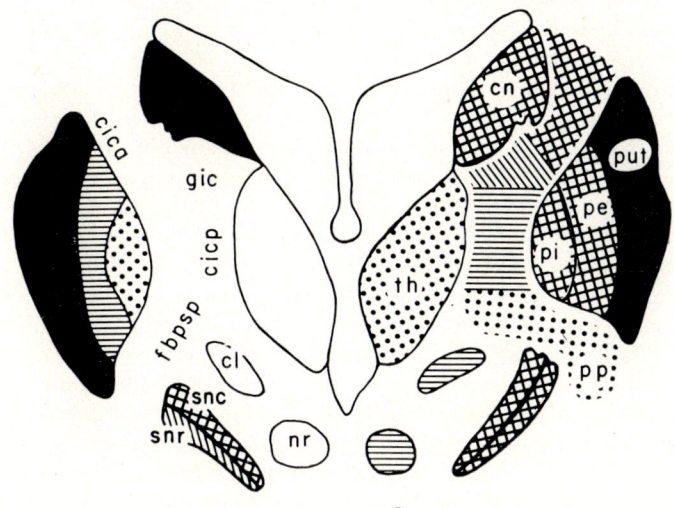

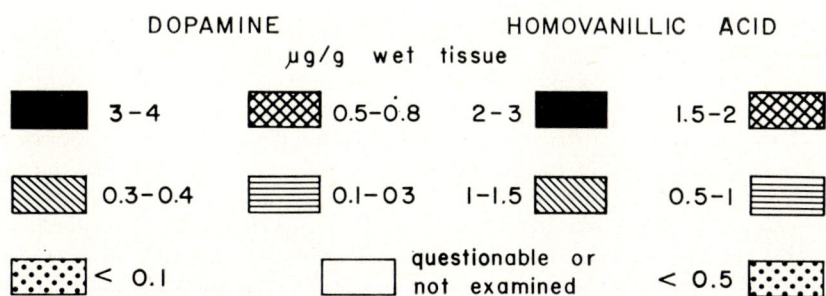

Figure 38.1 Dopamine and homovanillic acid in the normal human brain: Distribution pattern within the basal ganglia complex. Abbreviations: cica, cicp = anterior/posterior limb of the internal capsule; cl = subthalamic nucleus; cn = caudate nucleus; fbpsp = fibrae pallido-subthalamicae and pedunculares; gic = genu of the internal capsule; nr = red nucleus; pe, pi = external/internal part of the globus pallidus; pp = pes pedunculi; put = putamen; snc, snr = compact/reticular layer of the substantia nigra; th = thalamus.

the compact layer of the substantia nigra and the globus pallidus. Therefore we are justified in assuming that also in the human brain there exists a large nigro-striatal dopamine pathway. Homovanillic acid shows a distribution similar to that of dopamine, but in addition there is homovanillic acid present in the internal capsule. Within the internal capsule the homovanillic acid shows a caudo-rostral concentration gradient, with lowest concentration in the posterior limb, i.e. in the vicinity of the substantia nigra, and highest concentrations in the anterior limb between the caudate nucleus and putamen. This is compatible with the existence, between the substantia nigra and the striatum, of a fibre system which contains dopamine running through the internal capsule in the caudo-rostral direction.

The question which I should like to discuss now is: What is the functional role of the nigro-striatal dopamine system? In contrast to the meso-limbic and thalamic dopamine systems about which as I mentioned we don't have much information, we are in the fortunate position of knowing quite a bit about the functional role of the nigro-striatal dopamine system. This is so because the nigro-striatal system has its own chemistry, its own pathology, and in addition its own pathological neurochemistry.

Therefore, damage to the nigro-striatal dopamine system produces definite morphological changes as well as chemical changes, and changes in function of the basal ganglia.

In laboratory animals interruption of the nigro-stratal dopamine system or direct damage to the substantia nigra, by means of electrocoagulations placed in the ventro-medial tegmentum of the midbrain, produces a dopamine deficiency in the striatum and akinesia as the main symptom. In man, Parkinson's disease represents a brain disorder which is associated with degeneration of the neuronal population in the compact layer of the substantia nigra. It is therefore not surprising that Parkinson's disease is characterized neurochemically by a marked deficiency of dopamine and homovanillic acid in the striatal nuclei which normally are 'innervated' by dopaminergic fibres from the substantia nigra. This is shown in Table 38.2 which also shows that, as expected, in Parkinson's disease there is a marked decrease in dopamine and in homovanillic acid in the substantia nigra (cf. Hornykiewicz, 1972).

There is little doubt that it is the degeneration of the substantia nigra that causes the deficiency of striatal dopamine in Parkinson's disease. As can be seen in Figure 38.2 there exists a satisfactory correlation between the degree of substantia nigra lesion and the dopamine and homovanillic acid decrease in the caudate nucleus of patients with Parkinson's disease. This direct relationship between the morphological condition of the substantia nigra and the striatal dopamine has been confirmed in animals with experimental nigral lesions.

The dopamine deficiency in Parkinson's disease is quite specific for all Parkinsonian syndromes regardless of their aetiology. Over the last 10 years we have been able to examine the brains of patients with Parkinsonian syndromes of varying aetiologies, namely postencephalitic, idiopathic, arteriosclerotic and manganese Parkinsonism. In all of these cases there was a more

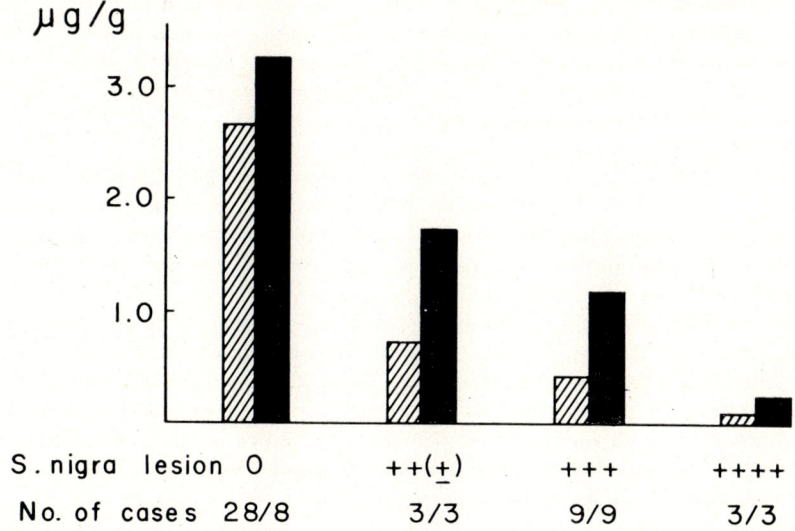

Figure 38.2 Human Parkinsonism: Correlation between the degree of nerve cell loss in the substantia nigra and deficiency in dopamine (hatch bars) and homovanillic acid (black bars) in the caudate nucleus and putamen. Data taken from: Bernheimer, Birkmayer, Hornykiewicz, Jellinger & Seitelberger (1965).

or less severe deficiency of dopamine in the caudate and putamen. The results are shown in Table 38.2.

Table 38.2 Dopamine and homovanillic acid in the basal ganglia in human Parkinsonism.

	Aetiology of Parkinsonism							
	Postencephalitic		Idiopathic		Arteriosclerotic		Controls	
	n	mean (μg/gm)	n	mean (μg/gm)	n	mean (μg/gm)	n	mean (μg/gm)
Caudate nucleus								
dopamine	4	<0·06	5	0·40	6	0·63	28	2·64
homovanillic acid	4	0·05	5	1·10	6	1·28	8	3·23
Putamen								
dopamine	4	<0·05	5	<0·03	6	0·20	28	3·44
homovanillic acid	4	0·58	5	1·07	6	1·28	8	4·29
Globus pallidus								
homovanillic acid	6	0·24	12	0·77	4	1·48	8	2·12
Substantia nigra*								
dopamine	10	0·07	—	—	—	—	5	0·49
homovanillic acid	9	0·41	—	—	—	—	5	1·79

*For this region no distinction was made between the different varieties of Parkinsonism. Data taken from: Bernheimer, Birkmayer, Hornykiewicz, Jellinger & Seitelberger (1965).

In addition to experimental lesions and those caused by a disease process in the substantia nigra, it is possible to produce a dopamine deficiency in the striatum by drugs. All of these drugs produce essentially the same main symptom (which also characterizes Parkinsonism), namely akinesia. These drugs are (a) reserpine and reserpine-like compounds which deplete the striatum of its dopamine, or catecholamine synthesis inhibitors such as α-methyl-p-tyrosine: these drugs cause an actual dopamine deficiency in the striatum; and (b) phenothiazines or butyphenones (e.g. chlorpromazine or haloperidol) which block dopamine receptors in the striatum and therefore cause a functional dopamine deficiency at the level of the striatal dopamine receptors. Drugs producing striatal dopamine deficiency, either actual or functional, are interesting from many points of view especially since most of these compounds belong to the group of neuroleptic drugs, that is to say drugs which are used in the treatment of certain schizophrenic manifestations. It is tempting to hypothesize that the 'antipsychotic' effectiveness of the anti-dopaminergic drugs may be related to their influence on the functioning of the dopamine-containing mesolimbic and thalamic systems. In my opinion this possibility deserves serious consideration in future studies.

Akinesia is apparently a symptom directly associated with dopamine deficiency in the striatum. In Parkinsonian patients the degree of dopamine deficiency in the striatum was found to be significantly correlated to the severity of akinesia: The more severe the akinesia was, the lower were the dopamine levels in the caudate nucleus (Bernheimer, Jellinger, Seitelberger, Birkmayer & Hornykiewicz, manuscript in preparation).

The direct relationship between striatal dopamine deficiency and the symptom of akinesia is proven, in my mind, by the fact that drugs which have a central dopaminergic activity, have a prompt and strong effect on akinesia. Such drugs are able to abolish akinesia, be it drug-induced or in genuine Parkinsonism. Most important among these dopaminergic drugs is, at present L-dopa. In animal experiments, it is possible to show directly that the anti-akinesia effect of L-dopa (e.g. in reserpinized animals) is paralleled by an increase of the dopamine concentration in the striatum. An analogous mechanism can be assumed for the strong and specific antiakinesia effect of L-dopa in patients suffering from Parkinson's disease. In patients receiving L-dopa therapy, the effect of the drug can be correlated with an increase in dopamine concentrations in the striatum. Recently we have examined a series of brains of Parkinsonian patients treated chronically with large doses of L-dopa until death (Davidson, Lloyd, Dankova & Hornykiewicz, 1971). The results of this study are shown in Table 38.3.

It can be seen from Table 38.3 that dopamine in the caudate nucleus increases on the average from 0·5 μg/g in untreated patients to about 2 μg/g in the L-dopa treated patients; the latter value is close to the normal level. A similar trend is also seen in the putamen. For homovanillic acid the differences between non-dopa and dopa-treated patients are even larger. From this it can be concluded that the L-dopa therapy is able to replenish, in principle, the missing dopamine in the Parkinsonian striatum.

Table 38.3 Chronic L-dopa therapy (2–6 g daily) in Parkinson's disease: effect on brain levels of dopamine, homovanillic acid, dopa and 3-o-methyl-dopa (in μg/g fresh tissue).

Treatment	Dopamine	Homovanillic acid	DOPA	3-o-methyl-DOPA
		Caudate nucleus		
NonDOPA treated	0·47 ± 0·33 (3)	1·18 ± 0·10 (3)	nd (3)	nd (3)
DOPA treated	2·22 ± 0·93 (4)	8·16 ± 3·10 (4)	0·24 ± 0·14 (4)	1·66 (4)
		Putamen		
NonDOPA treated	0·26 ± 0·09 (3)	0·67 ± 0·27 (3)	nd (3)	nd (3)
DOPA treated	2·06 ± 0·71 (4)	11·46 ± 3·28 (4)	0·25 ± 0·18 (4)	3·00 ± 2·43 (4)
		Temporal cortex		
NonDOPA treated	nd (2)	nd (2)	nd (2)	nd (2)
DOPA treated	nd (3)	3·01 ± 0·92 (4)	1·01 ± 0·54 (3)	3·28 ± 2·56 (3)

Data taken from: Davidson, Lloyd, Dankova & Hornykiewicz (1971): nd = not detectable. Number of cases in parentheses.

From all these data the conclusion suggests itself that striatal dopamine is essentially a 'kinetic' substance and that lack of this substance in the basal ganglia is related to the symptom of akinesia. Consequently, also L-dopa can be assumed to be primarily a kinetic substance in terms of its overall effect on the extrapyramidal motor function. This is not so puzzling since it is known that in normal laboratory animals L-dopa causes locomotor hyperactivity. And it can be shown that this hyperactivity is correlated with an increase in dopamine levels in the striatum. In addition, it can be shown that this 'kinetic' action of L-dopa is of striatal origin. Thus, in animals (mice) with bilateral striatal lesions, L-dopa's hyperkinesia-inducing activity is significantly less than in control animals.

B. NORADRENERGIC MECHANISMS

Although all the available evidence demonstrates that striatal dopamine is of crucial physiological importance for the extrapyramidal motor activity, the role played by noradrenaline, another major monoamine found in the brain, should not be overlooked.

Fluorescence microscopic observations indicate that most of the subcortical noradrenergic neuronal systems have their origin in cell bodies located in the lateral parts of the pons-medulla (cf. Fuxe, Hökfelt & Ungerstedt, 1970). These cell bodies project short as well as long axons both in the caudal and rostral directions. Thus noradrenaline-containing terminals can be found scattered throughout the central nervous system. Of special physiological interest is the occurrence of high amounts of noradrenaline within the reticular formation of the brain stem, including the hypothalamus.

In contrast to dopamine, brain noradrenaline does not seem to be directly involved in the activation of the extrapyramidal motor mechanisms. Thus, preferential increase of brain noradrenaline (by means of threo-3,4-dihydroxyphenylserine(=dops) which is decarboxylated directly to noradrenaline) does not produce a L-dopa-like locomotor hyperactivity. However, recent observations show clearly that dopaminergic drugs lose their kinetic effectiveness if brain noradrenaline synthesis is inhibited and the amine's levels are low (e.g. by treatment with diethyldithiocarbamate). Under these conditions, the kinetic effectiveness of the dopaminergic drugs can be easily restored by increasing brain noradrenaline concentrations (by means of dops) or by concomitant direct stimulation of central noradrenaline receptors (by means of clonidine). From this the idea suggests itself that the noradrenergic subcortical systems determine, in a critical way, the sensitivity of the extrapyramidal motor effectors to dopamine. Although we do not know anything about the anatomical substrate of such a noradrenergic control mechanism, it is tempting to assume that the reticular activating system is involved. This noradrenaline-containing system is known to increase in an 'unspecific' manner the responsiveness of a number of specific brain mechanisms; anatomical connections between the reticular system of the brain stem and the basal ganglia are well established.

C. SEROTONINERGIC SYSTEMS

Finally, I would like to turn to the third major monoamine system in the brain, namely the serotonin-containing subcortical system. In this presentation I will confine myself only to a small portion of the brain, and discuss briefly some aspects of serotonin metabolism in the human hindbrain. Fluorescence microscopic evidence shows that most of the serotonin cell bodies are located in the raphe area of the midbrain, pons, and medulla. These cell bodies project in a diffuse manner to practically all forebrain structures, and also to the spinal cord (cf. Fuxe, Hökfelt & Ungerstedt, 1970). There exist apparently also short interneurones within the reticular system of the raphe which contain serotonin. It is obvious that the wide distribution of the serotoninergic neurones makes it rather difficult to attribute any specific function to such a diffuse system. This is quite in contrast to the nigro-striatal dopamine system which is clearly defined, and therefore much easier to understand from a functional point of view. Despite the extensive literature on the fluorescence microscopy of the serotoninergic raphe system in the animal brain, no quantitative data seemed to be available for the human brain.

The preliminary results of our recent study of the human hindbrain disclosed a rather interesting aspect of brain serotonin (Farley, Lloyd and Hornykiewicz, in preparation). There are especially two areas in the human hindbrain which contain the highest amounts of serotonin—concentrations between 2 and 3 $\mu g/g$ (which is about five times more than the serotonin content of, for example, the hypothalamus or the amygdala). These two areas are the dorsal raphe area of the mesencephalon, the area which contains the dorsal raphe nucleus, and the area containing the central superior nucleus of the tegmentum. Although some other raphe areas of the pons-medulla are also rich in serotonin, their serotonin content is considerably lower than that of the areas of the central superior and the dorsal raphe nucleus.

This finding is quite interesting in view of the fact that many years ago, Dr Nauta (Nauta, 1958) had shown that it is exactly these two nuclei which are interconnected with the forebrain limbic structures, thus representing the mesencephalic extension of the limbic system. This is an important relationship in my mind because at least here we have a more or less well-defined neuronal system, a circuit, into which these two serotonin-rich nuclei of the human hindbrain are interplaced. Therefore these findings offer us a possibility to study the behaviour of serotonin in a more narrowly circumscribed neuronal system.

Since mental depression has been repeatedly postulated to be related to brain serotonin metabolism, we have focused our attention, at present, on the behaviour of serotonin in the different hindbrain raphe nuclei in suicidal cases with a background of depression. Some of our very preliminary results seem to indicate that the serotonin concentration in the dorsal raphe nucleus may be significantly reduced in such cases (Farley, Lloyd, Deck & Hornykiewicz, in preparation). These observations are, however, of a very preliminary nature.

If confirmed in a larger case material, what would this finding mean? There is no question that the raphe areas which contain the highest amounts of serotonin are part of the reticular formation of the brain stem. From the point of view of its functional-anatomical organization, the reticular formation is the most widely 'open' system of the brain, thus being very suitable to play the role of a major homoeostatic control system; as Dr Nauta has put it, the reticular formation '. . . in a sense . . . assumes the significance of an internal adjustment system of the brain itself. . .' (Nauta, 1972). Therefore it may be not too unjustified to assume that within the reticular formation the role of the raphe nuclei which represent the midbrain extension of the limbic system is specifically related to homoeostasis in respect to affect, being thus responsible for the stabilization of the affective level. Disturbances of serotonin metabolism in these nuclei might therefore render this special part of the reticular system vulnerable to external or internal stressful stimuli thus disturbing the homoeostatic control of affect, with the result of excessive (pathologic) mood reactions.

It is obvious that this is a hypothesis which has to be treated with due caution and reservations but I hope that within the foreseeable future we will be able to collect enough hard data so as to prove or disprove this possibility.

REFERENCES
Bernheimer H, Birkmayer W, Hornykiewicz O, Jellinger K & Seitelberger F (1965). In: *Proceedings of the 8th International Congress of Neurology*, Vol. IV, p. 145. Vienna: Wiener Medizin. Akad.

Davidson L, Lloyd K, Dankova J & Hornykiewicz O (1971). *Experientia*, **27**, 1048
Falck B, Hillarp N-Å, Thieme G & Torp A (1962). *J. Histochem. Cytochem.*, **10**, 348
Fuxe K, Hökfelt T & Ungerstedt U (1970). In: *International Review of Neurobiology* (Eds Pfeiffer CC & Smythies JR), **13**, 93–126. New York: Academic Press.
Hornykiewicz O (1966). *Pharmacol. Rev.*, **18**, 925
Hornykiewicz O (1971). In: *Biogenic Amines and Physiological Membranes in Drug Therapy*, Medicinal Research Series (Eds Biel JH & Abood LG), **5**, 173–258 New York: Dekker.
Hornykiewicz O (1972). In: *Handbook of Neurochemistry* (Ed Lajtha A), **7**, 465–501 New York: Plenum Press.
Nauta WJH (1958). *Brain*, **81**, 319
Nauta WJH (1972). In: *Limbic System Mechanisms and Autonomic Function* (Ed Hockman CH) pp. 21–33. Springfield, Ill.: C C Thomas Publ.

CHAPTER 39

Connections of the frontal lobe with the limbic system
WALLE J H NAUTA

In his extensive review, Dr Powell repeatedly referred to connections of the frontal cortex with the limbic system. In the following account I shall try to deal in some detail with these connections and the neural circuits with which they are associated. But first of all, it is necessary to consider briefly the meaning of the term, limbic system.

The connotation of this term is undeniably vague. Its origin lies in the term, *the great limbic lobe*, introduced by Broca to indicate a somewhat prominent zone along the medial margin of the mammalian cerebral mantle, a zone composed of the gyrus fornicatus (gyrus cinguli and the parahippocampus gyrus including the olfactory cortex of the uncus) and the hippocampus proper (Ammon's horn, dentate gyrus, and fimbria fornicis). The only subcortical component, the amygdala, became included in the great limbic lobe because of its close association—and, indeed, local fusion—with the olfactory cortex. The term, limbic lobe, thus came to subsume a great diversity of neural structures ranging in architecture from neocortical (gyrus cinguli) and allocortical (olfactory cortex and most of the remainder of the parahippocampal gyrus) to subcortical (amygdala). Despite this structural heterogeneity, and almost despite the fact that the term, limbic lobe, originally referred merely to a superficially apparent gross-anatomical entity, a need for a collective name for this vast complex in the medial wall of the hemisphere remained even after Broca's term fell into disuse. One such collective designation—the long-lived term, rhinencephalon—was based on the widely held assumption that all components of the limbic lobe subserved the sense of smell. When later this functional notion proved untenable, or at least too restrictive, the nomenclature gradually returned to a modification of Broca's original, functionally non-committal term (MacLean, 1952). Thus, the present designation, limbic system, no longer hints at an association with any specific sensory modality in particular. Instead, the notion has developed that the unifying trait that justifies a collective name lies in the circumstance that all components of the limbic system of the cerebral hemisphere are collectively implicated in neural circuits linking the complex to a fairly well-defined subcortical neural continuum that extends from the septal region and hypothalamus into a paramedian zone of the midbrain sometimes referred to as the 'limbic midbrain area' (Nauta, 1958). This highly differentiated subcortical apparatus is known to be centrally involved in the regulation of endocrine and visceral effector mechanisms; moreover, there is reason to believe that its functional patterns express themselves in the spectrum of affects ('mood') and behavioural motivations. As schematically illustrated by Figure 39.1, its relationship with the limbic system of the cerebral hemisphere is reciprocal, that is to say, it both receives the downward discharge of the limbic structures—in particular from the hippocampus and amygdala by way of the fornix, the medial forebrain bundle and the stria terminalis—and projects forward to these structures, in part by way of the thalamus, in part by a thalamic bypass that ascends in the medial forebrain bundle. Studies by the recently developed histofluorescence method (Andén et al., 1966) have shown that this ascending thalamic bypass is made up in part of serotonin-containing fibres originating from cell bodies in the limbic midbrain area; it also contains norepinephrine-carrying fibres presumably arising from neurones lying outside that area in more lateral regions of the brain-stem tegmentum.

It seems certain that the functional state of the septo-hypothalamo-mesencephalic continuum is not affected solely by neural afferents from the limbic structures of the cerebral hemisphere. The viscero-endocrine periphery constitutes another important source of modulation, exerted in part by way of—anatomically as yet ill-defined—visceral-sensory pathways ascending from the spinal cord and medulla oblongata, in part also by blood-borne agents such as the gonadal and adrenocortical steroids. Thus, the limbic hemisphere, its subcortical correspondent the septo–hypothalamo–mesencephalic continuum, and the peripheral viscero-endocrine effector apparatus together appear to compose a functional chain, each link of which affects both others.

On the basis of the foregoing considerations it is only natural to assume that any central-nervous mechanism that has efferent connections with either the limbic system or the septo–hypothalamo–mesencephalic continuum, or both, is potentially a modulator of viscero-endocrine function and, beyond that, of the central experiential state symbolized by the term, affect. In the context of this assumption the question becomes significant, whether regions of the cerebral cortex can be identified that have such connections. As will be emphasized in the following account, the frontal lobe, although by no means the only cortical region having access to the limbic organization, entertains the greatest variety of cortico-limbic connections.

1. FRONTO-LIMBIC CONNECTIONS

(a.) Efferent connections of the frontal cortex with the gyrus fornicatus
The earliest experimental evidence that the frontal cortex projects to the gyrus fornicatus (i.e. the 'limbic cortex', composed of the gyrus cinguli, retrosplenial cortex and parahippocampal gyrus) was reported by Adey & Meyer (1952) from a study by the Glees method in the monkey. In that study, Adey and Meyer traced fibre degeneration from lesions involving the medial surface of the frontal lobe caudalward in the cingulum bundle as far as the

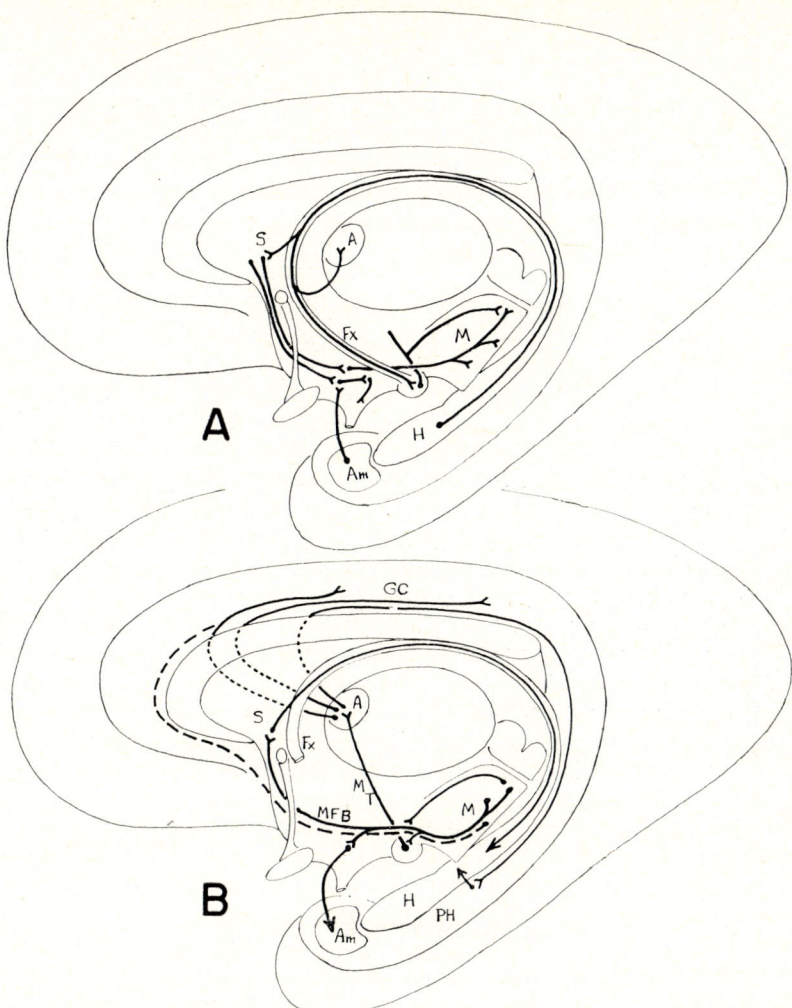

Figure 39.1 Schematic representation of (A) some of the major fibre projections from the limbic structures of the cerebral hemisphere (hippocampus and amygdala) to the septo–hypothalamo–mesencephalic continuum, and (B) pathways ascending from that subcortical continuum towards the limbic structures. Note in B that the subcortico-limbic connection is established in part by way of the mammillo-thalamic tract and anterior thalamic nucleus, in part also by a thalamic by-pass system that follows the medial forebrain bundle and contains, among other components, serotonin fibres (dashed line) originating in the midbrain tegmentum and apparently ascending directly to the cingulate gyrus. Note also the initially rostral orientation of the thalamo-cingulate radiation here drawn in accordance with Domesick's (1970) observations in the rat; as a result of this fibre disposition, relatively rostral transsections of the fasciculus cinguli may disconnect from the thalamus most or all of the limbic cingulo-parahippocampal cortex behind the lesion. Abbreviations: *A*: anterior thalamic nuclei; *Am*: amygdala; *Fx*: fornix column; *GC*: gyrus cinguli; *H*: hippocampus; *M*: paramedian zone of midbrain tegmentum; *MFB*: medial forebrain bundle; *MT*: mamillo-thalamic tract; *PH*: parahippocampal gyrus; *S*: septum.

presubiculum and entorhinal area of the parahippocampal gyrus. Adey and Meyer's fronto-limbic pathway was observed again in several later studies (Nauta, 1964; Pandya & Kuypers, 1969; Jones & Powell, 1970), none of which, however, could confirm a connection with the entorhinal area. Findings in one of these later studies (Nauta, 1964) suggest that this association system in the monkey originates mainly in the dorsal part of the frontal convexity, perhaps also from the medial frontal cortex, and is distributed to the cortex of the cingulate gyrus, to the retrosplenial cortex and the presubiculum; its longest fibres even appear to extend into the subiculum immediately grading into Ammon's horn. That this fronto-limbic pathway connects with the circuitry of the hippocampus via the presubiculum and subiculum seems almost certain, even though technical difficulties so far have made the last link in the connection inaccessible to exact experimental analysis. Moreover, there is evidence from experiments in the cat that the presubiculum independently contributes to the major subcortical projection system of the hippocampus, the fornix bundle (Karten, 1963). A second conduction route from the frontal cortex to the hippocampus has been demonstrated by Van Hoesen and co-workers (1971) in a recent study in the monkey. This pathway in contrast to the one described by Adey and Meyer, originates in the caudal part of the cortex covering the orbital surface of the frontal lobe, and extends from there caudalward over a ventral route to the entorhinal area, a uniquely structured cortical region immediately behind the olfactory cortex of the uncus. Because the entorhinal area has long been known to project massively to the hippocampus, it seems certain that this fronto-entorhinal association constitutes a route by which the

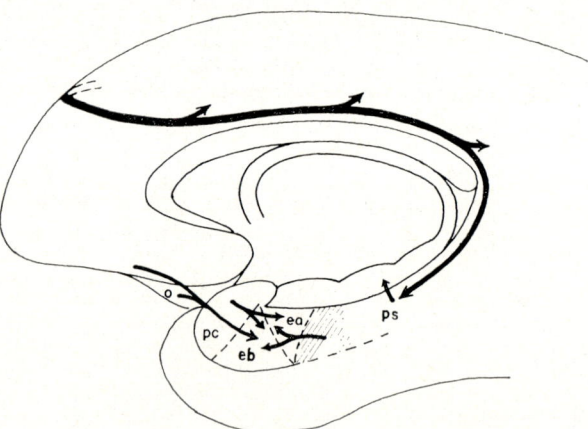

Figure 39.2 Schematic indication of the two conduction routes leading from the frontal cortex into the hippocampal mechanism. The dorsal pathway originates in a dorsal convexity region and follows the fasciculus cinguli as far as the presubiculum (*ps*). The ventral path (Van Hoesen, Pandya & Butters, 1971) arises in the posterior orbito-frontal cortex (*o*) and terminates in the rostral half of the entorhinal area (*eb*). Note that both subdivisions *ea* and *eb* of the entorhinal area receive afferents from the olfactory cortex (pc) of the uncus and from field TH of von Bonin and Bailey (shaded).

caudal orbito-frontal cortex can affect the neural mechanisms of the hippocampus.

The two fronto-hippocampal pathways discussed in the foregoing account are illustrated schematically in Figure 39.2.

(b.) Connections of the frontal cortex with the amygdala

No direct projections from the frontal cortex to the amygdala have been reported. Strictly speaking, the frontal lobe's association with the hippocampus cannot be considered direct either, since it involves intermediary processing stations. Indirect frontal lobe connections with the amygdala can be inferred from the observation that, in the monkey, the convexity of the frontal lobe is associated with the superior and middle temporal gyri by way of the uncinate fasciculus; the rostral parts of the middle and inferior temporal gyri which, as Dr Powell pointed out, also receive a massive association from the peristriate cortex, are known to project directly to the lateral and basal nuclei of the amygdaloid complex (Whitlock & Nauta, 1956). This potential conduction route to the amygdala differs from the two known fronto-hippocampal pathways in the sense that its intermediary processing station forms part of the temporal isocortex, and thus lies outside the boundaries of the limbic cortex. The association of the frontal cortex with the amygdala would therefore seem to be somewhat more remote than the fronto-hippocampal association. It seems none the less likely that the frontal cortex, by modulating certain mechanisms of the temporal cortex, can affect the functional state of the amygdaloid complex.

2. FRONTAL-LOBE PROJECTIONS TO THE SEPTO–HYPOTHALAMO–MESENCEPHALIC CONTINUUM

Dr Powell's impressive account of the systems of cortico-cortical association—which he and his colleagues have done so much to clarify—was organized around the question, at which points these systems lead into subcortical circuitry involving the hypothalamus. For the purpose of my account, I have found it necessary to amplify the term, hypothalamus, to a wider term denoting not only the hypothalamus as traditionally defined but also the subcortical grey-and-white regions with which the hypothalamus is continuous rostrally (the preoptic and septal regions) and caudally (the paramedian 'limbic midbrain area' that includes the ventral tegmental area of Tsai, Bechterew's composite nucleus centralis superior tegmenti, Gudden's nucleus tegmenti profundus, and the ventral part at least of the central grey substance containing, among others, Gudden's nucleus tegmenti dorsalis). This amplification is based not so much on the accident of tissue continuity as, rather, upon the circumstance that the three major components of this septo–hypothalamo–mesencephalic continuum are interconnected by a fairly distinct intrinsic circuitry (Nauta, 1958), into which lead afferent systems from the amygdala and hippocampus as well as from the spinal cord and lower brain stem, and from which emerge channels to the hypophysial complex and visceral motor system. As will be discussed below, the septo–hypothalamo–

mesencephalic continuum has additional efferent connections with the thalamus.

Of the whole extent of the cerebral isocortex, only the frontal lobe is known to project directly to the septo–hypothalamo–mesencephalic continuum. The first evidence suggesting direct fronto-hypothalamic connections came from studies by the method of strychnine-neuronography (Ward & McCulloch, 1947; Sachs, Brendler & Fulton, 1949). Anatomical support for the notion of direct fronto-hypothalamic connections came from Legros Clark & Meyer's (1950) and Wall, Glees & Fulton's (1951) studies by the Glees method. As Dr Powell already mentioned, the evidence upon which these early anatomical reports were based later became the subject of much controversy and doubt. None the less, later studies in the monkey by other silver techniques have led to the identification of two direct frontal-lobe projections to the septo–hypothalamo–mesencephalic continuum. One of these originates in the caudal part of the orbito-frontal cortex and passes caudally in part in the medial edge of the internal capsule, in part along a ventral extracapsular route that leads through the sub-striatal grey matter (substantia innominata), to its distribution in the septum (Johnson, Rosvold & Mishkin, 1968) and lateral hypothalamic region (Nauta, 1962). A second projection of this category has been found to arise in the dorsal region of the frontal convexity (i.e. dorsal to the monkey's sulcus principalis) and to extend caudally in the medial part of the internal capsule not only to a rostral part of the lateral hypothalamus but also to the dorsal hypothalamic area; in its caudal extent this pathway distributes numerous fibres to Bechterew's nucleus centralis tegmenti superior (Figure 39.3).

In summary, the present evidence suggests that two widely separate regions of the monkey's frontal cortex project directly to the septo–hypothalamo–mesencephalic continuum. It indicates the caudal orbito-frontal cortex as the source of fibres to the septal area and the lateral hypothalamus, whereas a region in the dorsal part of the frontal lobe's convexity (presumably composed of parts of areas 9 and 46) is the origin of a projection to lateral and dorsal districts of the hypothalamus and to the paramedian zone of the mesencephalic tegmentum. No projections of this sort have been found to originate in any other sub-field of the frontal cortex, but it must be stressed in this case in particular that absence of evidence does not equal proof of absence. The fronto-fugal fibres to the septo–hypothalamo–mesencephalic continuum identified so far all appear to be of very small calibre and could be demonstrated only in cases of exceptionally successful silver impregnation. It is by no means unlikely that further studies employing silver methods, or better perhaps, the recently developed technique of autoradiographic fibre tracing, will reveal that such projections have a wider origin.

In accordance with the title of this paper, the foregoing account has emphasized those cortico-limbic connections that originate from the frontal cortex. However, the frontal lobe is not the only district of the cortical mantle that entertains such connections. As we heard Dr Powell explain, further cortico-limbic connections are known to originate from certain regions of the

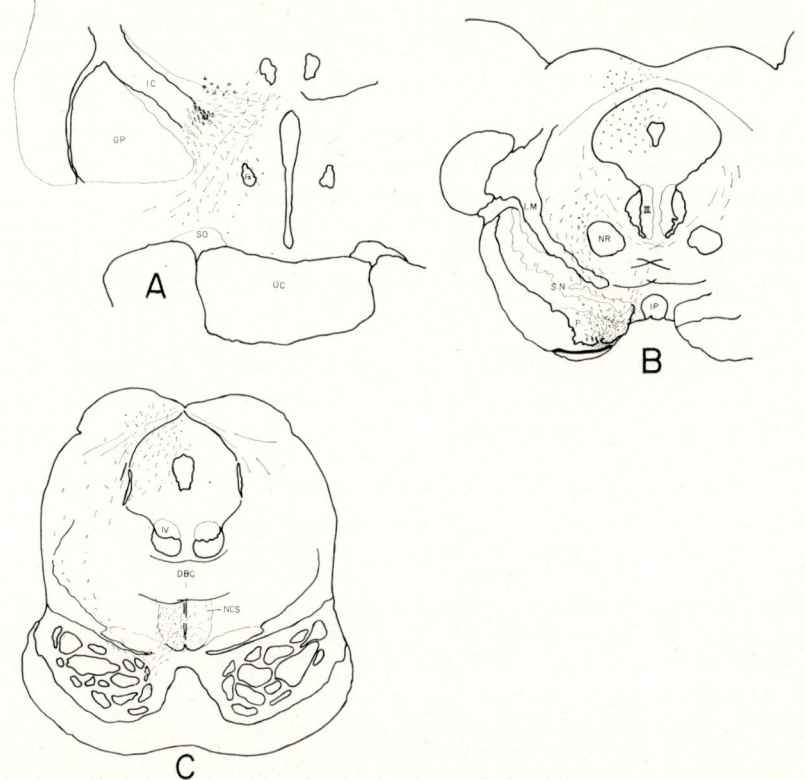

Figure 39.3 Fibre degeneration elicited by a lesion of the monkey's frontal convexity dorsal to the principal sulcus. Degenerating fibres are indicated by stippling. Note in particular the spread of degenerating fibres from the internal capsule to the lateral and dorsal hypothalamus (A), and from the cerebral peduncle to the nucleus centralis tegmenti superior (NCS), a component of the 'limbic midbrain area' (C).

parietal and temporal lobes. Of these extra-frontal projections to the limbic system, however, only two appear rather immediately comparable to the apparent general plan of the fronto-limbic connection: a rostroventral region of the temporal cortex projects *directly* to the amygdala, and the inferior parietal lobule has *direct* efferent connections with the cingulate cortex. No cortical regions other than the frontal cortex have been shown to project directly to either the entorhinal area or the presubiculum. The access routes of other cortical regions to these two pre-hippocampal stations all appear to involve a 'funnelling' through perirhinal transition areas (Bailey and von Bonin's field TH, indicated in Figure 39.2 by shading, appears to be such a way-station for the conduction routes from the temporal cortex to the entorhinal area). In fact, from a certain point of view the two frontal fields maintaining direct efferent connections with the parahippocampal cortex (entorhinal area, subiculum and presubiculum) could appear directly comparable to these perirhinal transition areas. Judging by the same score, with respect to its relationship with the amygdala the frontal lobe appears to be overshadowed by the rostroventral temporal cortex, but it is possible that the caudal orbito-frontal cortex at least may have additional, subcortical routes of access to the amygdala by way of the medio-dorsal nucleus of the thalamus, the septum, and the hypothalamus (Nauta, 1962).

Quite apart from the associative fronto-limbic connections reviewed above are the subcortical projections that link the frontal cortex to the mechanisms of the limbic system. As explained in the foregoing account, the frontal cortex is the only isocortical region that is known to project directly to the septo–hypothalamo–mesencephalic continuum, the subcortical region that also receives the major part of the fibre bundles originating from the limbic system. This circumstance adds considerable weight to the contention that the frontal cortex of all cortical regions is most closely related to the limbic system: it suggests that at least two of its sub-fields stand in a position not only to affect the functional state of the limbic system itself but, in addition, to modulate the effects of limbic-system discharge upon its subcortical target sites.

2. LIMBICO-FRONTAL CONNECTIONS

The problem of limbico-cortical connections is of interest in view of the possibility that certain affective disorders of ideation might have their primary cause in some functional disturbance in either the limbic system or the septo–hypothalamo–mesencephalic continuum.

Fibre connections from the cortex to deep brain structures generally have been easier to demonstrate than their opposites. In particular, the search for limbico-cortical connections has been hampered by the difficulty of finding means of surgical access to the limbic structures that spare both the cerebral cortex and the major fibre systems associated with the latter. Only the gyrus cinguli has proven a ready target for experimental lesions. It is interesting that such lesions in the monkey have been found (personal communication from Dr Deepak Pandya) to result in fibre degeneration leading to the region of the frontal cortex immediately dorsal to the principal sulcus, a region corresponding in part at least to the field that is known to project to both the gyrus fornicatus and hypothalamus. The gyrus cinguli is projected upon by the anterior thalamic nuclei which in turn receive their major afferents from (a) the mammillary body by way of the mammillo-thalamic tract, and (b) the hippocampus over the fornix column (see Figure 39.1). As shown in studies by the histofluorescence method (Andén et al., 1966), it also receives direct projections from groups of serotonin-containing neurones in the caudal pole of the septo–hypothalamo–mesencephalic continuum (see Figure 39.1). It seems reasonable to assume that the cingulo-frontal association could serve to provide the frontal cortex with various forms of information concerning the functional state of both the hippocampus and the septo–hypothalamo–mesencephalic continuum. Since both these mechanisms are rather directly accessible to neural and blood-borne signals emanating from the viscero-endocrine periphery, the cingulo-frontal connection could be viewed, in part at least, as an afferent route by which the frontal cortex monitors—and is affected by—the organism's internal milieu.

Further pathways by which the frontal cortex could receive information related to the functional state of the limbico-subcortical axis may lead over the medio-dorsal nucleus of the thalamus. The nature of the input to the medio-dorsal nucleus so far has been difficult to ascertain. Unlike several other thalamic cell groups this nucleus does not receive a circumscript single lemniscus. Instead, it is converged upon by a remarkable variety of fibre systems, namely: (*a*) a projection from the olfactory cortex of the uncus (Powell, Cowan & Raisman, 1965), (*b*) a projection from the septum (Guillery, 1959), (*c*) fibres ascending along the fasciculus retroflexus from a ventro-medial region of the midbrain tegmentum (Massopust & Thompson, 1962), and possibly (*d*) a direct projection from the amygdala (Figure 39.4). All of

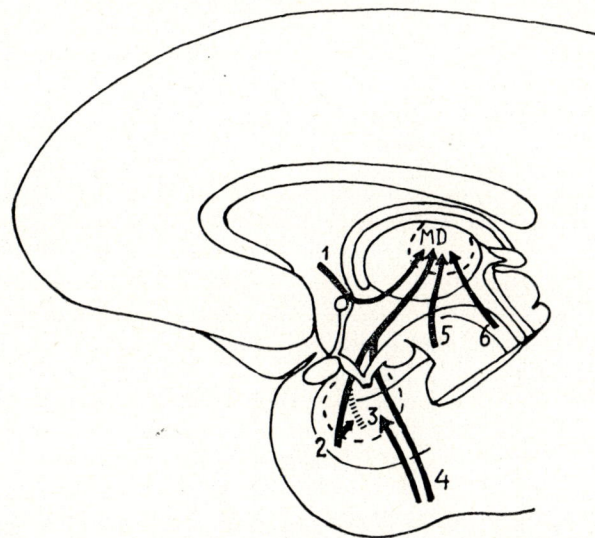

Figure 39.4 Schematic indication of afferent pathways to the medio-dorsal thalamic nucleus. 1: afferents from the septum (Guillery 1959); 2: afferents from the olfactory cortex (Powell *et al.*, 1965); 3: afferents from the amygdala (Nauta, 1962; not definitively demonstrated); 4: afferents from the inferior temporal cortex (Whitlock & Nauta, 1956); 5: afferents from the ventromedial tegmentum (Massopust & Thompson, 1962.)

these fibre systems terminate nearly exclusively in the medial, magnocellular subdivision of the medio-dorsal nucleus, i.e. that subdivision that is known to project to the orbital surface of the frontal lobe. These relationships suggest that the posterior orbito-frontal cortex, itself projecting to the hippocampal mechanism, the septum, and the hypothalamus, by way of the medio-dorsal nucleus receives neural afflux representing the olfactory sensorium and the functional state of the septo–hypothalamo–mesencephalic continuum.

DISCUSSION

It seems evident from the foregoing review of the known and suspected connections of the frontal lobe that at least two subdivisions of the frontal cortex entertain close and apparently reciprocal connections both with the limbic structures of the cerebral hemisphere and with the subcortical expanse of grey-and-white matter (the septo–hypothalamo–mesencephalic continuum) with which the limbic structures are reciprocally associated. The functional significance of the limbico-subcortical axis at present can be expressed only in rather general terms. It appears certain that this multipartite mechanism by way of its effector channels to the pituitary complex and the preganglionic visceral motor neurones plays a leading role in the brain's control of the organism's internal milieu, and that it monitors the neural and chemical signals arising from that milieu. There is strong circumstantial evidence that the fluctuating functional states of the limbico-subcortical axis manifest themselves not only in the viscero-endocrine domain but also in the organism's motivational 'set', i.e. his affects.

It is with this complex mechanism that two separate regions of the frontal cortex are associated by efferent and, as it would seem, also by afferent connections. The impressive evidence that Dr Powell reviewed for us strongly suggests that the external environment as reported to our sensory cortices by all our exteroceptive sensory systems finds some form of re-representation in our frontal lobes. It seems highly probable that the frontal cortex, or at least its two subdivisions known to be associated with the limbico-subcortical axis, has a very similar significance with respect to the *internal* milieu.

The two areas in question in the monkey are the caudal orbito-frontal cortex and a dorsal convexity region probably corresponding to areas 9 and 46 of Brodmann. By their fibre connections, both these frontal regions would appear to be equipped to transmit to the limbico-subcortical axis neural codes representing the perceptual and ideational processes of the cerebral cortex. Conversely, any changes in the functional state of the limbico-subcortical axis caused by such cortical signals could be reported back to the frontal cortex either via the anterior thalamic nucleus and cingulate cortex as in the case of the dorsal convexity field, or, in the case of the caudal orbito-frontal cortex, via the medio-dorsal nucleus. Elsewhere (Nauta, 1971) I have suggested that this interaction between the frontal cortex and the limbico-subcortical axis could be, among other things, an important prerequisite for the normal human ability to compare alternatives of thought and action plans. This suggestion attributes to the limbico-subcortical axis the function of a 'sounding board' or 'internal test-ground' enabling man to preview the affective consequences of any particular action he might consider, and thus, to permit him a choice between alternatives of thought and action. Such a view would seem compatible with at least some of the behavioural changes more commonly associated with massive impairment of frontal-lobe function ('flatness' of affect, instability of intent, loss of ability to foresee the outcome of one's actions, socially inappropriate behaviour, etc.).

The severity of these losses have rightly led psychiatrists and neurosurgeons to abandon the massive frontal leucotomies and lobotomies of the 1940s, and to resort to far more limited interventions on the frontal lobe in their efforts to deal with drug-resistant chronic depressive and obsessive-compulsive disorders. It is remarkable that each of the two psychiatric-surgical procedures that have resulted from these efforts—stereotaxic transsection of the fasciculus cinguli (or, alternatively, decortication of a rostral part of the cingulate gyrus) and undercutting of part of the posterior orbitofrontal cortex—would seem certain to affect one of the two known major channels of interaction between the frontal lobe and the limbico-subcortical axis. The former of these interventions unavoidably interrupts (*a*) the supracallosal route by which the frontal lobe is connected with the hippocampal mechanism (Figure 39.2), (*b*) a large part of the thalamic radiation to the gyrus cinguli and parahippocampal gyrus (Figure 39.1 B), and (*c*) the only direct route for impulse conduction from the gyrus cinguli rostralward to the frontal lobe. Undercutting of the orbital cortex is certain to interrupt all of the fibre connections of the affected area, and therefore must involve (*a*) the ventral of the two pathways known to connect the frontal lobe with the hippocampal mechanism (Figure 39.2), and (*b*) one of the two known direct projections from the frontal cortex to the septo–hypothalamo–mesencephalic continuum. It seems certain from this accounting that the two surgical procedures affect different components of the fronto-limbic association. It could therefore be expected that their effects, although comparable in more general terms, are not identical.

In closing this discussion I should like to point at the admonition that emerges from a review of the present evidence. If it now seems obvious that the frontal lobe and the limbico-subcortical axis encompass neural mechanisms that allow man to be human, then it also must seem inconceivable that surgical interventions upon these brain structures could have only beneficial effects. There are few exceptions to the rule in medicine that therapeutic benefits to the patient are obtained at the cost of some or other loss. In psychiatric surgery as in all of medicine there is a great need for criteria by which to judge whether or not the benefits of any one of its practices outweigh the associated losses, criteria that may forever remain open to new challenges in the context of man's ever-changing views of himself and his society.

ACKNOWLEDGEMENTS

The studies upon which this review is based were supported by US Public Health Service grants MH22697 and NS 06542 to the author.

REFERENCES

Adey WR & Meyer M (1952). Hippocampal and hypothalamic connexions of the temporal lobe in the monkey. *Brain*, **75**, 358–84.

Andén N-E, Dahlström A, Fuxe K, Larsson K, Olson L & Ungerstedt U (1966). Ascending monoamine neurons to the telencephalon and diencephalon. *Acta physiol. scand.*, **67**, 313–26.

Domesick VB (1969). The fasciculus cinguli in the rat. *Brain Res.*, **20**, 19–32.

Guillery RW (1959). Afferent fibers to the dorsomedial thalamic nucleus in the cat. *J. Anat. (Lond.)*, **93**, 403–19.

Johnson TN, Rosvold HE & Mishkin M (1968). Projections from behaviorally-defined sectors of the prefrontal cortex to the basal ganglia, septum and diencephalon of the monkey. *Exp. Neurol.*, **21**, 20–34.

Jones EG & Powell TPS (1970). An anatomical study of converging sensory pathways within the cerebral cortex of the monkey. *Brain*, **93**, 793–820.

Karten HJ (1963). Projections of the parahippocampal gyrus of the cat. (*Abstr.*) *Anat. Rec.*, **145, No. 2**, 247–8.

LeGros Clark WE & Meyer M (1950). Anatomical relationships between the cerebral cortex and the hypothalamus. *Brit. Med. Bull.*, **6**, 341–5.

MacLean PD (1952). Some psychiatric implications of physiological studies on fronto-temporal portion of limbic system (visceral brain). *EEG Clin. Neurophysiol.*, **4**, 407–18.

Massopust LC and Thompson R (1962). A new interpedunculodiencephalic pathway in rats and cats. *J. comp. Neurol.*, **118**, 97–105.

Nauta WJH (1958). Hippocampal projections and related neural pathways to the midbrain in the cat. *Brain*, **81**, 319–40

Nauta WJH (1962). Neural associations of the amygdaloid complex in the monkey. *Brain*, **85**, 505–20

Nauta WJH (1964). Some efferent connections of the prefrontal cortex in the monkey. In: *The Frontal Granular Cortex and Behavior* (Eds Warren and Akert) pp. 397–409. New York: McGraw-Hill.

Nauta WJH (1971). The problem of the frontal lobe: a reinterpretation. *J. Psychiat. Res.*, **8**, 167–87

Pandya DN & Kuypers HGJM (1969). Cortico-cortical connections in the rhesus monkey. *Brain Res.*, **13**, 13–36.

Powell, TPS, Cowan WM & Raisman G (1965). The central olfactory connexions. *J. Anat. (Lond.)*, **99**, 791–813

Sachs E Jr, Brendler SJ & Fulton JF (1949). The orbital gyri. *Brain*, **72**, 227–40

Van Hoesen GW, Pandya DN & Butters N (1971). Cortical efferents to the entorhinal cortex of the Rhesus monkey. *Science*, **175**, 1471–3

Wall PD, Glees P & Fulton JF (1951). Corticofugal connexions of posterior orbital surface in Rhesus monkey. *Brain*, **74**, 66–71

Ward AA & McCulloch WS (1947). The projection of the frontal lobe on the hypothalamus. *J. Neurophysiol.*, **10**, 309–14.

Whitlock DG & Nauta WJH (1956). Subcortical projections from the temporal neocortex in Macaca mulatta. *J. comp. Neurol.*, **106**, 183–212

CHAPTER 40

Morphological plasticity of the synapse
KONRAD AKERT & ROBERT B LIVINGSTON

> The starting point of bone, flesh and all substances of the body, was the formation of nervous marrow. For the bonds of life, as long as the soul is bound up with the body, were made fast in the marrow, constituting the roots of mortality. For the marrow itself, the god set apart from their several kinds those triangles which, being unwarped and smooth, were originally able to produce fire, water, air and earth of the most exact form. Mixing these in due proportion he made out of them the marrow....
> And he moulded into spherical shape the ploughland, as it were, to contain the divine seed, and this part of the marrow he named 'brain'.
> *Timaeus* Plato

From the time of establishment of the neurone doctrine by Waldeyer in 1891, a great deal of attention has been focused on the mechanisms by which nerve cells signal to one another. In 1897, Sherrington introduced the term *synapse*, derived from the Greek notion of clasping, to designate the locale for such interneuronal signalling.

By means of light microscopy it was possible to identify axonal endings on dendrites and cell bodies, presenting the appearance of bulbous synaptic contacts. Electron microscopy revealed further that the synaptic junctions where, presumably, neurotransmitter substances are released, occupy only small areas within the overall territory of the synapse. It then became possible to raise the question as to whether synaptic junctions undergo morphological changes in relation to different functional states. As a crude beginning, might it be possible to identify differences between tissues taken from anaesthetized and unanaesthetized animals?

This study on the differences between anaesthetized and unanaesthetized rats was undertaken by a group of investigators working at the Brain Research Institute of the University of Zürich in collaboration with members of the Electron Microscopy Laboratory at the Swiss Federal Institute of Technology in Zürich. Reports on this investigation have recently been published (Akert *et al.*, 1972; Streit *et al.*, 1972). The experiments consisted of applying the techniques of thin-section electron microscopy and freeze-etch electron microscopy to tissues extracted under the same conditions from the ventral horn of the lumbar spinal cord of rats, anaesthetized and unanaesthetized. Quantitative determinations were undertaken to test the reliability of certain subjective impressions that seemed strikingly different when viewing synapses in these two functionally distinct states.

INTERPRETATION OF FREEZE-ETCHED ELECTRON MICROSCOPY

The freeze-etch process can be applied to tissues with or without fixation prior to the freezing. Aldehyde fixation does not appear to alter the appearance of membranes, including synaptic membranes. Since it is more convenient to work with fixed tissues, the identical procedures for the two experimental conditions could be pursued up to the point of freezing for freeze-etch purposes and staining for thin sections. The process of fracturing the frozen specimen is conceived as splitting the unit membrane, the bilayer, along the hydrophobic interior of the membrane. This means that a cell membrane, only 75 Å thick, can be split into two halves! It would be virtually impossible to construct a microtome that would follow the undulations along such an unimaginably thin channel, but the fracture line, running ahead of the microtome, separates the tissue along its weakest cleavage plane. This evidently, is between the methyl ends of the hydrocarbon chains, pliant and disordered, in the core of the membrane bilayer.

Since one half of the fractured surface is discarded and a platinum-carbon replica of the remaining half is preserved, the observer at the electron microscope can look at only one or the other of the two inner surfaces thereby exposed. Practice enables identification of all four leaflets belonging to two unit membranes of adjoining cells. By searching for synaptic junctions, the investigator can give an accounting for the hydrophobic interiors of the four leaflets engaged in the important business of synaptic transmission. Comparisons between thin-section and freeze-etch electron microscopy permit evaluations of membranes cut across or seen in panoramic view, revealing complementary aspects of similar structures.

Studies of synapses by these two methods have already been considerably advanced by Moor *et al.*, 1969; Akert *et al.*, 1969; Akert *et al.*, 1972; Pfenninger *et al.*, 1972; Streit *et al.*, 1972; Akert, 1973.

ULTRASTRUCTURE OF THE SYNAPSE

Present insight into the structure and function of the synapse is well summarized by Peters, Palay & Webster (1970); Cooper, Bloom & Roth (1970); Bloom (1970); Pfenninger *et al.* (1972). From studies such as these, the following interpretations appear warranted. The presynaptic ending is characterized by synaptic vesicles and an elaborate presynaptic grid. The vesicles are presumed to contain neurotransmitter substances. The grid apparently acts as a guide or attractant agency to bring the vesicles into contact with the presynaptic membrane at specific locations. Vesicular movement is apparently initiated by the arrival of nerve impulses at the nerve terminal and is a calcium-dependent process. Once the vesicle is in the vicinity of the presynaptic membrane, it evidently fuses with the presynaptic membrane so that the two membranes become co-extensive. This opens the contents of the vesicle into the synaptic cleft. The process is probably like that of exocytosis elsewhere.

The act of the membrane fusion and fission, as modelled *in vitro* takes practically no energy and is nearly instantaneous. Fission involves the reverse process by which the two membranes, vesicular and presynaptic, become disengaged. The vesicle is conceived as pinching off to restore integrity of the presynaptic membrane and returning to the cytoplasmic pool of synaptic vesicles. If fusion and fission do take place, as conjectured, three contingent problems are thereby solved. First, synaptic transmitter is literally poured into the synaptic cleft. Second, the return of the same synaptic vesicle precludes the accumulation of redundant synaptic membrane that would be formed if there were repeated additions of vesicular to presynaptic membrane. Third, return of the vesicle to the cytoplasmic pool permits re-uptake of a considerable fraction of neurotransmitter, a process that is known to occur. The whole act of neurochemical delivery by quantal (vesicular) release would thus be accomplished by the ubiquitous process of *pinocytosis*, including both exocytosis and endocytosis, perhaps the commonest means of delivery of bulk substances across cell membranes in any tissue. The fact that the synaptic vesicle is smaller than most pinocytotic vesicles and that a specialized junction with an elaborate grid structure is involved does not alter the general principle of chemical transport.

Once admitted to the synaptic cleft, the neurotransmitter substance is believed to act upon specific receptor sites and through them to have its effect upon the postsynaptic cell. Probably the enzyme systems for degradation of the neurotransmitter are closely associated with the receptor sites. Postsynaptic particles clustered around the postsynaptic region have been identified morphologically and may be intramembraneous portions of the receptor and/or enzyme system (Sandri *et al.*, 1972).

The exact location of neurotransmitter release through the presynaptic membrane is evidently controlled by the dense projections of the presynaptic grid. These have been identified on thin-section electron micrographs by means of special staining techniques (Gray, 1959; Akert *et al.*, 1969; Pfenninger *et al.*, 1969). The dense projections have a triagonal arrangement, permitting neurotransmitter release by vesicular exocytosis in a hexagonal configuration (Pfenninger *et al.*, 1969; Pfenninger *et al.*, 1972). The dense projections are thought to be made up of neurofilaments which may manifest motility, perhaps sufficient to contribute to vesicular manoeuvring and also to stabilize the presynaptic membrane during the processes of membrane fusion and fission.

Release of neurotransmitter substance into the synaptic cleft is therefore the key event in the process of signalling between neurones. Many of these assumed steps are still somewhat conjectural because the evidence is mostly indirect, and it is not compellingly simple. Obvious questions remain open: how does this synaptic machinery operate in normal conditions? Can the process be visualized? The investigation of synaptic junctions by means of electron microscopy has been concerned mainly with thin sections. And it has dealt almost exclusively with material obtained from deeply anaesthetized preparations. Is it possible that synaptic junctions in unanaesthetized neuropile would look different? Can 'waking' as compared with 'anaesthetized' synapses provide clues that might confirm or deny various hypotheses relating to synaptic transmission? How 'plastic' are synapses?

ANAESTHETIZED AS COMPARED WITH UNANAESTHETIZED SYNAPSES

The following interpretations are based largely on evidence for synaptic plasticity obtained recently by Streit, Akert, Sandri, Livingston and Moor and represented in summary form in Figure 40.1.

The appearance of the synapse in the quiescent state of barbiturate anaesthesia is represented in the upper part of Figure 40.1. A nerve terminal and synaptic cleft are depicted. The terminal contains a number of synaptic vesicles, a mitochondrion, and, along the presynaptic membrane are seen the pyramidal dense projections. The presynaptic and postsynaptic membranes are parallel, smooth and flat. The synaptic vesicles are not especially aggregated towards the junction between the two cells.

The waking state, in contrast, shows vesicles that are closely packed or congregated in the neighbourhood of the presynaptic membrane. The presynaptic and postsynaptic membranes are arched upward, towards the cytoplasmic side of the nerve terminal. The presynaptic membrane is undulating, departing from being strictly parallel to the postsynaptic membrane. Two 'omega figures' are seen where vesicular and presynaptic membranes are depicted as fused and where vesicular contents are thereby exposed to the synaptic cleft. Synapses containing such omega forms have only very rarely been seen in electron microscopy. David Bodian told us that he has seen only two or three such figures in all of his years of examining thin sections. Neither he nor others, to our knowledge, have sought to examine synapses in unanaesthetized preparations.

Figure 40.2 provides views of comparably prepared thin section and freeze-etch material from neuropile in the ventral horn of the spinal cord of the rat. unanaesthetized, sacrificed by perfusion with gluteraldehyde fixatives. In each half of the figure can be identified two omega figures, presumably synaptic vesicles which were fused with the presynaptic membranes at the moment of fixation. The advantage of freeze-etch material is evident in this figure which reveals a larger expanse of membrane than can be studied with thin sections by any means other than painstaking serial section reconstructions. Note also in Figure 41.2 how the presynaptic and postsynaptic membranes are arched.

Figure 40.3 provides a freeze-etch micrograph illustrating a point of view from *inside* of an unanaesthetized presynaptic ending. Loci where the synaptic vesicles have been close to the presynaptic membrane or perhaps have actually fused with it can be seen as protuberant undulations of that membrane. Because of the splitting of the unit membrane, the most extensive panorama of presynaptic membrane, seen from this point of view, is the inner surface of the outer leaflet. The protuberances represent the fracture line cutting off the necks of vesicular attachments to the presynaptic membrane. There are evidently both partial and complete hexagonal arrays of such protuberances, confirming Pfenninger *et al.* (1969, 1972) that vesicular attachments occur in relation to the geometric organization of the presynaptic dense projections. Three general regions of presynaptic membrane modulations suggest that there are three active synaptic junctions at this location.

Freeze-etch view from *outside* the presynaptic nerve terminal shows a complementary array of membrane modulations (Figure 40.4). This per-

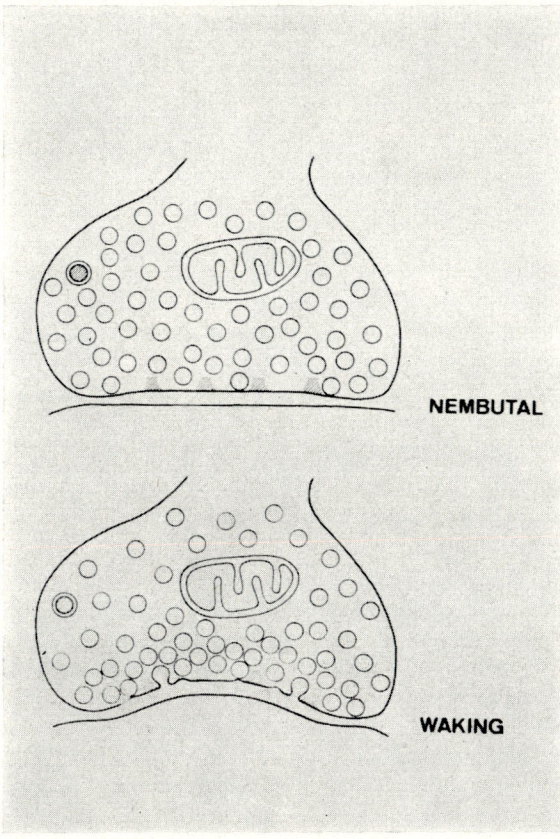

Figure 40.1. Drawing schematizing distinctions between an anesthetized (top drawing) and unanesthetized synapse. In each case, a presynaptic ending with its synaptic vesicles is seen abutting the synaptic cleft and a postsynaptic membrane. With nembutal, synapses show little arching of the presynaptic and postsynaptic membranes, the synaptic vesicles are not aggregated close to the presynaptic membrane, and there are almost never seen any "omega" figures formed by the attachment of vesicular and presynaptic membranes, yielding exposure of the synaptic contents to the synaptic cleft. Without anesthesia, synapses show arching of the presynaptic and postsynaptic membranes with convexity pointing in the direction of the presynaptic cytoplasm, with crowding of the vesicles toward the presynaptic membrane, and, occasionally, with "omega" figures.

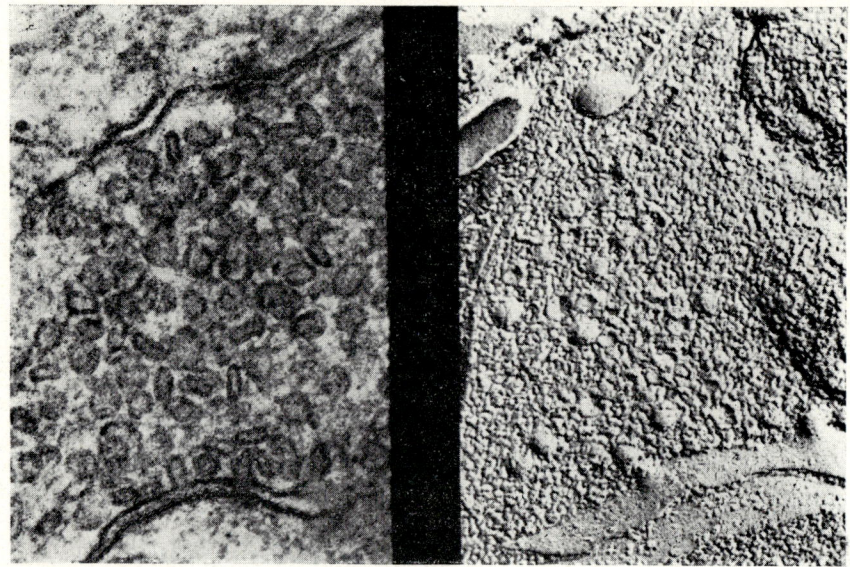

Figure 40.2. Comparison between thin section and freeze-etching exposures of unanesthetized synapses. On the left is seen a thin section with strongly arched presynaptic and postsynaptic membranes, vesicles crowded close to the presynaptic membrane, and at least one and perhaps two "omega" figures indicative of fusion of vesicular and presynaptic membranes, exposing the vesicular contents to the synaptic cleft and vice versa. On the right is seen in freeze-etched form a synaptic region with synaptic vesicles two of which have apparently fused with the presynaptic membrane. Original magnification × 80,000.

spective reveals not craters but dimples or pits that are orientated so as to funnel towards the cytoplasmic side of the nerve terminal. If it were supposed that the membrane disruptions seen in freeze-etched material were due to some artifact of the freezing process, or to the sublimation of water from the surface exposed by the fracture, it would have to be assumed additionally that such artifacts would be diametrically opposite in direction on the two leaflets, bursting out of the outer leaflet and imploding into the inner leaflet. It is much more economical to suppose that the membrane modulations of the two leaflets are orientated in the same direction (towards the cytoplasmic side) and that the 'craters' will point up towards the cytoplasmic viewpoint and that the pits will descend away from any point of view outside the presynaptic membrane. Moreover, it is hardly credible that artifactual events opposite in direction on the two companion leaflets would each be arranged in a similar-sized hexagonal pattern. The pattern itself conforms to the triagonal arrangement of dense projections as seen on thin-section electron microscopy of presynaptic terminals.

Figure 40.4 reveals clear evidence for synaptic activity: curvature of membranes, and membrane modulations in partial or complete hexagonal configuration.

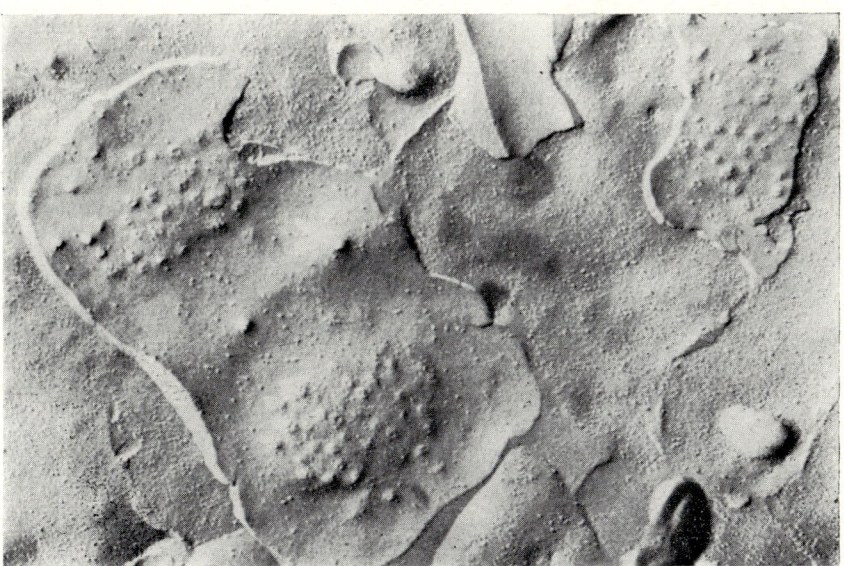

Figure 40.3 A freeze-etched panorama revealing the outer leaflets of one or more presynaptic membranes riding like islands on a larger portion of a single postsynaptic membrane. Three active sites can be identified within which a number of crater-like protuberances stand up from the presynaptic membrane surface. Some of these show partially completed and, more rarely, fully completed hexagonal arrays. Original magnification ×40,000.

Figure 40.5 is from a replica obtained from a deeply anaesthetized rat. There are faint traces of shallow, presumably non-penetrating indentations where synaptic vesicles might be presumed to attach if the nerve terminal became more active. Figure 40.6 is from a comparable-appearing area in an unanaesthetized rat. Obvious signs of synaptic activity are presented, notably arching of the membranes, wrinkling, and disruptions of the membrane characteristic of synaptic vesicular pinocytosis.

Figure 40.7 is from a rat in agonal stages following lethal dosing with tetanus toxin. Dr Pfenninger prepared such animals and followed them through recurrent generalized tonic convulsions and signs of toxaemia. Specimens taken after the seizures had ceased and the animals were obviously in agonal stages, revealed extensive panoramas, similar to Figure 40.7 in which although synaptic sites could be inferred, they were flattened, there were relatively fewer membrane modulations than even during deep nembutal anaesthesia, and neither craters nor dimples could be seen on the respective outer and inner leaflets over vast regions of synaptic endings. The sequence, then, of waking-to-anaesthetized-to-agonal constitutes a span of three different levels of activity as expressed in morphological differences in the presynaptic membranes examined in these three functionally distinguished states.

The Zürich group has found evidence for morphological changes similar

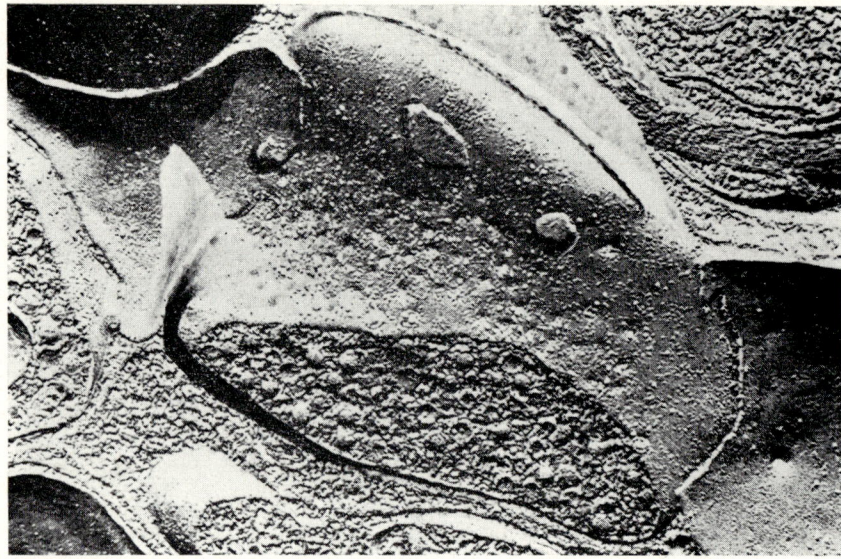

Figure 40.4. A freeze-etched panorama from a point of view outside the presynaptic terminal, hence revealing the inner leaflet. Note, in comparison with Figure 40.3, that this membrane shows pits or indentations instead of elevated crater-like protuberances. The two leaflets, seen from opposite sides of the original membrane, present evidence for a through and through penetration of the membrane in the same direction. In the fractured profile of the terminal cytoplasm can be seen numerous synaptic vesicles. A small portion of another synaptic ending can be seen to the left. Original magnification ×40,000.

to those seen with nembutal when different anaesthetic agents have been employed. With both ether and chloralose anaesthetics, the normally 'active' synaptic sites become relatively flattened, show fewer bold membrane modulations, and exhibit fewer open craters and deep pits. The effects seen are in the same directions of morphological alteration as seen with nembutal, but they are not so clearly pronounced. What is even more interesting is that if an agent that counteracts the anaesthetic effects of nembutal (Megimid) is administered to an animal deeply anaesthetized with nembutal, the synaptic junctions are restored towards normal in parallel with the restoration of wakefulness and active alert behaviour.

Given the similar morphological characteristics of synaptic sites in conditions of anaesthesia with three different anaesthetic agents, we may suppose that most of the effects are the direct or indirect results of the general anaesthetizing properties of these three agents. Nevertheless, the barbiturate may have additional direct membrane effects. Perhaps this accounts for the greater distinctiveness of alterations seen with this anaesthetic agent. Blaustein (1968) observed that there is an increase in transmembrane resistance to electrical perturbations and an accompanying reduction in maximum sodium and potassium conductances. He suggested that the non-polar part of the barbiturate molecule may penetrate the lipid region of the membrane bilayer and thereby induce the changes in resistance and conductances. It is also clear that the barbiturates tend to increase calcium binding to membranes. If they do so at the presynaptic membrane that might interfere with the aggregation of the synaptic vesicles and with the processes of fission and fusion between vesicular and presynaptic membranes. Perhaps the fact that nembutal seems to be more distinctive in its morphological effects is due

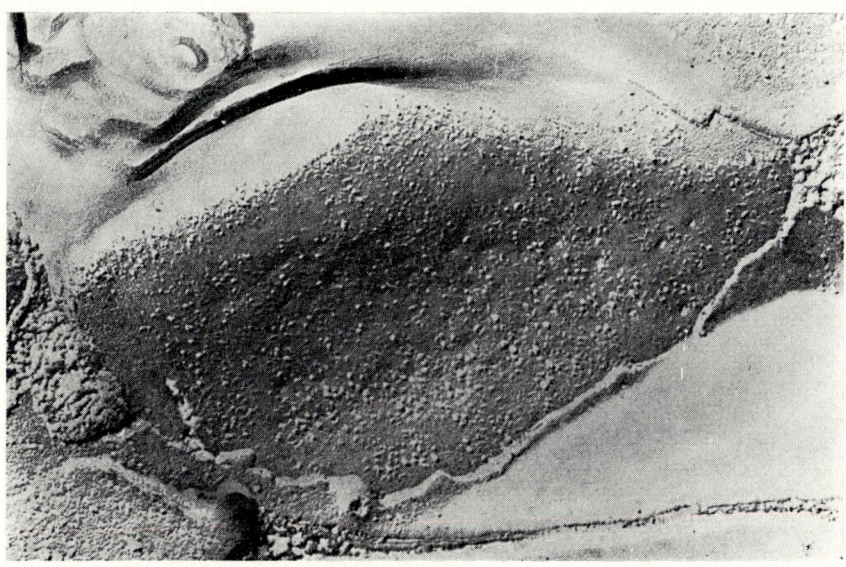

Figure 40.5. Presynaptic inner leaflet from a rat deeply anesthetized with nembutal. There is a modest curvature suggestive of an active synaptic junction, and shallow membrane indentations, but few signs of deeply penetrating pits. Original magnification × 40,000.

partly to factors common to all general anaesthetics, perhaps indirectly resulting from the state of being anaesthetized, plus some additional direct effects on the presynaptic membrane.

QUANTITATIVE EVALUATION OF SYNAPTIC PLASTICITY
Criteria that distinguish active from inactive synaptic junctions were tested by asking naïve observers to sort photographs of freeze-etch and thin section materials according to whether there appeared to be more or less curvature of the membranes, smooth or wrinkled surfaces, and open or closed craters as seen on freeze-etched outer leaflets. The observers compared a random assortment of photographs relating to waking and anaesthetized specimens.

One obvious question is whether there may be differences in density per unit area of presynaptic membrane modulations when comparing inner and outer leaflets. If there were notable differences, this would cast doubt on the notion that delivery of neurotransmitter involves through and through penetration of the membrane, thereby affecting both leaflets. Grids were prepared to facilitate quantitative measurement of the number of membrane modulations, perforated or not, per 0·01 μm^2 of well exposed synaptic sites. There were no significant differences between inner and outer leaflets in terms of density of occurrence of membrane modulations in either anaesthetized or

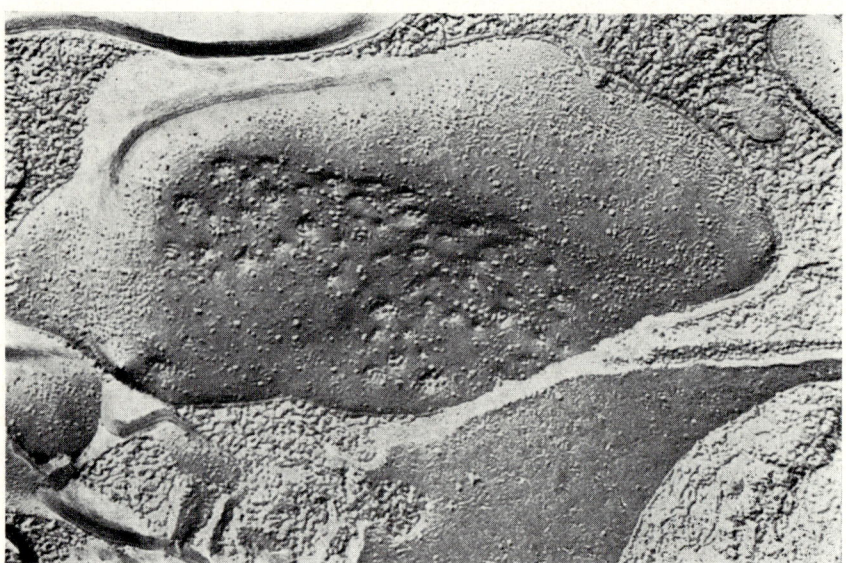

Figure 40.6. Presynaptic inner leaflet from an unanaesthetized rat. There is more conspicuous arching and more definite indentations or pits, suggesting frequent fusion of synaptic vesicles to the cytoplasmic side of the presynaptic terminal. Compare Figures 40.5. and 40.6. Original magnification × 40,000.

unanaesthetized states. The density of presynaptic membrane modulations ranges from about 0.4 as a minimum to over 4.0 maximum per 0·01 μm^2, with peaks in the neighbourhood of 1.5–3.0. Since the inner and outer leaflets had corresponding densities of modulations in each functional state, the membrane perturbations must involve both leaflets equivalently, thus giving strong support to the idea of pinocytosis for neurotransmitter release.

There was also no significant difference in concentration of presynaptic membrane modulations identified between specimens taken from anaesthetized and unanaesthetized preparations. This means that faint signs can be made out, even in the anaesthetized state which reveal the synaptic site and that the modulations are as concentrated there as in the waking state even though the markings in the latter condition are far more obvious. This suggests that the presynaptic membrane may be characteristically distinguished at each point of potential vesicular attachment, bearing faint but enduring witness indicative of fusion sites.

The number of open as compared with closed craters, as tested by naïve observers sorting photographs of outer presynaptic leaflets, was significantly greater in unanaesthetized as compared with anaesthetized synaptic junctions (Figure 40.7). Under anaesthesia, there was no significant difference between the number of open and closed modulations. The number of open as compared with closed craters was significantly greater when comparisons between those two conditions were confined to the unanaesthetized preparations.

In both thin-section and freeze-etch specimens, there were significant differences between flat and curved leaflets, the latter being more common,

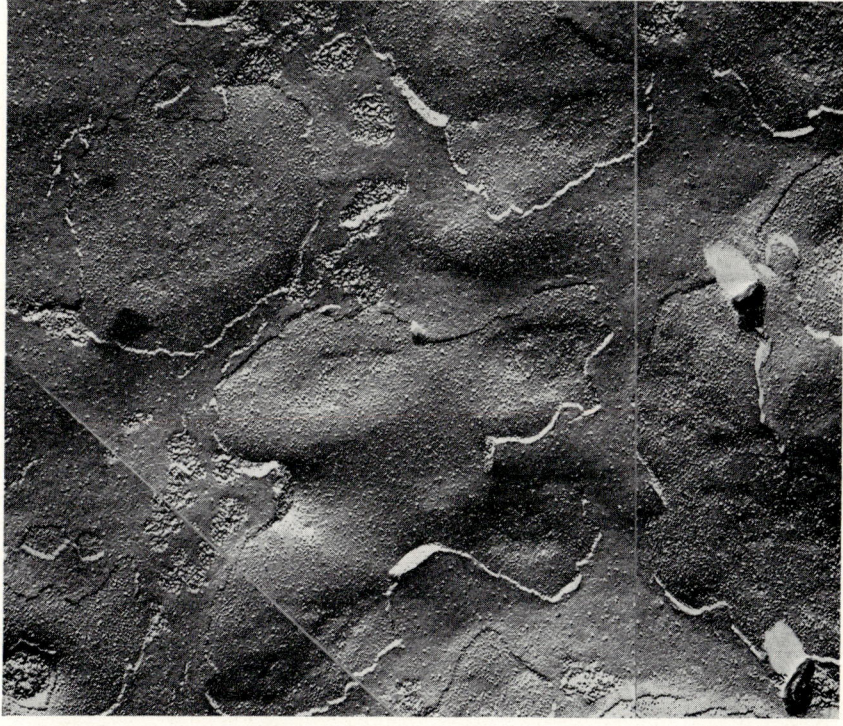

Figure 40.7. Broad panorama of a considerable number of presynaptic terminals attached to an extensive postsynaptic membrane that has the appearance of continental masses and isthmuses resting on top of the presynaptic endings. Many shallow "footprint-like" indentations are suggestive of synaptic junctions but these surround indentations that are relatively flat and do not have the pitted appearance typical of through penetration. This panorama was obtained from the ventral horn area of the spinal cord of a rat that had been treated with tetanus toxin and was agonal after cessation of seizures. Many such fields were encountered and were apparently characteristic of this state in the several animals so treated. Original magification $\times 8,000$.

with confidence beyond the 0.01 level, in the unanaesthetized state. This same strong tendency was found in thin sections for terminal endings that contained either spherical or flattened types of synaptic vesicles. This point is of interest because flattened vesicles have been considered a morphological characteristic of inhibitory synapses (Uchizano, 1965). The implication is, therefore, that the direct and indirect effects of nembutal anaesthesia may be similar on both excitatory and inhibitory endings.

SOME SPECULATIVE INTERPRETATIONS

On the basis of information obtained by two radically different electron-microscopic techniques there is a remarkable nicety of correspondence of the evidence that distinguishes synaptic junctions between two functional states, 'waking' and anaesthetized. Since most of the pictures we have of 'normal' synaptic junctions are based on materials obtained from anaesthetized animals, we need to revise our impressions of what is their 'really normal' appearance.

It is clearly established that the control of signalling between neurones must relate to the events taking place at the synapse. The morphological differences found with each of these two complementary techniques not only dramatize the plasticity of synapses but confirm in substantial further detail the conception of pinocytotic delivery of neurotransmitter substances.

The synapse is a crucial junction for all the normal traffic essential for the support of life, for the regulation of visceral well-being and the management of everyday behaviour. It is also obvious that the synapse is an important junction for higher nervous processes as well. Synapses thus represent a nodal point for the control of neuronal transmission not only at the reflexive level but at the level of thought regulation, dreams and even of creativity. It must play a role in all sorts of modifications of behaviour, in the development of sensorimotor and perceptual skills, and probably as well in memory storage and forgetting. Undoubtedly, the synapse plays its part in whatever processes are involved in alterations of neuronal circuitry in both health and disease, in learning, in epilepsy, in intractable pain, in neuroses and psychoses.

The supposition is that when circuits are strengthened there is a functional improvement of impulse penetration through synaptic sites along that pathway. This may result from some changes in the metabolic engines that operate at the neurotransmitter or neuroreceptor sites, but the expression of increased activity along that pathway must be manifested by an increase in synaptic activity: there is no alternative to this link. It may be possible to develop sufficiently refined means for estimating very subtle gradations of synaptic activity level on a morphological basis and thereby to witness many additional dynamics of circuitry, in health and disease, in increasingly comprehensive patterns. It is possible that only the size or number or density of synaptic junctions may be affected and that individual junctions may appear approximately the same. It may also be that traffic density can change without there being a readily appreciable morphological indicator reflecting this change.

Although impulse traffic along axons is 'all-or-none', the response at synaptic junctions is 'graded'. The 'quantal release' of synaptic transmitter substances is apparently overwhelmed during nerve impulse traffic by the large number of synaptic vesicles that release neurotransmitter. What we are witnessing in the freeze-etch panoramas of presynaptic membranes is the cascade or bombardment of vesicles in a quick succession of pinocytotic release phenomena. The fact that we seldom see all six penetrations of the presynaptic membrane at a given roundel of hexagonal pattern implies that the release of neurotransmitter around a single presynaptic dense projection seldom engages all of the six vesicles at once. It also suggests that the duration of penetrating figures may be relatively brief.

In pursuit of the entrancing problem of synaptic transmission, morphologists naturally intend to push their entry into the problem as far as possible. It is only a first step towards full understanding of what takes place to have identified morphological changes in the presynaptic membrane that are correlated with the blanketing effects of central anaesthesia. The path beckons for exploration of what additional signs of plasticity of synapses, on the presynaptic or postsynaptic membranes, may be correlated with what kinds of alterations in interneuronal communication.

ADDENDUM

We would like to celebrate with you the significant revelations of Graham Goddard and his colleagues as communicated in the literature and at this meeting. The stimulation of selected sites in the brain leads to a progressive increase in excitability affecting the local and increasingly remote elements of a circuit. There must be operating some kind of 'feed-forward' effect, what Goddard calls a 'kindling effect', that augments itself enough to engulf larger and larger domains into its dominating control. This effect obviously has some bearing on temporal lobe epilepsy but perhaps also on any of a wide variety of 'vicious circle' disorders such as are commonplace in medicine and psychiatry.

We cannot help but wonder whether Goddard's kindling may be accompanied by morphological changes at synaptic junctions. This speculation is made more worthy because of the potential importance of identifying the morphological as well as physiological and chemical parameters of *any process that strengthens synaptic transmission*. But there is something of even more general interest and this stems from the fact that Goddard's kindling is obtained from intermittent stimulation of parts of the *limbic system*. An animal with electrodes in such a location is readily entrained to self-stimulation (Olds & Milner, 1954; Olds, 1956). There is much literature on the relationship between the limbic system, particularly the hippocampus, and mechanisms of learning and memory (see Ojemann, 1966). The limbic system appears to be a mechanism that provides intrinsic or central reinforcement. It has been suggested that activation of this system leads to the strengthening of those circuits that have been just recently active (Livingston, 1964; Livingston, 1969; Kety, 1969, 1970). Whether the mediating agency operates by activation of the diffusely projecting systems or through some widely circulating neurotransmitter is moot, but the end result must be a conditional strengthening of the specific pathways that were just recently active.

Perhaps Goddard's kindling can lead not only to strengthening of local pathways, as he has demonstrated so elegantly, but remote pathways as well. If one were to associate on a regular basis a remote conditioned stimulus, in the Pavlovian paradigm, that is, just prior to and overlapping with the limbic kindling stimulation, the conditioned event might be similarly strengthened. Until now, presumably, Goddard's kindling stimuli have not been linked regularly to any other artificial neurological event. Hence, even if he were getting remote reinforcement of synaptic connections, this would occur against a random background of events and therefore would not yield evidence of conditioning.

So it would appear desirable to test Goddard's kindling experiments with an added conditioning stimulus, using the kindling stimuli as the reinforcement. It is tempting to speculate that there would not only be an appreciable strengthening of local synapses but also synaptic strengthening in the region of conditional stimuli as well, and, hopefully, not elsewhere! That is what everyone would like to see, morphological evidence for learning and memory!

SUMMARY AND CONCLUSIONS

Most notions of synaptic structure are based on electronmicroscopic evidence obtained from anaesthetized animals. Using two distinctly different but complementary techniques of electron microspy, thin-section and freeze-etch, it has been possible to establish that there are morphological changes in the presynaptic membrane between waking and anaesthetized conditions. In the waking state, both presynaptic and postsynaptic membranes are more deeply arched upward towards the presynaptic terminal cytoplasm. The presynaptic membrane shows quantitative differences in signs attributed to pinocytosis that are significantly greater in the waking state. In agonal conditions, the presynaptic membrane is even smoother, flatter and less disrupted or rumpled by signs of pinocytosis than in the anaesthetized condition. The morphological effects of anaesthesia are similar for nembutal, ether and chloralose, but they are more pronounced in the case of the barbiturate anaesthetic.

> The composition of the living creature is so ordered as to have a regular period of life for the species in general; and each individual by itself is born with its allotted span . . . since the triangles in every creature are from the outset put together with the power to hold out for a certain time, beyond which life cannot be prolonged. . . . And at last, when the conjoined bonds of the triangles in the marrow no longer hold out under the stress, but part asunder, they let go in their turn the bonds of the soul. And she, when thus set free, flies away with joy, for that which happens according to nature is pleasant, and that which happens contrary to nature is pain.
>
> *Timaeus*   Plato

ACKNOWLEDGEMENTS

An earlier version of this communication was presented at the invitation of Professor Manfred Eigen at the Max Planck Institute for Biophysical Chemistry in Göttingen on June 19th, 1972 and in the same city on September 14th, 1972 as the Schloss Hardenberg Lecture before the European Brain and Behaviour Society (Akert 1973.) The authors are indebted to Professor Hans Moor, Dr Peter Streit, Dr Karl Pfenninger and Miss Clara Sandri for their participation in the original research; we are all most grateful to Miss Cynthia Berger for preparing the freeze-etched replicas, to Miss Louise Decoppet for the photography, to Misses R. Emch and E. Schneider for the drawing and to Mr A. Fäh for his help in the operative procedures. The research was supported by grants from the Swiss National Foundation for Scientific Research Nr. 3.133.69, 3.134.69 and 3.336.70 and by the Dr Eric Slack-Gyr Foundation, Zürich.

REFERENCES

Akert K. (1973). Dynamic aspects of synaptic ultrastructure, Brain Res., **49**, 511–518
Akert K, Moor H, Pfenninger K & Sandri C (1969). Contributions of new impregnation methods and freeze-etching to the problem of synaptic fine structure. In: *Mechanisms of synaptic transmission, Progress in brain research* (Eds Akert and Waser), **31**, 223–40. Amsterdam: Elsevier.
Akert K, Streit P, Sandri C, Livingston RB & Moor H (1972). Synapsen im Zeichen erhöhter und erniedrigter Aktivität; eine elektronenmikroskopische Analyse. *Schweizer Archiv. Neurol. Neurochir. Psychiat.*, **111**, 227–36
Blaustein MP (1968). Barbiturates block sodium and potassium conductance increases in voltage-clamped lobster axons. *J. gen. Physiol.*, **51**, 293–307
Bloom FE (1970). Correlating structure and function of synaptic ultrastructure. In: *The neurosciences second study program* (Ed Schmitt FO), 729–47. New York: The Rockefeller University Press.
Bodian D (Personal communication).
Cooper JR, Bloom FE & Roth RH (1970). *The biochemical basis of neuropharmacology*, viii + 220p. London: Oxford University Press.
Gray EG (1950). Axo-somatic and axo-dendritic synapses of the cerebral cortex; an electron microscope study. *J. Anat. (Lond.)* **93**, 420–33
Kety SS (1967). The central physiological and pharmacological effects of the biogenic amines and their correlations with behavior. In: *The neurosciences, a study program* (Eds Quarton, Meknechuk and Schmitt), 444–51. New York: The Rockefeller University Press.
Kety SS (1970). The biogenic amines in the central nervous system, their possible roles in arousal, emotion and learning. In: *The neurosciences second study program* (Ed Schmitt FO), pp. 324–36. New York: The Rockefeller University Press.
Livingston RB (1964). Cited (pp. 25–7) in: Nauta WJH. Some brain structures and functions related to memory. *Neurosci. Res. Program Bull.*, **2**, 1–35
Livingston RB (1967). Brain circuitry relating to complex behavior. In: *The neurosciences, a study program* (Eds Quarton, Melnechuk and Schmitt), pp. 499–515. New York: The Rockefeller University Press.
Livingston RB (1967). Reinforcement. In: *The neurosciences, a study program* (Eds Quarton, Melnechuk and Schmitt), pp. 568–77. New York: The Rockefeller University Press.
Moor H, Pfenninger K & Akert K (1969). Freeze-etching of synapses. *Science*, **164**, 1405–7

Ojemann RG (1966). Correlations between specific human brain lesions and memory changes: a critical survey of the literature. *Neurosci. Res. Program Bull.*, (Suppl.) **4**, 1–70

Olds J & Milner P (1954). Positive reinforcement produced by electrical stimulation of septal area and other regions of rat brain. *J. comp. physiol. Psychol.*, **47**, 419–27

Olds J (1956). A preliminary mapping of electrical reinforcing effects in the rat brain. *J. comp. physiol. Psychol.*, 281–5

Olds J (1958). Self-stimulation of the brain. *Science*, **127**, 315–24

Peters A, Palay SL & Webster H deF (1970). *The fine structure of the nervous system; the cells and their processes*, xvi + 198 pp. New York: Harper and Row.

Pfenninger K, Akert K, Moor H & Sandri C (1972). The fine structure of freeze-fractured presynaptic membranes. *J. Neurocytol.*, **1**, 129–49

Pfenninger K, Sandri C, Akert K & Eugster CH (1969). Contribution to the problem of structural organization of the presynaptic area. *Brain Res.*, **12**, 10–18

Sandri C, Akert K, Livingston RB & Moor H (1972). Particle aggregations at specialized sites in freeze-etched postsynaptic membranes. *Brain Res.*, **41**, 1–16

Streit P, Akert K, Sandri C, Livingston RB & Moor H (1972). Dynamic ultrastructure of presynaptic membranes at nerve terminals in the spinal cord of rats; anesthetized and unanesthetized preparations compared. *Brain Res.*, **48**, 11–26

Uchizono K (1965). Characteristics of excitatory and inhibitory synapses in the central nervous system of the cat. *Nature (Lond.)*, **207**, 642–3

Index

A

Acetylcholinesterase activity, 225
Active avoidance, 253
Activation, 245
Acute schizophrenic episode, 198
Adaptive Behaviour Scale, 148
Adjective Self-Inventory, 53
Affective psychosis, 197
Affective symptoms, 51
After-discharge, 109
Aggressiveness, 66, 70, 122, 125, 129, 135, 138, 144, 182, 189
Alcoholism, 47, 118
Amines, 14
Ammonshorn sclerosis, 118
Amphetamine, 15
Amygdala, 110, 183, 190, 225, 266
   electrical stimulation of, 184, 226
   electrical stimulation of septum, 116
   telemetric stimulation, 226
   chemical stimulation, 225
   responses to stimulation, 184
   personality changes, 111
   lateral part, 184
   medial part, 184
Amygdalotomy, 33, 125, 129, 136, 138, 142, 184
   assessment of, 141, 143, 148, 151
   biochemical studies of, 147
   case reports, 139
   complications of, 127
   effects in animals, 225, 230
   effects in cat, 254
   lateral target, 129, 254
   medial target, 129, 254
   results of, 127, 139, 151
   results on behavioural disorder, 129
   results on EEG paroxysms, 129
   technique, 138
Antipsychotic drugs, 14
Anxiety, 78, 101, 159, 167, 182
   pathophysiology, 78
   treatment, 78

B

Barrat Impulsiveness Scale, 40
Basal cortex, 6
Basolateral limbic circuit, 248
Beck Scale, 167
Behavioural disorders, 182
Bender-Gestalt Test, 52
Biological psychiatry, 13
Brain, 215
   electrical stimulation of, 215
Brain stem reticular core, 247

C

Capsulotomy, anterior, 159
   complications, 162
   effects; immediate, delayed, 162
   effects; clinical, psychological, 162
   technique, 160
Catatonia, pathophysiology, 78
   treatment, 78
Catecholamines, 147
Cenesthiopathy, 197
Centrencephalic epilepsy, 237
Cerebral localization, of emotions, 194
   of personality, 194
Cerebrovascular accident, 118
Cholinergic hippocampal afferents, 284
Cholinergic-monoaminergic balance, 288
Cholinergic pathways, 282

Chronic neurosis-like schizophrenia, 200
Chronic pain, 63
Cingulate cortex, 268
Cingulate undercutting, 29
Cingulectomy, 69, 174
    clinical effects, 177
    psychological effects, 177
Cingulotomy, stereotactic, 32, 39, 41, 59, 65, 69, 101, 165, 174
    clinical results, 40, 102, 177
    complications, 4
    failure of operation, 102
    psychological results, 40, 177
Cingulum, 39, 51, 68, 102
    anatomy of, 72
    electrical stimulation of, 43, 65, 74
    electrical stimulation of lower medial quadrant, 166
    autonomic effects of electrical stimulation, 166
    responses to stimulation, 44, 66
    affective responses, 46
    behavioural responses, 67
    consciousness responses, 45
    correlation of stimulation response and clinical result, 46
    motor responses, 67
    psychological responses, 67
    sensory-motor responses, 46
    speech responses, 44
    temporal lobe responses, 44
    vegetative responses, 66
    implanted electrodes, 65
    lesion of, 190
Conditioned emotional response, 111
Corpus callosum, 74
    electrical stimulation of, 74
    responses to stimulation, 75
Cortical dysplasia, 122
Cortical undercutting, 6, 97
    results of, 97
Corticosterone level in plasma, 253

D

Depersonalization syndrome, 197
Depression, 23, 97, 101, 168, 180, 191
Depth EEG recording, 216, 229, 231
    telemetric, 216
Diencephalic instability, 237
Dominant temporal lobe, 22

Dopamine, 17, 233
Dopamine pathways, 293
Dorsal tegmental pathway, 284
Draw-A-Person Test, 52

E

Electrical stimulation in animals, 109
    risks of repeated stimulations, 112
Electrical stimulation of brain, 215
    telemetric, 216
    transdermal, 217, 220
Emotion, 245
Emotional behavioural homeostasis, 249
Entorhinal area, 306
Epilepsy, 22, 66, 125, 129, 197, 224
    limbic, 224
    psychomotor, 224
    temporal lobe, 118, 136, 144
Epileptic activity, 109
Epileptic after-discharge, in cats, 115
Erethism, 125
Extrapyramidal subcortical centres, 293
Extraversion, 26, 168, 174
Eysenck Personality Inventory, 78

F

Face Recognition Test, 152
Feedback control, 246
Formaldehyde-fluorescence, 282
Fornix-fimbrial system, 267
Freeze-etch electron microscopy, 315
    interpretation of, 316
Frontal pole, 269
Fronto-hippocampal pathways, 307
Fundus of the stria terminalis, 135
    complications, 136
    function of, 135
    hyperphagia, 136
    hyperpyrexia, 136
    results of treatment, 136
    stereotactic lesions to, 135

G

Gibson Spiral Maze, 150
Gilles de la Tourette syndrome, 210
Gyrectomies, 4
Gyrus cinguli, 303

H

Hallucinations, 138, 140
Hamartoma, 121
Hamilton Scales, 167, 168
Hargreaves Nursing Rating Scale, 148
Hippocampectomy, complications, 34
Holtzman Inkblot Test, 77
Homeostasis, 301
Homovanillic acid, 293
Hostility and Direction of Hostility Questionnaire, 152
Hypothalamotomy, 125
  complications of, 127
  results of, 125
  posteromedial, 136, 185
  ventromedial, 185
Hypothalamus, 225

I

Inferior quadrants, 4
Impulsive behaviour, 238
Intelligence, 177
Interhemispheric cingulostriate fibres, 78
Internal capsule, anterior, 159
  electrical stimulation, 159
  emotional function, 159
Internuncial pool, 245
Interpretive cortex, 248
Intractable psychiatric illness, 250
Intralaminar thalamotomy, 208
  complications, 210
  results of, 210
Introversion, 174

K

Kindling effect, 327
Kindling of epileptic seizures, 109
Korsakoff-like syndrome, 70

L

Learning, 245, 253
Leucotomy, selective, 69
  limbic, 166
  multiple lesions, 166, 189
  orbital, 69
Limbic brain, 224
Limbic-forebrain circuits, 246
Limbic lobe, 61, 303
Limbic midbrain area, 304
Limbic system, 3, 17, 19, 109, 328
Limbic system model, 245
Limbico-subcortical axis, 311
Lobotomy, paramedian, 238
  standard, 3
  temporal 122
  unilateral, 4
Localization of emotional illness in brain, 18
Location of lesions, 33
Loss of recent memory, 33

M

Manic-depressive psychosis, 22
Maudsley Personality Inventory, 167
Mechanism of psychosurgery, 19, 34
Medial limbic circuit, 247
Medial quadrants, 5
Memory, 245
Mental retardation, 125
Mesencephalon, 301
Mesial temporal sclerosis, 121
Meso-limbic dopamine system, 294
Mesoloviotomy, anterior, 75
  clinical effects, 78
  indication to, 75
  psychological effects, 76
Methionine, 13
Midbrain, 62
Midbrain reticular formation, 284
Middlesex Hospital Questionnaire, 167
MMPI, 53, 179
Monoaminergic systems, 282
Monoamines, 293
Multiple lesions, 102, 125, 166, 182

N

Neuroleptics, 298
Neuroticism, 76, 167, 174
Nigro-striatal dopamine pathway, 294
Non-dominant temporal lobe, 22

O

Obsessional neurosis, 168
Obsessive–compulsive neurosis, 176, 182
Obsessive–compulsive symptoms, 51, 96, 101, 208
  early onset, 99
  insidious onset, 99

Obsessive–compulsive symptoms—*continued*
  late onset, 99
  sudden onset, 99
Obsessive–compulsive syndrome, 159
Offensive–defensive reactions, 227
Oligophrenia, 65, 182
Orbital leucotomy, 69
  in aggression, 70
  in depression, 70
  in obsessive symptoms, 70
  in schizophrenia, 70
  psychological assessment, 72
  side effects of, 70
Orbito-frontal cortex, 307
Orbito-frontal tractotomy, 90
Orbito-frontal undercutting, 90
Orbito-ventromedial undercutting, 197
  long-term assessment of results, 197

P
Pain mechanisms, 61
Pallidothalamic connections, 263
Pallidotomy, 179
  dominant, non-dominant hemisphere, 179
  psychological effects, 179
Pallidum, 257
  electrical stimulation of, 257
  electrophysiological study, in cat, 257
  non-specific cortical activation, behavioural change, 263
Papez circuit, 247
Parahippocampal gyrus, 306
Paramedian lobotomy, 238
Paraphrenia, 200
Parietal cortex, 268
Parkinsonism, 179, 296
Passive avoidance, 253
Pedophilia, 182
Perirhinal area, 269
Phobia, pathophysiology, 78, 208
  treatment, 78
Pinocytosis, 317
Postoperative organic psychosyndrome, 20
Postoperative personality changes, 20
Postoperative psychological changes, 20

Presubiculum, 306
Psychiatric 'dis-ease", 246
Psychomotor seizures, 123
Psychosis, 176
Psychosomatic mechanisms, 8
Psychotropic drugs, 7, 234
Putamen, 257
  electrical stimulation of, 257
  electrophysiological study, in cat, 257
  non-specific cortical activation, behavioural charge, 263

Q
Quadrants, inferior, 4
  medial, 5

R
Radioactive lesions, 102
Rage reaction, 227
Raphe nuclei, 300
Reticular activating system, 245
Reticular formation, 301
Rey-Davis Pegboard Test, 152
Rorschach Test, 52

S
Scalp EEG recording, 238
Schizo-affective psychosis, 198
Schizophrenia, 13, 23, 118, 125, 139, 169, 189
  'atypical', 196
Sensory convergence, 266
Septo-hippocampal inhibition, 116
Septo–hypothalamo–mesencephalic continuum, 304
Serotonin, 300
Sixteen Personality Factor Questionnaire, 152
Sociopathy, 50, 189
Somatic symptoms, 51
Specificity of operations, 20
Standard lobotomy, 3
Stereotactic tractotomy, 101
Stereotaxic operations, 5
Stereotypia, 139
Steroids, 147
Stress, 253
Subcaudate region, 84, 102
Substantia innomata, 84, 102
Substantia innomata lesions, 97, 190
  results, 97, 191

Synapses, 315
  anaesthetized, 318
  unanaesthetized, 318
  ultrastructure of, 316
Synaptic junctions, 315
Synaptic plasticity, 323
  quantitative evaluation of, 323

T

Taylor Scale, 168
Temporal-limbic dysfunction, 22
Temporal lobe epilepsy, 118, 136, 144
  and depressive states, 122
  and psychosis, 122
  and schizophrenia, 122
Temporal lobe scars, 121
Temporal lobe gliosis, 121
Temporal lobectomy, 122
  results of, 122
  social adaptation, 122
Temporal pole, 271
Tension, 238
  pathophysiology, treatment, 78
Thalamotomy, 125, 179, 185
  dominant, non-dominant hemisphere, 181
  dorsomedial, ventromedial, 185
  intralaminar, 185, 208
  complications, 127, 210
  psychological effects, 179
  results of, 127, 185, 210
Thalamus, 61
Thin-section electron microscopy, 315
Thiocholine method, 282
Tics, pathophysiology of, 208
Topectomies, 4
Tractotomy, 97
  lower medial frontal quadrant, 170
  results of treatment, clinical, 167

  psychological, 167
  psychiatric assessment, 167
  orbito-frontal tractotomy, 83, 90
  stereotactic tractotomy, 101
Transneuronal degeneration, 266

U

Uncotomy, 33
Undercutting, cingulate, 29
  cortical, 6, 97
  results of, 97
  orbito-frontal, 90
  orbito-ventromedial, 197
  long-term assessment of results, 197

V

Ventral tegmental pathway, 284
Viscero-endocrine functions, 304

W

WAIS, 52
Wechsler-Bellevue Scale, 52, 176
Wechsler Memory Scale, 52
Williams Memory Scale, 152

X

X-ray emission microanalysis, 283

Y

Yttrium implantation, 83, 90
  accuracy of surgery, 83, 90
  anatomical localization, 85
    bony landmarks, 84
    ventricular landmarks, 86
  autopsy findings, 86, 90
  neuropathological findings, 92
  secondary degeneration, 94